Loving Yourself to
GREAT HEALTH

ALSO BY LOUISE HAY

All of the above are available at your local
bookstore, or may be ordered by visiting:

Hay House USA: www.hayhouse.com®
Hay House Australia: www.hayhouse.com.au
Hay House UK: www.hayhouse.co.uk
Hay House South Africa: www.hayhouse.co.za
Hay House India: www.hayhouse.co.in

Louise's Websites: www.LouiseHay.com® and www.HealYourLife.com®

Loving Yourself to
GREAT
HEALTH

Thoughts & Food—the Ultimate Diet

LOUISE HAY
AHLEA KHADRO
HEATHER DANE

HAY
HOUSE

HAY HOUSE, INC.
Carlsbad, California • New York City
London • Sydney • Johannesburg
Vancouver • Hong Kong • New Delhi

Published and distributed in the United States by: Hay House, Inc.: www.hayhouse.com® • *Published and distributed in Australia by:* Hay House Australia Pty. Ltd.: www.hayhouse.com.au • *Published and distributed in the United Kingdom by:* Hay House UK, Ltd.: www.hayhouse.co.uk • *Published and distributed in the Republic of South Africa by:* Hay House SA (Pty), Ltd.: www.hayhouse.co.za • *Distributed in Canada by:* Raincoast Books: www.raincoast.com • *Published in India by:* Hay House Publishers India: www.hayhouse.co.in

Cover design: Amy Rose Grigoriou
Interior design: Tricia Breidenthal

Interior illustrations: Courtesy of the authors
Indexer: Jay Kreider

Library of Congress Cataloging-in-Publication Data

Hay, Louise L.
  Loving yourself to great health : thoughts & food-the ultimate diet / Louise Hay, Ahlea Khadro, and Heather Dane.
    pages cm
  Includes index.
  1. Self-actualization (Psychology) 2. Self-care, Health. 3. Nutrition--Psychological aspects. 4. Mind and body. I. Khadro, Ahlea. II. Dane, Heather. III. Title.
  BF637.S4H3794 2014
  615.8'52--dc23

                    2014028652

ISBN: 978-1-4019-4286-1

11 10 9 8 7 6 5 4 3
1st edition, October 2014
2nd edition, October 2015

Printed in the United States of America

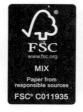

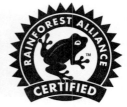

CONTENTS

PART I: 7 STEPS TO EAT, THINK, AND LOVE YOUR WAY TO GREAT HEALTH

Discover why symptoms, illness, and dis-ease occur and how to create a whole new perspective on your ability to create health, happiness, and longevity.

The truth about food, weight loss, and dis-ease, and the loving steps you can take to heal your body and mind.

Learn how your digestive system works and how your body was perfectly designed to support your wellness.

Find out how to listen to your body, so you can allow inner guidance to take the lead if decisions about your health, wellness, and nutrition become confusing.

Learn the foods to eat and avoid for your best health.

PREFACE

Start Your Own Love Story

by Louise Hay

At 88 years of age, I can say that health and happiness are the most important tenets of my life. Many of you who have read my books know that I did not have an easy childhood, nor any of the advantages of money or education for much of my life.

Then I discovered the one thing that changed the course of my health and my life: the belief that every thought we think is creating our future. This one little idea shifted the direction of my life. I found that if I could create peace, health, and harmony in my mind, I could create the same in my body and in my world.

This book is not about the latest trend or fad. It's about how to craft a life that will nourish and support you. It's about all the ways you can love yourself more. It's about ancient healing wisdom that will work with your busy schedule. And it's about learning that you matter. Somewhere in all the stress, noise, and to-do lists, there is still space for you. My fellow authors and I are going to show you how to find that space so you can feel good now and long into your future.

Over the years, there have been some key points to my philosophy on life, happiness, and health that have remained timeless. I am going to share them with you right now because they will help set the stage for this book you're about to read.

What I Believe

- Life is really very simple. What we give out, we get back. Every thought we think is creating our future.

- It is only a thought, and a thought can be changed. I believe this is true for your health, too.

- We create every so-called illness in our body, and we have the power to change our thoughts and begin to dissolve it.

- Releasing resentment and negative thoughts will help dissolve even the most "incurable" health conditions.

- When you don't know what else to do, focus on love. Loving yourself makes you feel good, and good health is really about feeling good.

- When we really love ourselves, everything in our life works, including our health.

This book is a love story. It's about loving yourself as a way to create health, happiness, and longevity. Yes, you will learn tips, menus, recipes, affirmations, and exercises that have worked to keep me healthy, vibrant, and strong throughout my life. But more than that, your heart will be opened to new ways to love and support yourself on this incredible journey.

Over the years, I have taught ways to eliminate the negative thoughts in your mind and to replace them with positive affirmations. To practice forgiveness and to dissolve resentment. To learn to really love who you are. To do mirror work. Those of you who have followed these lessons have seen your lives turn around for the better. Now it is time for the next step.

I have had so many of you say to me, "You look so young and vibrant." Or, "I want to be healthy like you when I get older." In this book, I will be sharing exactly what I do. For me, this is the next step in changing your thoughts. It's changing your way of life to one that focuses on nourishing and treating your body with love.

♥

I have always loved learning new things, and I believe that every hand that touches me is a healing hand. In this way, I have found many wonderful people doing extremely good work, and I often like to share what I've learned from them with the rest of the world. For example, years ago I met Esther and Jerry Hicks (who present the teachings of the Non-Physical entity Abraham). They were doing phenomenally good work, but their very loyal audience was relatively small. I wanted to get as many people as possible to know them—it took me two years, but now, a decade later, their audience covers the globe.

In this book, I am introducing two people who have transformed my life: Ahlea Khadro and Heather Dane. I would like them to transform yours as well, if you are willing. In this book, the three of us will share the things I do to feel my best while working, traveling, writing, and having an active social life. Some of the secrets we share will be new to you, while others may remind you of what you would like to reaffirm.

As I look back and think about why I feel so good at age 88, I truly believe it's because of the way I live. My thoughts from morning until I go to sleep at night are mostly a stream of positive affirmations. I firmly believe that Life loves me and everything I need comes to me at the right time. I also believe that I am a big, strong, healthy girl! Then I leave it to Life to bring my thoughts into manifestation so that this comes true for me.

When you expand your thinking and beliefs, your love flows freely. When you contract, you shut yourself off. Can you remember the last time when you were in love? Your heart went *ahh!* It was such a wonderful feeling. It is the same with loving yourself, except that you will never leave once you have that love. It's with you for the rest of your life, so you want to make it the best relationship that you can have.

It has been such a pleasure to work with Ahlea and Heather on this book, and I know you will enjoy it as much as I have.

I love you,
Louise

♥ ♥

INTRODUCTION

How We Came Together to Write This Book

by Ahlea Khadro and Heather Dane

Louise has brought to the world such a profound and incredible gift with her affirmation work, and this book takes those teachings to the next level. One of the most significant secrets to Louise's personal success is how she eats and cares for herself every day, in the small moments. When people say that affirmations don't work for them, she always asks them, "What did you have for breakfast?" In this book, we are going to share the many reasons why this simple question reveals great wisdom about how you think and feel.

We all want to feel our best every day. We want to wake up energized and excited for the adventures ahead. We want to enjoy life, at every stage. And this is our natural state. Unfortunately, what we are seeing too often today are habits, beliefs, and messages that separate people from their health and happiness. We wrote this book to unravel the messages that separate you from feeling your best, to reveal how much nature is here to offer you everything you need, and to remind you that everything you need for health and healing is within.

Having worked successfully to bring hundreds of clients back to their natural state of wellness, we both were overjoyed to meet a shining example of the secrets of health, happiness, and longevity that have seemed to be mostly forgotten. This shining example is Louise Hay. She came into our lives because she has a commitment to feeling her best at every stage of her existence. One of the ways she does this is by surrounding herself with experts who become part of her wellness team. She is a true partner in her health and, therefore, a true team member. Louise models her commitment to health in the way she thinks, eats, exercises, and enjoys life. She is one of the most balanced people we know, and believe us—we've seen her blood tests and traveled the world with her—she is definitely the "big, strong, healthy girl" she says she is!

Over the decade we've known her, we've watched her move through her 70s and 80s with strength, grace, and a joy for life. She celebrates everything from waking up in a comfortable bed, to starting her car ("Hello, baby, we're going to have a great ride!"), to eating healthy meals. These may seem like little things, yet it's thousands of simple, little things that make up a life worth living. She is our inspiration, and we are thrilled to share her secrets, our knowledge, and a whole lot of delicious fun in the pages of this book.

Allow Us to Introduce Ourselves

Ahlea: Over 15 years ago, I started my business, Soulstice, a center for optimal living and rehabilitation, specializing in yoga, reformer Pilates, meditative practices, holistic nutrition, craniosacral therapy, and visceral manipulation. Almost 11 years ago, I got a call from Louise Hay about working with me. You can imagine how exciting that was! From the start, I could see that Louise was willing to do whatever it took to love and support her healthy body. What I didn't expect was that we'd spend so much time laughing! And yet that's what makes Louise special—she brings a sense of fun to the serious work of healing.

I don't think Louise realized that in addition to Pilates and bodywork, she was going to experience the part of my work that keeps my clients coming back for more. You see, for most of my life, I could see the stories that lie beneath the surface of people's lives and under the layers of the human body. I can hear the stories that people's organs, tissues, and bones want to tell. It's listening to these stories and sharing them with my clients that has such a profound effect on their health. Responding to the stories with love is how healing begins.

My deepest desire is to serve others, so I am grateful to be a conduit for the body's messages. My mission is to support others in learning to listen to the body, so that they can lovingly respond to its needs. You will learn that here in this book.

Heather: I started my career in the corporate sphere, specializing in identifying and resolving patterns that got in the way of people and companies performing their best. Whenever there was a team in crisis or a problem that no one could figure out, I was the one whom senior management called to find out what was happening and how to fix it. I found that I had a unique ability to discover the root cause of large-scale human and organizational performance issues because of a passion for what they called "systems thinking" in my graduate program—not to mention a love of detective work!

Systems thinking is about looking at symptoms as part of a whole system, rather than pieces and parts. It's not unlike the call for "holistic" health, where we view a person as a whole being and assess health from that level in order to promote wellness. One of the most challenging issues I saw in my 15 years in the corporate world was a buildup of stress and overwork that was having an adverse effect on people's health. I was swiftly climbing the corporate ladder when I came to the realization that no one around me from the vice president level and above was healthy. People were collapsing in stairwells, missing work due to major surgeries, coming to the office exhausted, and suffering from chronic health conditions. And honestly, I was one of them. That's when I decided that my own health had to be more important than the job, the to-do list, and everything else.

In this book, you'll learn the journey I took to heal myself of so-called incurable illness and addiction, and how I used my knack for identifying the root cause of symptoms to transform my health. A decade ago, I left my corporate career; became a certified professional coach; and received additional certifications in nutrition, digestive health, yoga, and energy healing. I have had the great fortune of researching with and writing hundreds of articles for some of the top experts in nutrition, medicine, digestive health, and energy medicine. And I was blessed to find two soul-sister health experts, Louise Hay and Ahlea Khadro, who were living and practicing similar lifestyles that enabled them to not only achieve their best health, but to help millions of others achieve theirs, too.

I met Louise eight years ago at a nutrition seminar in Los Angeles. We bonded over how delicious healing food could be and a love for learning all we could about health. A year later, Louise introduced me to Ahlea, and it was like finding my giggling and wellness soul mates. We have been giggling ever since, all while unlocking the secrets—both ancient and new—that help people heal. Having these two amazing women come into my life has been the greatest gift.

About This Book

When you're passionate about something, it tends to find its way to the center stage of your life. The three of us are passionate about health, and we've often found our way into deep conversations with each other about how simple good health could be with the right ingredients. Two of them, as Louise has always taught, are thoughts and food. If you get both right, good health follows.

The three of us have spent years together in continuous discovery, studying things like homeopathy, genetics, nutrition, cooking, and energy healing. We work as a team on Louise's health, and we both have busy practices working with clients. You'll hear several of our clients' stories here in this book, so that you can see how strong the human body and mind are, even when it looks like the chips are down.

A couple of years ago, while Ahlea was pregnant, we birthed the idea for this book. As we talked about how to bring a new life into the world and nurture its health and happiness, we had so much to say that we felt compelled to write it down. From the beginning to the end of life, good health—feeling good—gives us the foundation we need to work with our thoughts, to grow, to develop, to live, and to love. And in the center of good health is one key principle: *loving yourself.* If you can start there, everything else is so simple.

The three of us gathered over nettle tea and bone broth and shared our experience, wisdom, and love for life and each other in this beautiful and rich book. While there are many "diet" books available, this one is unique in its scope—inviting you to listen to your body and tune in to your unique wisdom, while having the support of affirmations, recipes, practical lists, and an education about how your body works.

What makes our book different is it's a health book that addresses how to heal the body and the mind and how both really matter (in Louise's words, "getting your thoughts and food right"). We gently teach you why making better, loving choices is your greatest tool for health and healing. We focus on ancient yet time-proven health tips that are dogma-free and transcend fads.

Most people are confused about what to eat, especially if diagnosed with illness, such as an autoimmune disease. We teach you to listen to your body, first and foremost, and to make more loving food choices. We teach you that nourishing your body makes affirmations, good moods, willpower, and better decision making much easier.

We have separated this book into two parts. Part I teaches you 7 steps to eat, think, and love your way to good health. And each chapter begins with a quote from Louise that sets the tone for that chapter:

Chapter 1 invites you to rethink what health really means and create a perspective that embraces your innate power to heal. We take the mystery and fear out of illness and share tips on tapping into your body's natural healing process.

Chapter 2 teaches you how and why making more loving choices is key to your ability to feel your best. If you haven't been able to make changes in the past, we give you simple exercises to take those small steps that produce big results.

Chapter 3 educates you about how your digestive system works and why it's so important for every system in your body, including your brain health, moods, ability to sleep, ability to maintain a healthy weight, and even your willpower and decision making! You will learn why Louise always says, "If it doesn't grow, don't eat it!"

Chapter 4 supports you in learning how to listen to your inner voice, or as Louise calls it, your "inner ding." Learn about intuition, gut feelings, and other symptoms and sensations you can become aware of and what these signals can mean. Find out how they can help you have better health and a better life.

Chapter 5 takes you on a journey of food. You will find out about the psychology, deceit, and trickery the manufactured-food industry uses to get you to eat more; the toxic additives in processed food; and which foods to avoid and which foods to emphasize for your wellness and longevity. You'll even learn tips for eating healthy on a budget, how to reduce or eliminate cravings, and the kind of sweet treats that are simultaneously loving toward your body *and* taste buds.

Chapter 6 reveals some home remedies, supplements, and natural practices that can help dissolve common ailments—as well as improve your overall health!

Chapter 7 gives you a road map for moving forward with your new, healthy habits. By this time, you will be ready to take the first step and continue to build, one small step at a time. Or maybe you'll be ready for giant leaps . . . either way, we have some practical tips for you wherever you are in your journey.

In Part II, we give you everything you need to start loving your body with delicious, home-cooked meals, snacks, and desserts. You'll get kitchen tips and suggested tools to make things easier, sample menus, shopping lists, and a whole bunch of our favorite easy recipes that taste delicious and nourish your body.

The three of us wrote this book because, most of all, we want to support your best health. Like Louise said, we love you!

— Ahlea and Heather

♥ ♥

7 Steps to Eat, Think, and Love Your Way to Great Health

Chapter 1

Step #1: Create a New Perspective on Health

We all have a story about our life and our health—where we've been, where we are, and where we think we're going. We may have told this story to ourselves or others a thousand times. But what if where you are right now or what challenges you have faced in the past don't matter? What if you knew the truth—that your body was designed to heal? What if your story was a love story?

You've probably been taught that you have to go outside yourself, to doctors and experts, to be "fixed." What if instead you knew that while doctors and experts can provide insightful guidance, *you* have a great power inside of you? Well, it's true— you do!

> "Perfect health is my Divine right, and I claim it now."
>
> — Louise

You have the power to start listening to your body. Your body, like everything else in life, is a mirror of your inner thoughts and beliefs. Every cell responds to every thought you think and every word you speak, so continuous patterns of thoughts and beliefs can produce body behaviors and patterns of eases and dis-eases. The more you get to know your body and the better you listen to it, the more it will guide you to good health. We will talk more specifically about this throughout this book. Right now, though, just know this: *If you experience a health challenge, Life is inviting you to love yourself.* In other words, no matter what your problem is, there is only one answer: loving yourself.

Whenever you deal with a health issue, your body is asking you to be kinder to yourself, and that starts with loving yourself a little more each day. Think about the person or the animal you love the most—how do you feel when you think of them? Settle into that for a moment, and really feel it. Loving yourself means you can feel that same amount of love you just felt for them. If it feels too hard to love yourself that much, know that you're not alone.

As you start loving yourself more, you'll easily give yourself what you need, without waiting until you've done everything else on your to-do list. Sometimes, though, you may not even know what you need. As you read this book, you will learn the tools to help you recognize what your body needs most from you to feel healthy, happy, energized, and strong.

The fact that you have found *Loving Yourself to Great Health* means that you are ready to love yourself and make a positive change in your health. We acknowledge you for this, and we invite you to acknowledge yourself as well!

And now, what if you could craft a new story? In this chapter, we want to share some new ways to write your love story.

What Is Health?

To answer this question, we felt it was important to look briefly at how science views health, including the biggest issues we see today. (Don't worry—we will be brief and promise not to get too technical!) Because in the middle of this science, there is a deeper story here that we want to highlight.

You see, two facts came out of our quick look at how science views health:

1. Lifestyle choices play a major role in the biggest health issues faced today.

2. A large and growing population of people are being diagnosed with an illness for which science can find no root cause and no cure.

These two facts, to us, mean two very important truths:

1. You have the power to create good health.

2. When no one has the answers, it provides the perfect opportunity to create a new perspective on health.

A Quick Peek at How Science
Views the Current State of Health

At one time, the biggest health concern was infectious diseases that you could catch from others, such as tuberculosis and HIV. By 2008, however, the World Health Organization reported that the trend in health had shifted from infectious disease to what they called "noncommunicable diseases." Such diseases—like cancer, heart disease, and diabetes—are largely considered chronic and are not contagious.[1]

What's interesting about this shift is that noncommunicable diseases have four major contributors based on our lifestyle:

1. Tobacco use

2. Poor diet

3. Lack of exercise

4. Alcohol abuse

What we are seeing now is that the choices we make each day affect our health. Instead of a danger being "out there," the opportunity we have every day is to choose to love our bodies and treat them well. While the World Health Organization states it in more scientific language, they do report that if we make better lifestyle choices, we can impact our health tremendously.

Autoimmune Disease:
When the Body No Longer Recognizes Itself

One category of noncommunicable disease is autoimmune disease, which occurs when the immune system attacks healthy organs and tissue in the body. In other words, the immune system can no longer tell the difference between healthy tissue and harmful substances such as bacteria, viruses, and other pathogens.

To us, this feels like the body no longer recognizes itself, and the cells no longer recognize what is healthy. Think about this for a moment. *If one thinks negative, unloving thoughts about the body and oneself, how will the cells know not to similarly attack themselves?*

Research shows that there are at least 100 different autoimmune conditions. As of 2005, nearly 24 million Americans were diagnosed with autoimmune illnesses and the numbers are on the rise worldwide, particularly in Western, industrialized nations. Seventy-five percent of sufferers are women, often of childbearing age.[2] In fact, autoimmune conditions are one of the leading causes of death in young and middle-aged women, the second leading cause of chronic illness, and the third leading cause of Social Security disability (after heart disease and cancer).[3]

Some common autoimmune conditions are[4]:

- Celiac disease

- Crohn's disease

- Diabetes (type 1)

- Fibromyalgia

- Food allergies

- Hashimoto's thyroiditis

- Inflammatory bowel disease

- Lupus

- Multiple sclerosis

- Pernicious anemia (severe lack of B_{12})

- Psoriasis

- Rheumatoid arthritis

- Scleroderma

- Vitiligo (a skin disorder)

Examples of disorders also thought to be related to autoimmune conditions are autism, chronic fatigue syndrome, eating disorders[5], Lyme disease, and narcolepsy.

Autoimmune symptoms often involve pain, fatigue, fever, and general lack of well-being; most are considered chronic and incurable. A perplexing aspect to autoimmune conditions is that most people show no outward signs that they are sick and appear perfectly healthy to their friends and loved ones. In fact, until someone is diagnosed, they are often told that the symptoms are "all in your head" or a result of anxiety. Unfortunately, many with autoimmune illness have been viewed as hypochondriacs.

Scientists around the world have been baffled by the rising numbers of autoimmune diagnoses and can find no cause. The current theory is that the environment, genetics, and lifestyle could be contributing to the increase in these types of conditions.

Stress: Chronic Negative Thoughts Become Beliefs and Habits

Most experts will agree that stress is at the heart of all illness and disease.

To find out how science sees stress, we looked to the American Psychological Association (APA). They describe it as a feeling of being worried, overwhelmed, or run-down.[6] In their 2012 report on stress in America, they found that instead of decreasing, stress was either staying the same or increasing for 80 percent of survey respondents. In addition, 20 percent of respondents felt that they were experiencing "extremely high" stress.[7]

Where do these feelings of being worried and overwhelmed come from? How do you get to the point where you feel run-down? It all starts with a thought. Over time, chronic negative thoughts turn into beliefs and habits. Pretty soon, your lifestyle is based on these negative thoughts, beliefs, and habits, creating chronic stress—and chronic stress has a devastating effect on your health.

If you're overwhelmed, what are you thinking about? You are likely thinking about everything you have on your to-do list. The more you think about how much you have to do and how little time there is to do it, the more overwhelmed you feel.

What about if you're worried? Worrying is often about going over the past and wishing you could change something, or fixating on the future and what could happen.

And if you are run-down, like so many people today, it could likely be that you have said yes to so many things that you aren't giving yourself time to rest and replenish. Perhaps you know that you would benefit from setting boundaries, but it feels too difficult to say no.

The habit of negative thinking can absolutely contribute to endless cycles of chronic stress, which has a direct and profound effect on your health. While some stress is actually good for the body, chronic stress creates challenges. Studies show that emotions are not just something in your mind—your body is impacted by emotions as well.[8] For example, when you're angry, your body tenses up, your digestive organs become rigid, your heart rate increases, and your jaw and facial muscles contract.

We'll talk more about the mind and body connection in Chapter 3; for now, we want to share what happens to your body when you're under stress. When stress becomes chronic, it sends a danger signal that stops blood from rushing to your brain, immune system, and digestive system and instead directs it to your limbs so that you can outrun the danger.[9, 10] This means that your body cannot digest properly, your immune system cannot protect you, and your brain cannot think straight. Studies show that brains can even shrink under prolonged stress.[11]

Under chronic stress, your nervous system is no longer in balance. What was once a harmonious relationship between the sympathetic nervous system (which mobilizes your nervous system's fight-or-flight response) and parasympathetic nervous system (which helps you rest, sleep, digest, and heal) is now tipped toward the sympathetic nervous system. In effect, chronic stress keeps you revved up and hypervigilant, making it hard for you to rest, replenish, and nourish your body.

If you are experiencing chronic stress, know that you are not alone.

Perhaps, like so many today, you have learned that life is not safe. No matter what you've been taught or what you believe in this moment, though, we want you to know that as you step into your love story, you will see how safe and supported you are. We are going to show you how to shift from chronic stress to thoughts and beliefs that support your health and happiness. This book is chock-full of ways you can reduce the stress felt by your mind and body. No matter where you are now when it comes to stress, you can always come back and heal.

Disconnection = Dis-ease

The Blue Zones by Dan Buettner examines the top solutions for living longer and better from some of the world's longest-living communities. Three of the nine solutions that he recommends have to do with connection: (1) connection to a spiritual community, (2) connection to family, and (3) connection to an inner circle or "tribe" of friends. Interestingly, while Buettner didn't include this as one of his "Power 9," all of the "Blue Zone" populations he studied also had a connection to the earth. They all gardened and ate fresh, whole foods.

These days, priorities have shifted because lives have become busier. We don't connect as much as we used to, and when we do, there is often a barrier of technology between us. While many people joke about it, seeing people eating dinner together and checking their phones, texting, and posting on Facebook has become more common than being in the present moment and relating to one another.

The concept of family dinner is becoming a rarity in most homes. On top of this, we see a lot of people eating on the run: in their cars, at their desks, or while watching TV or surfing the web. This shows not only a disconnection from others during meals, but also a disconnection from ourselves. We are no longer connected to the loving and sensory act of nourishing our bodies.

Over time, as our habits changed as a society, our food system has also changed. The fast- and manufactured-food industries grew as a way to allow people to eat quickly, on the run, and with minimal effort. Science has found ways to make "food-like" chemicals so that meals would cook faster, taste better, and make people come back for more.

Manufactured foods are not food at all. In fact, we believe that synthetic, manufactured foods are the final disconnection: They disconnect us from the earth and nature. They deny who we are and what we need to function optimally as the natural beings we are.

Vikas Khanna, a top chef from India, tells a story about food and connection in his book *Return to the Rivers: Recipes and Memories of the Himalayan River Valleys:* "My latest stay in Bhutan in 2011 reminded me of how much my life in New York was disconnected from that world. When I am living and traveling in the Himalayas I feel intimately tied to nature in a way that I don't anywhere else."[12]

Vikas goes on to talk about how when he walks to his friend's home, he goes through fields where the food he eats is growing. When he looks through the window of his bedroom, he sees the sheep that provided the wool in his blanket. And in the town where he goes to the farmers' market, he knows everyone selling and bartering their goods.

What Vikas realizes in Bhutan is that he knows everyone who produces the food he eats. This not only creates connection among the community and nature, but it also creates a system of accountability, where people care about creating healthy and satisfying products for others. They feel responsible for one another's well-being. He describes something many of us have never experienced—the deep connection that the Blue Zones communities have.

We believe that good health is about connection: to ourselves and our bodies, to nature, and to other people. And the most important step you can take to build your connection is establish a relationship with yourself. This is in fact also the key to reducing stress and eliminating dis-ease. So let's take a look at how you can do this.

A New Perspective on Health: Your Health Is a Mirror of Your Relationship to Self

The growing "epidemic" of stress, lifestyle diseases, and autoimmune diseases has no root cause according to mainstream medicine, yet that root cause seems simple to us: it's really an epidemic of not loving the self.

This is a new perspective on health. It's actually not so mysterious, and it brings the power back into your hands. Your health is a mirror of your relationship to yourself and your body. We don't believe in incurable dis-eases; we believe that illness is an invitation to change your relationship with yourself for the better.

Interestingly, new findings in science seem to agree. For example, Bruce Lipton, Ph.D., is an internationally recognized cell biologist who performed pioneering studies at Stanford University's School of Medicine. In his book *The Biology of Belief,* he talks about a new paradigm of health based on the science of epigenetics.

Bruce conducted some groundbreaking experiments showing that our genes do not control biology. The idea that genes control biology is a faulty scientific assumption that was debunked by the Human Genome Project around the year 2003, a finding that fit very well with experiments Bruce was doing with cells in the lab. His experiments showed that it was not the genes that controlled the cells, but how the cells *responded to the environment they were in.* Bruce explains that since human beings have brains, our response to our environment is much more complex than that of a cell. We have beliefs, and it is through these beliefs that we respond to our life situation (or environment).[13]

What message are you giving to your cells right now?

If you believe that you are a bad person, your cells are listening. If you believe that you are sick, your cells are listening. Likewise, if you believe that you are a beautiful being worthy of love and that you are healthy, your cells are listening.

What kind of relationship do you think you are creating with yourself and your body if you're sending negative messages and embracing negative beliefs about yourself?

Loving Yourself Is about Taking Care of Yourself

When you love yourself, you take care of your own needs. Yet too often today, people (especially women) believe they must take care of other people or other responsibilities before themselves. For example:

- Do you find yourself saying yes when you really want to say no? Are you helping others so often that you have little time to rest and relax? Do feel like you'll rest once you retire, or once your kids are grown up?

- Do you find yourself saying, "I just need to get through this, and then I will rest/take a break"?

- Do you feel like a people pleaser or do you fear others' disapproval of you? Are you constantly feeling like you give and give, while not getting much back from others (or possibly not being able to receive support, gifts, or compliments from others)?

- Are you often trying to set boundaries and failing?

We believe that the real health epidemic is a disconnection from self. We think that the immune system gets a little confused when you put yourself last.

Science states that the root cause of nearly every chronic disease—inflammation—happens when the immune system can no longer tell the difference between what is good and bad for the body.[14] Metaphysically, we feel that inflammation and chronic disease are really about your body loving you enough to give you a wake-up call. It's an *invitation* to listen to your body and return to a state of self-love.

When babies are born, they love everything about themselves. They are fascinated by their hands and feet, and even their feces. Over time, we are taught that things about us are wrong and bad. Too often, we become ashamed of our bodies or characteristics about ourselves, and we come to feel like we're not good enough. We learn that "the rules," expectations of others, and proven evidence are more important than how we feel or what we want. We are taught to listen to everyone else so much that we feel we cannot trust ourselves.

It's no surprise that under those circumstances, we'd disconnect from our inner guidance system, which Louise calls her "inner ding." We all have one, although most of us have not been taught to listen to that inner voice, feeling, or signal that guides us.

The most beautiful thing about your body is that it has a deep knowing about what you truly need for health and happiness. In fact, one of Ahlea's specialties is listening to what people's bodies are asking for. She can see into the body or touch near an organ and hear what the organ is saying. She often hears what a person's body has been trying to tell them through symptoms.

Over the past ten years of working with clients, the biggest pattern Ahlea has seen is a message of fear in the kidneys. She says that the kidneys are saying they are sad and afraid because they don't feel protected, and that overall, bodies do not feel heard. This led us to a discussion about the child inside all of us. Too often, the inner child is forced into situations it does not want to go into, which creates a great deal of discomfort. While you may make a plan to "get through it" when you really don't want to do something, your inner child suffers, and your organs tend to suffer as well. In order to push through things you don't really want to do, you often have to disconnect from yourself, your inner child, or your inner guidance in some way.

The power to achieve your best health goes beyond your immune system. It all starts with a little-known secret: loving yourself. We believe that as you start to listen to your inner guidance with love, your kidneys, your immune system, and your entire body will start to feel safe. When your body feels safe, it can heal. Just remember that your body *wants* to heal.

Client Stories

Catherine: Fibromyalgia

Catherine, a woman in her 50s, came to Ahlea after having been to many doctors and receiving a diagnosis of fibromyalgia. Fibromyalgia is an autoimmune disease characterized by all-over muscle and joint pain, tender points in the body, and fatigue; it often leads to depression.[15]

Catherine was understandably scared about her condition and how to treat it. Ahlea started slowly by teaching her some deep-breathing exercises to get more oxygen in her body, and stretching exercises to get some circulation in her tissues. She began to notice that she could breathe easier, and within a month, she felt calmer and her pain started to go away. Her nervous system was beginning to move out of fight-or-flight and into "rest and digest" mode, which allowed her body to start healing. This gave her the confidence to move forward with her health protocol.

The next step was for Ahlea to work with her on removing old physical and emotional trauma from a car accident, which happened just before the fibromyalgia showed up. As Catherine started releasing this trauma, she felt ready to move on to Ahlea's suggested nutrition protocol.

The first thing Ahlea recommended was for Catherine to give up sugar. Within a couple of weeks, Catherine felt good enough to start doing Pilates, which allowed her to develop muscle and abdominal strength. This new strength helped to support her joints, and the pain dropped away.

The best part about Catherine's symptoms resolving was that she started to dance. She had always wanted to do so and felt she had an inner ballerina. Pretty soon, she'd show up for her healing sessions in a leotard and dance across the room with great joy. Ahlea saw that Catherine's inner child was thrilled to feel playful again, and that the adult Catherine trusted this newfound freedom in her body.

Stacey: Lyme Disease

Lyme disease is caused by the bacteria *Borrelia burgdorferi* and transmitted by the bite of an infected tick. The symptoms are flulike: achy joints, headache, fever, and fatigue. Experts are unsure as to whether chronic Lyme disease is autoimmune or nervous-system related, and some feel that it doesn't even exist.[16]

However, patients are well aware of the symptoms, including Stacey, a woman in her 50s who came to see Ahlea. Stacey had been to doctor after doctor and finally received a diagnosis of Lyme disease. To treat it, Stacey was prescribed large doses of antibiotics.

The first thing Ahlea did was to work with the messages Stacey's body was telling her. It was important for this woman to learn that her body was not attacking her; rather, it was speaking to her with love and asking her to make some changes.

The changes Ahlea had Stacey make were slow and steady. She had her client schedule some hyperbaric-chamber sessions, a type of therapy that brings more oxygen into the blood. As Stacey started feeling better, Ahlea had her focus on nutrition so that she could improve her gut health. The main nutritional focus was to add probiotics to Stacey's diet to cultivate more good bacteria that would help her digest and heal. Ahlea also taught Stacey to do proper food combining, which is a way of eating certain foods together to make them very easy to digest.

In the year that followed, Stacey felt well enough to start walking and doing Pilates, which strengthened her body. She let go of emotions that were being held in her body, along with beliefs that were limiting her health and happiness. Within the year, Stacey felt completely recovered from Lyme disease.

♥

With autoimmune and other dis-ease conditions, we often see that the physical symptoms are accompanied by emotional trauma. When you work on both the body and the mind, the benefits increase exponentially. Later in the book, we will teach you how to listen to your body, so you can hear the story of your organs, listen to your inner child, and learn to protect yourself so that your body does not have to take on dis-ease from lack of protection. We will also share tips and techniques that you can use to love your body to good health, including many of those that Ahlea used to help Stacey to heal from Lyme.

We want you to know that if you are experiencing a chronic health condition, it is really an invitation to come back to love. We are going to share many gentle tips with you to reconnect to yourself and your body. This is a miraculous, joyful, and loving process. It is as beautiful as coming home.

Now, when you think about coming home, you can't help but think about family and community. The thing is, you don't have to do this alone. Reconnection to self is also about reconnecting with others—finding your tribe, your community of like-minded, supportive people. It's important to learn to love and protect yourself. It's just as important to have people you can lean on. People you feel have your back.

Whether or not you have a supportive community of friends and family, one thing you do have on your side is Life. Part of reconnecting is knowing that Life loves you. Life has your back. When you trust Life to support you, you are never alone. Life will always support you as you take the power of your health and happiness back into your own hands!

A Simple Health Assessment

As we've shown in this chapter, science is proving what we have known for a long time: *you have the power to heal.*

We believe that health is a reflection of your inner self. Take a moment to assess your health by checking off the statements that are true for you:

- You feel good about yourself just the way you are.
- You feel good about your body—you are not always feeling like you want to fix or change something about it.
- You are not concerned by any symptoms; that is, you don't have chronic aches, pains, addictions, or low moods.
- You like yourself and you like other people—you are not complaining about life and the people around you.
- There is an ease to your life, and things seem to flow easily.
- You feel connected to nature and to other people.
- You choose food and beverages that are healthy for your body and that make you feel good.
- You are not taking any medications.
- You have a sense of balance in your life—you feel comfortable and are not overwhelmed with work, to-do lists, or stress.
- You give and receive in a balanced way; in other words, you are not feeling as if you give and give and never get anything in return.
- You have good relationships with people you trust and whom you feel you can count on.
- You feel that you take care of yourself very well.
- You have an inner guidance system that you trust.

How did you do? If you checked off one or more items, congratulations! And chances are, you noticed some opportunities for improvement. Everyone has areas where they can improve their lives, and each chapter of *Loving Yourself to Great Health* will show you how to do just that.

Exercises to Create a New Perspective on Health

Health, just like life, is simple. What we give out, we get back. Our beliefs comprise years of thinking the same thoughts. What we think and believe about ourselves, about life, and about our health becomes our reality. The good news is, you can change your thoughts and your beliefs! These exercises will help get you started.

1. When You Don't Know What to Do, Focus on Love

In 1985, Louise started the Hayrides, support-group meetings for people living with HIV/AIDS, along with their families and loved ones. In the '80s, everyone was terrified of AIDS. Doctors didn't know what to do, and people feared even touching anyone with the dis-ease. People diagnosed with HIV or AIDS lived in guilt, fear, shame, and secrecy, and often felt that death and suffering were inevitable. There was so much fear.

No one knew what to do at the time. But as author and speaker David Kessler said, "When everyone else was taking a step back, Louise Hay took a step forward."

Louise didn't know what to do either, but she knew one thing for certain: *love heals*. Her message then and now is clear: "When you don't know what else to do, focus on love."

In 2013, Louise had a Hayride reunion. Many of the men from the original group attended and attested to the fact that focusing on love changed everything for them. And for the men who did die during that time, attending the Hayrides made it easier to face death. They had a chance to drop their shame and experience love, connection, and forgiveness. This made the dying process more gentle and peaceful for them.

In the nearly three decades since Louise first started those meetings, so much has changed. Today, we know that people can live with HIV. We know that we can touch and hug people with HIV or AIDS and not be afraid of catching it. Yet in a society so focused on modern medical technology, it can be easy to forget that love does in fact heal. That love fosters connection. And that love breeds more love.

If you have a chronic condition or even a stressful situation and you don't know what else to do, take a moment right now to focus on love:

Put your hands on your heart and feel your heart beating. Take deep breaths. Feel into your body. Breathe deeply into your body and invite it to relax . . . every muscle, every cell, relax. Now focus on the feeling of love. If you aren't sure where to start, think of a pet or a loved one and notice how that feels. Bring that feeling right into your body. As you take deep breaths, breathe that feeling into every cell. Imagine that feeling surrounding you. Give it a color if you like—maybe green, pink, or white, or whatever feels good to you.

Feel yourself becoming enveloped in the feeling of love. Do this for five minutes each day when you wake up and before you go to bed. Start with one minute if that is all you have at first, then build up.

We also invite you to remind yourself each day to focus on love if something feels difficult or overwhelming. Notice how that shifts things for you.

2. Mirror Work and Affirmations: Sweet and Loving Thoughts Begin the Healing Journey

Mirrors reflect back to us our feelings about ourselves. They clearly show us the areas to be changed if we want to create a loving, fulfilling life. The most powerful way to do affirmations is to look in the mirror and say them out loud.

When people from all over the world who have followed Louise's teachings were asked about their success with affirmations and mirror work, hundreds of them responded. They reported so many positive changes in their health, such as losing up to 100 pounds, dissolving autoimmune disease, overcoming addiction and eating disorders, eliminating pain, relieving stress and post-traumatic stress disorder, overcoming anxiety and insomnia, and much more. It's amazing what can happen when you are kind and loving to yourself!

While you read this book, we suggest that you have a mirror close by so that you can use it for all of the affirmations in this book. Doing your affirmations in the mirror will allow you to look into your own eyes and notice if you are seeing resistance or love.

Let's start with an important affirmation. Look in the mirror and say to yourself: *I am willing to change.*

Notice how you feel. Do you feel any resistance to change? Do you feel as if you can change? Do you even want to? Noticing how you feel about change is important, because when you're looking at self-growth, your willingness to change can make or break your own success. This is why we want you to start with assessing your willingness to change.

If you feel resistant, know that you're not alone. Heather used to work as a change-management expert, and part of her job was to understand such resistance —why it happens and how to support people through times of transition. Even when helpful, positive changes were introduced in companies, they could fail based on whether people embraced the change or not.

Resistance to change is actually common for several reasons. Most center around being afraid of what will be different. Human beings tend to live with the status quo because we fear what will be different about our lives if we change. Perhaps we fear we'll lose the identity we've built for ourselves or we'll have to face something that's not working in our lives.

A woman once told Heather, "I really don't like what I'm doing at work. I want to change my career, but my husband doesn't work and I have to keep my job." This woman desperately wanted to do something else and it was impacting her health, but she felt so locked into her job that she was afraid to leave. She was even afraid to hire a life coach because coaching could reveal that she would benefit from working at something entirely different. This woman was so afraid that she stayed in her job until she became so sick that she had to leave it after all.

If we let fear stop us from changing, we lose out on the opportunity to see how powerful we really are and how Life really loves us and is there for us!

Psychologists might recommend some things you can do to help with your willingness to change, such as "monitor your behaviors," "logically sequence events," and "examine the consequence."[17] However, we're going to keep it simple by sharing some really great tips that you can implement starting today:

— **Decide you are important enough.** Louise always teaches that once you try something and you see that it worked out for you, it makes change easier because it gives you permission to do it again. The thing is, you have to give yourself permission to try it in the first place. You have to feel you are important enough to give yourself that permission, to give yourself the space to change, to prioritize it in your life, and to support yourself in being successful with the rest of these tips!

Sometimes the best way to change is to just do it, just take that first step of knowing that your health and happiness are important. *You* are important.

— **Take baby steps.** Pick one small thing to do—it can be as quick and easy as you like, but do pick one thing and get started. For example, kiss your hand and say, "You are worth healing." You can just do that for as long as you like and then move on whenever you're ready. Remember the lesson from the tortoise and the hare: slow and steady wins the race.

— **Keep it simple and gentle.** The gentler you are with yourself, the better. This is not a "no pain, no gain" approach. Part of loving yourself is keeping things easy and being kind to yourself. Think about how this would feel. Remember how afraid the kidneys often are, remember your inner child, and be gentle. Here's an example of something gentle you can say to yourself: "You are safe with me."

— **Be consistent.** Keep in mind that the more you do your mirror work and practice your affirmations, the easier it will get. The more consistent you are, the more results you will experience. Think about the idea of practice—with any new skill, you don't start out an expert. The more you practice, the better you get!

— **Get helpers.** One great way to build connection and to make change is to create a support system. This could be a friend, spouse, coach, family member, or whomever you feel comfortable with. Some people find or create online support groups or Facebook groups. In any event, it really helps to find a like-minded person or group to support you in doing your affirmations and sharing any roadblocks and wins you have along the way.

— **Have fun!** Make the process fun in whatever way you can. Laugh at yourself; be silly. Louise walks by a mirror and says, "Hi, kid, you look great today!" It doesn't matter who's around and, inevitably, it makes everyone smile and love her even more. Ahlea winks at herself when she passes the mirror. Heather throws her arms up in the air and jumps around after her affirmations. One of the greatest things about Louise and Ahlea's health and bodywork sessions together is that they laugh all the time. They are doing serious work, yet it's also fun. Remember, change and healing can be joyous!

— **Celebrate even small successes.** As you start to change, give yourself credit for starting! You don't have to wait for major changes to celebrate; you can highlight the little successes you have along the way. Choose rewards that are meaningful to you, yet they can be as simple as giving yourself lots of hugs and kisses. Small children know the healing power of getting kisses from their mothers to make a "boo-boo" feel better. Kisses and hugs have great healing power, especially when you give them to yourself. It might feel silly at first, but it's a beautiful way to be sweet to yourself.

— **Think positive.** Psychologists understand what Louise has been teaching for decades: Change is easier when it's based on positive thinking, rather than guilt, shame, or fear. We have provided you with some affirmations on the next few pages so that you can reinforce your positive thoughts and beliefs!

While change can feel hard at first, there is something magical about trying out something new. It gives you the opportunity to see how strong you are. You must be strong—you wouldn't be here reading this book if you weren't. Or if you weren't curious about what change could be like.

When Heather was first learning to scuba dive, she didn't trust the breathing equipment. On her first ocean dive, the water was very choppy. By the time she swam around the boat to the front, she was already out of breath, which made her even more afraid to descend into the water. Her instructor looked her in the eyes and said, "You can go back if you want to, or you can just put your head underwater and see what you think. We'll come right back up if you want."

While Heather was so scared that she wanted to turn back, she felt comforted by this idea of just going under the water a small amount and deciding how she felt first. She and her instructor went under less than one foot and remained there a few minutes. This allowed Heather to see how easy it was to breathe with the equipment—it actually worked! So she agreed to go deeper very slowly, and once she felt comfortable, she proceeded to do her first dive.

After the dive, Heather felt exuberant! She overcame her fears and fell in love with scuba diving. She realized that if she hadn't taken a baby step, she would have missed out on the feeling of being able to fly underwater. While turning back would have been fine, the experience she had was ten times better.

As you can see, if you're wanting to try something that feels scary, being gentle with yourself and taking baby steps can help you build the courage for something bigger, and can help overcome fears about the next step and the next one after that.

Change is one of the greatest teachers. It scares us and asks us to reach deep inside ourselves for courage we didn't even know we had. It asks us every day to prove our commitment to ourselves. It leads us into the dark places and allows us to fill them with light. It shows us things about ourselves we never knew. It allows us to recognize that failure and success are two sides of the same coin. And before we know it, it shows us how powerful and strong we are. Change doesn't ask us to go faster or further than we are ready to go—it teaches us to listen to our hearts and take chances that will set us free.

♥

Try the following affirmations, picking one to begin with. You can choose more when you feel ready. Practice them throughout the day, whenever you feel that you need them.

Change

If you feel resistant to change, look in the mirror and affirm:

It is only a thought, and a thought can be changed.

I am open to change.

I am willing to change.

I greet the new with open arms.

I am willing to learn new things every day.

*Each problem has a solution. All experiences
are opportunities for me to learn and grow. I am safe.*

Loving and Accepting Yourself and Others

Look in the mirror and ask yourself: "How can I love and accept you more?" Be open and listen for an answer, a feeling, or whatever comes to you. Trust that if nothing comes to you in this moment, it will at another time. And affirm:

I accept myself and create peace in my mind and heart.

I am good enough just as I am.

I love and approve of myself.

*As I forgive myself, I leave behind all feelings of not
being good enough, and I am free to love myself.*

[Your name], *I love you. I really love you.*

I love myself.

I am special and wonderful.

I love my life.

I love this day.

It is wonderful to feel the love in my heart.

My heart is open, and I allow my love to flow freely.
I love myself, I love others, and others love me.

I forgive myself for not being the way I want me to be. I forgive myself,
and set myself free to be just the way I am. I love and accept myself as I am.

I bless you with love, and I bring harmony to this situation.
(This is a wonderful affirmation to use when someone is doing
something to disrupt the harmony of your life, as is the next one.)

I forgive you for not being the way I want you to be. I forgive you and set you free.

I cannot change another person. I let others be
who they are, and I simply love who I am.

I move beyond forgiveness to understanding, and I have compassion for all.

Health

Your health and happiness is a mirror of your relationship with yourself. Affirm:

My sweet and loving thoughts begin my healing journey.

I allow the love from my heart to wash through me, cleansing
and healing every part of my body. I know I am worth healing.

My body is always working toward optimal health.

My body wants to be whole and healthy. I cooperate
and become healthy, whole, and complete.

I now express health, happiness, prosperity, and peace of mind.

Taking Care of Yourself and Listening to Your Inner Guidance

Listening to your inner guidance and acting on it is the way to health and happiness. Remember, you are the first step in your health, and your immune system is learning from your ability to care for yourself. Your cells are learning from what you think and believe. Affirm:

I love and care for my inner child.

*I trust my inner wisdom. I say no when I want
to say no, and I say yes when I want to say yes.*

*I am guided throughout this day in making the right choices. Divine
intelligence continuously guides me in the realization of what is right for me.*

*As I go about my day, I listen to my own guidance. My intuition
is always on my side. I trust it to be there at all times. I am safe.*

I speak up for myself. I ask for what I want. I claim my power.

Trusting Life

You can ask Life to help you in any situation. Life loves you and is there for you, if only you'll ask. Look in the mirror and ask Life, "What do I need?" Listen for the answer, a feeling, or whatever comes up. If nothing comes up in that moment, be open to an answer coming at a later time. And affirm:

Life loves me.

I trust things to be wonderful.

I observe with joy as Life abundantly supports and cares for me.

I know that only good awaits me at every turn.

All is well. Everything is working out for my highest good.

Out of this situation only good will come. I am safe.

3. Meditation: Reconnecting to the Earth and All Things

Your health and happiness are bolstered by your connection to yourself, other people, the earth, and all things. As you disconnect on one level, you may feel yourself disconnecting on many levels. Over time, it can start to feel like you are all alone. You can forget that Life loves and supports you.

A common pattern that Ahlea sees in her practice is that people's bodies are crying for a connection to the earth. Humans once lived off the land; we touched the soil and understood plants and trees. Tribal communities used nature the way we use signs and Global Positioning Systems (GPS) to get from one place to another. This cry from the body that she hears is one of desperation. The less we connect to the earth and nature, the more our bodies cry out for this primal connection.

The following meditation is a way that Ahlea helps her clients reconnect to the earth, themselves, and all things. This is a very healing meditation:

> *Lie down in a quiet, comfortable place and close your eyes. Bring your attention into your body. Feel your breath and follow it as you breathe deeply, in and out. Continue to follow your breath until you feel your body relax.*
>
> *Now imagine yourself in a beautiful field, under the most beautiful tree. You are comfortably warm and the sun is shining. You are safe and the tree is providing you shelter and shade. See and feel that safe, beautiful, comfortable space.*
>
> *Feel your body sink deeper into the ground. Know that the ground is protecting and nourishing you. Feel your body growing roots right into the soil. As you continue to focus on your breath, allow the roots to get deeper and deeper, reaching into the core of the earth.*
>
> *As you continue to breathe deeply, gather the loving energy from the earth and breathe it right back up through those roots and into your body. Feel how deeply connected and loving this feels. You are protected, you are nourished, you are supported, you are loved.*
>
> *Feel that love and support . . . allow yourself to breathe it into every cell. Feel your cells respond to the connection to the earth. Now breathe deeply and feel that connection with everything around you. Breathe as if you are breathing with all of nature and all of life.*
>
> *Continue to feel that connection and the love, support, and nourishment it brings. Now gather up all this love and support and feel it in your body. Trust that this connection and this love is always there for you. Anytime you think of yourself in this space, under this tree, you will feel it. Anytime you think about your roots, connecting to the earth, you will feel it.*
>
> *Breathe deeply in and out for three more breaths and open your eyes.*

You can take your time with this meditation or do it in just three minutes. Some people benefit from doing it daily. Once you have done this meditation and have the memory of this feeling, we encourage you to think about and trust that this energy and connection is there for you anytime you need it. This way, if you are at work or going about your day, all you need to do is remember this feeling and it will help reinforce your connection.

4. Some Beautiful Ways to Reconnect

- **Garden**—Ahlea and Louise are avid gardeners, and you will see how gardening reconnects you to the earth in Chapter 5. We'll also give you some indoor gardening tips!

- **Eat whole foods**—nourishing your body with whole foods is very grounding. Likewise, touching foods from nature, like vegetables and fruits, is a great way to reconnect to nature.

- **Connect with nature**—hike in nature, walk barefoot in the sand or on the earth, or sit by the ocean or on a mountaintop.

- **Take breaks during your workday**—go outside and feel the sunshine on your skin. Maybe take your shoes off and walk barefoot on the ground. Stretch your body.

- **Spend time with friends and family**—focus on connecting with people in the present moment and agree to put away phones and electronics.

- **Seek out farms**—visit an organic farm, and if it's permitted, pet the animals. Visit your local farmers' market to reconnect with people growing and caring for your food.

- **Put your hands on your heart**—revisit the exercise earlier in the chapter.

- **Listen to your body**—we'll show you how in Chapter 4.

- **Affirm that you are a part of this process**—you have the power to reconnect to yourself and all things.

- **Practice compassion for yourself and others**—practice not judging or criticizing yourself and others. To help with this, take a look at the affirmations on love and acceptance in Step 2, earlier in the chapter. (We will provide more tips in Chapter 2.)

You Have the Capacity to Heal

It's an interesting question: why do people still look so good when inside, their bodies are suffering? Our feeling is that our society has been taught to "save face" under all circumstances. We learn to paint the picture we want people to see— to press on, even if we feel like we're dying inside. The more we do this, the more our bodies reflect that pattern.

We want you to see the other side of this coin as well. If your body is in a state of dis-ease and you still look healthy to everyone else, chances are you have a large capacity for health and resilience inside. And even if you feel you don't look healthy on the outside, the fact that you are reading this book tells us that you are committed to creating good health. You can take this commitment and capacity for health and trust that as you show your body tender loving care, you can nurture it back to wellness. You can shift the pattern of fear and hypervigilant protection that your body is using for survival into a pattern of love, where your body trusts that you are going to be there for yourself.

The more you lovingly protect and care for yourself, the more you come back into balance. This is the greatest love story of all, and you have the power to live it!

Now that you have a new perspective on health, we are going to show you some important tips for how to love yourself and your body.

Chapter 2

Step #2:
Love Yourself
and Your Body—
Food, Weight Loss,
Dis-ease, and More

We have established that health is a reflection of your relationship with yourself, and that health conditions are your body's way of asking you to come back to self-love. Now we think it's important to talk about why this is happening—why have so many people disconnected from themselves, and why does it seem so challenging to love oneself? As we've already mentioned, the lack of self-love comes from a feeling of not being good enough. Let's explore that a bit more.

> "Love is the great miracle cure.
> Loving ourselves works
> miracles in our lives."
>
> — Louise

How many of us have grown up learning how perfect we are? How everything about us is beautiful, unique, and wonderful? The truth is that most of us have been brought up with messages indicating the opposite: that there are many things wrong with us. Whether these messages came from family, school, religious institutions, friends, or the media, it seems that too many of us have grown up with a firm belief that we are not good enough. So how can we be who we really are or trust our inner guidance if we feel that we're not good enough?

In her best-selling book *You Can Heal Your Life*, Louise shares some very important exercises that we encourage you to do. Here are two of them that relate to what we've been talking about here:

1. Write down all of the negative beliefs you have about yourself and identify where they came from. Did they come from your parents, school, church, other authority figures, friends, or the media? Identifying where you learned these beliefs is one step toward realizing that these are just thoughts and they are not true. These beliefs stand in the way of your accepting and loving yourself. (Please note that at the end of this chapter, we are going to give you some affirmations to use for your mirror work anytime one of these beliefs comes up.)

2. Imagine a three-year-old child. Look at this three-year-old and think about what it would be like to yell all of those negative beliefs you carry at this tiny child. We all have a three-year-old inside of us, and when we continue telling this child that he or she is not good enough, it's no wonder that we don't feel well.

What if you told yourself how much you loved yourself instead of listing everything that is wrong? How do you think your life would be if you encouraged yourself and accepted yourself just as you are every day?

This is one of the greatest steps you can take toward creating good health.

The Media: Turning Off Negative Programming

Once you've committed to reconnecting to self-love, there is something you may become very aware of: messages in the media. Television and radio shows, magazines, and Internet sites are often geared to make money by reinforcing that you are not good enough. Advertising focuses on making you feel like less than the perfect person you are so that you will buy certain products or services. It plays into the part of you that believes the negative messages you learned growing up.

Since the 1800s, advertisers have used fear, guilt, and shame techniques to create emotional imbalance and compliance for their intended goal: to get you to purchase something.[1, 2] The end result is to disconnect you from yourself, so that you feel like you need something to make yourself acceptable or better in some way. In his book *Mind Programming,* Hay House author Eldon Taylor describes how advertisers spent $149 billion on market research in 2007 alone, using psychologists and other experts to find out what would make people buy products.[3] According to Taylor, they learn what makes us tick and how to manipulate our choices and behavior.

These messages of fear, guilt, and shame have shaped people's lives, decisions, and attitudes in many ways. These negative messages often reinforce choices that are not in alignment with good health. They sell a focus on the outside—on how you look or what others think of you—rather than the inside, on who you are and what makes you wonderfully unique.

In her 2014 San Diego TEDxYouth talk, Caroline Heldman, Ph.D., shared some startling facts from her study about what happens when media ads portray women as sexual objects[4]:

— The number of advertisements that the average person is exposed to has increased from 500 per day in the 1970s to 5,000 per day today. In modern advertisements, 96 percent of sexually objectified bodies are female.

— Children from the ages of 8 to 18 are attached to technology for an average of eight hours per day, where advertisers can get to them. These ads have become more hypersexualized to cut through the clutter of other ads competing for attention.

— The more women are conditioned to feel like sex objects, the more they:

- Have higher rates of depression.
- Engage in body monitoring, which means being hyperaware of how they're sitting, how their hair looks, who is looking at them, and so on. The average woman engages in body monitoring every 30 seconds.
- Develop body shame and eating disorders.
- Have sexual dysfunction.
- Have low self-esteem.
- Have a lower grade point average (GPA) in school.
- Compete with other women.

These are exceptional reasons to stop consuming damaging media and purchasing products that promote negative messages.

The good news is that you no longer have to be subject to this conditioning and can instead focus on love. As you move away from messages of shame and reconnect to your inner guidance, you get clearer about what you really want. You can choose to stop watching, reading, and listening to programming that only serves to reinforce negative thinking; instead, focus on cultivating positive thoughts that remind you that you are already perfect, whole, and complete in this moment.

The thing is, we are always in a state of growing, changing, and evolving, and it's much easier to grow when you can accept and love yourself where you are now.

Remember, you are perfect and lovable just as you are right now. The most stable foundation from which to change is a foundation of love and acceptance.

For 16 years, Heather searched for answers to help her recover from bulimia. And while she was successful on the surface and very optimistic, she held back some happiness and self-acceptance because of the shame and guilt she felt for having an eating disorder. She kept this secret locked away, worried that people would not accept her if they knew.

One day, she realized that the shame, guilt, and lack of self-acceptance kept her from fully enjoying her life. She began to wonder, *What if I never recover? Could I accept myself anyway? Could I maybe just enjoy precious moments in my life anyway? What if I could love myself just as I am?* As you can imagine, it felt a little scary to think these thoughts because most of us are taught that in order to change, we can't accept where we are. However, this was the beginning of Heather's recovery. The moment she decided to accept herself just as she was, something inside her shifted. She began to look at life from a more open, loving perspective. Within about a year, she was able to connect the dots that led to her recovery. Accepting herself did not stop her from looking for answers—it allowed her to love herself and her life more fully, which led her to a recovery that felt miraculous and simple.

Change implies that things are shifting and moving, and it often requires you to move out of your comfort zone. It is much harder to do this if you are constricted and bound by fear, guilt, or shame. You might take action from these places, but it's rarely sustainable.

It's time to put aside all messages that ask you to do anything other than love yourself and focus on creating a stable foundation for lasting change. Self-acceptance is an expansive feeling that can open you up to finding your own answers, beyond what "they" told you. The more you love yourself, the more you are guided to what is truly right for *you*.

Diets, Weight, and Health: When the Outside Is More Important Than the Inside

If you were to ask the average person what good health is, what do you think they'd say? Unfortunately, most of us have been taught that how a person looks determines whether they are healthy or not. And all too often, weight is the number one focus when it comes to health.

In 2013, the weight-loss market in the United States alone was projected to be $66.5 billion—and 83 percent of that market is geared toward women, many of whom make four to five attempts to diet each year.[5] At the same time, obesity rates are growing worldwide and the World Health Organization (WHO) estimates that over 1 billion adults are overweight—at least 300 million of them are in fact clinically obese, with the numbers continuing to grow.[6]

With all of this spending and all of these diet attempts, why are the obesity rates increasing?

Because of the weight-loss industry, the fashion industry, and other media messages, many women find this to be their main mantra: *I am not good enough. What's the use?* This kind of thinking can lead to them using their bodies as a focal point for self-hatred. Underneath all of this may be the thought *If I were only thin enough, they would love me.*

If this sounds familiar to you, perhaps you grew up hearing your mother judging her body or watching your friends go on extreme diets. Maybe, like Ahlea, you were a gymnast or in a competitive sport that would send you home if you weighed too much. Perhaps you noticed how people complimented others on weight loss or openly judged women because of weight or looks. It's not surprising that some part of you would feel like weight is an all-important goal.

But the truth is, nothing works when one's focus is solely on the exterior. Approximately 80 percent of all dieters regain the weight they lost.[7] Embracing self-acceptance and self-love is the true key to both weight loss and lasting health. And here's the other secret, the one that the advertisers don't really want to tell you: what you eat matters (and we're not talking about packaged food), because what you eat is a form of self-love.

Diets based on calorie restriction, packaged foods, and "no pain, no gain" mentalities are not sustainable.

The Only Diet that Works: A Media Diet

If you want to go on a diet, we recommend a media diet! Here, you'd abstain from any form of media that separates you from the lovable person that you are. The same principle is true for things you hear other people saying, or when you hear others judging one another based on looks. We invite you to surround these people with the energy of love. They are responding automatically to what they learned growing up, and they are likely judging themselves just as harshly, too. What others think is never as important as what you think and how you feel. It's the only thing you have control over, and it's a direct route to making choices that support your highest good.

Health is not a measure of what you weigh. It's not about going through something painful for a number on a scale or a size of clothing. It's not an outside job; it's an inside job. Health starts with how you think and ends with how you feel. It's about taking good care of yourself with the thoughts you think and the food you eat. And all of the little, loving things you do for yourself in between.

If weight loss is your goal, we'll show you gentle, natural ways to achieve it and share some inspiring stories of people who lost weight naturally with a few simple changes. First, we want to share some better measures for health than weight. Please answer the following:

- How do you feel?
- Does your body move with ease?
- Does your body support the life you want?
- Does your brain function well? Are your moods stable?
- Do you have the energy you want?
- Are you sleeping well at night?
- Do you trust your body's guidance?
- Are you comfortable in your own skin?

Your answers to the questions above are a better gauge on health than numbers on a scale.

Food Matters: If It Doesn't Grow, Don't Eat It

In the book *The Hundred-Year Lie: How Food and Medicine Are Destroying Your Health,* journalist Randall Fitzgerald details how he began seeing research and patterns that led him to investigate the relationship between manufactured food (or processed food) and health.

Fitzgerald found that three groups have great influence over what we eat: the processed-food industry, the pharmaceutical industry, and the chemical industry. Their goal is to convince us that their chemically created, synthetic foods are better than food grown in nature.[8] Unfortunately, they've been very successful in reinforcing this belief. Some important historical occurrences have also spurred them on, like food shortages during the Great Depression and World War II, and in more recent times, busy working families.

Margarine is a great example. In the 1930s and 1940s, the Great Depression and World War II caused food shortages in the U.S. Since there was a shortage of butter, "oleomargarine" was a popular replacement. Louise remembers this white substance that came in a plastic bag with a yellow dot of liquid—she would sit at the table and squeeze the two together to get the yellow color of butter.

Over time, manufacturers made margarine with a yellow color so that it would look more appetizing; you may recall the advertising that came along with it. Margarine was touted as much healthier than butter, and many people bought into this belief. Then, decades later, the truth about margarine came out: this synthetic fat is actually a "trans fat" (we will talk more about trans fats in Chapter 5), one of the most harmful fats for your health.[9] Experts are now agreeing that butter is better than margarine.

Below are some of the statistics that got Fitzgerald's attention when researching *The Hundred-Year Lie.* Over the past 100 years[10]:

- Cancer deaths have increased from 3 percent to 20 percent of all deaths.

- Diabetes has increased from 0.1 percent of the population to 20 percent.

- Heart disease went from being almost nonexistent to killing more than 700,000.

- Health-care costs have risen greatly.

- From 1974 to 1997, the incidence of death from brain diseases, like Alzheimer's and Parkinson's, tripled in nine Western countries, including the U.S.

Experts from a variety of industries can argue over why these health issues have been on the rise at the same time as synthetic, manufactured foods have been introduced into our food supply. However, in the study on brain diseases mentioned above, researchers speculated that the results are thanks to a combination of eating processed foods and food sprayed with toxic pesticides.

Fast food and packaged food are thought of as convenient and often inexpensive ways to feed ourselves and our families. Many of us grew up eating these foods. They are made to taste delicious and last a long time; they're packaged to look fun and exciting; and psychologists, scientists, and researchers have been employed to make sure that we'd want to eat more and more of them.

In the book *Fat Land: How Americans Became the Fattest People in the World,* author Greg Critser tells us that food manufacturers were having trouble because the size of the American population was not growing fast enough for their profits to increase. So what they did is focus on getting the average American to eat at least 200 calories more each day—by doing so, they could continue to make more money.[11] In order to increase their profit margin, processed-food companies also add toxic chemicals to make food more addictive, change packaging sizes and colors, and use advertising and other sneaky techniques.

Every cell, tissue, organ—*everything* in your body—relies on nutrients from food. Without the proper nutrients, your body and brain no longer function at their optimal levels. One important message that Louise has shared for years is: "If it doesn't grow, don't eat it." If you follow this guideline, you will be giving yourself a huge leg up on health.

Our bodies were designed to function using food and water found in nature. At one time, food from the land and ocean were all we ate. While manufactured food may have been created 100 years ago, modern humans have been around for 200,000 years. Our bodies have not changed, so what happens when synthetic foods are taken into a body that was made for foods found in nature? The body does its best, but we put it under a much greater burden and deny it what it needs to function optimally.

Client Stories

We believe that symptoms are the body's way of expressing a deficiency of some kind. And your body is longing to be heard. Looking at diet, lifestyle, thoughts, and beliefs is where we always start.

Jennifer: Severe Acne and Rash

Jennifer, a woman in her 30s, came to Ahlea with acne and a rash on her back, face, neck, and torso. This condition had been going on for ten years and was devastating for Jennifer. She had been to every type of doctor and had everything from her skin to her kidneys examined. She had been prescribed various drugs and steroid creams, yet nothing worked.

Interestingly, Ahlea was the first practitioner to discuss diet with Jennifer. When asked about her diet, Jennifer said that she was eating a lot of dairy and that her favorite breakfast was granola with berries and milk, which she thought was healthy. Yet when Ahlea looked at the ingredients of this breakfast, she pointed out how much hidden sugar was present.

Because Jennifer was worried about making big changes, Ahlea asked her if she was willing to switch from conventional milk to organic almond milk as a first step. Ahlea also taught her how to add some healing herbs, turmeric (a spice that is wonderful for healing inflammation and the skin), and some kidney cleansing to her routine.

Within a week, the rash and acne were visibly reduced; within a month, Jennifer no longer even had acne or the rash on her face, neck, and torso. This really opened her eyes to the value of nutrition and organic food. She began to make more dietary changes, and the rash and acne completely resolved. Now if Jennifer gets stressed or starts eating too much junk food, the acne and rash may start to come back just a bit. After working with Ahlea, however, she knows that this is just her body loving her by reminding her to take care of herself. Jennifer now sees that she can adjust her food, thoughts, and habits and get right back on track with her health.

James: Alcoholism and Depression

James, a man in his 40s, started working with Heather because he had been diagnosed with depression, for which he had been prescribed medication. On top of this, he had a daily habit of drinking one or sometimes two bottles of wine after work. He had been in a high-stress job for many years and felt the wine helped him relax. When he started working with Heather, he was concerned about what he felt was quickly becoming alcoholism, and he wanted to recover from his depression.

Heather noticed that James was energetically sensitive and also very driven, a type A personality. She started by showing him how to create more of a work/life balance, and teaching him how to work with his intuition and sensitivity. He began to notice patterns in the way he was thinking, the food he was eating, and how he was working that triggered blood-sugar imbalances and alcohol cravings. This motivated him to implement a nutrition protocol that Heather designed to strengthen his blood sugar, heal his digestion, and balance his moods.

After two weeks, James showed up at his appointment with Heather and announced that he was off his antidepressants and feeling great. He was surprised that changing his diet could have such a strong impact on how he felt. Within the next five months, he reduced his alcohol intake from two bottles of wine to one, and then to the occasional glass. Within a year, he had stopped drinking alcohol altogether; was sleeping more soundly; and found that his moods, energy, and vitality were better than ever.

Most alcohol and addiction issues are related to severe blood-sugar and gut imbalances. Blood sugar becomes imbalanced when you are not fueling your body properly or have issues with digestion. (We'll talk more about digestion, gut health, and blood sugar in the next chapter.)

You Are Worth It: Why You Can Afford to Eat Healthfully

Manufactured-food and beverage companies aim to increase profits by creating low-cost, quick, convenient products. Too often these days, it's cheaper to buy packaged items than to purchase healthy whole foods, like produce and foods that are minimally processed, unrefined, and without chemicals. However, there are hidden costs associated with packaged foods. In fact, experts who care about the health of our worldwide population and of the planet are analyzing the true cost of junk food, fast food, and processed food. We'd like to share some of their findings with you.

In 2013, the Sustainable Food Trust conducted an international conference on the theme of "True Cost Accounting in Food and Farming." The goal of the conference was: "Bringing together world-leaders from across food, farming, conservation, research, finance and government policy . . . to investigate why our current economic system makes it more profitable to produce food in ways that damage the environment and human health, instead of rewarding methods of production that deliver benefits."[12]

While it may seem as if the United States has the worst food-related health issues, it is actually a worldwide concern. The Sustainable Food Trust conference highlighted many international food-related health challenges, including these statistics from the United Kingdom[13]:

- Food-related diseases (cardiovascular disease, diabetes, and cancer) account for 125,000 premature (under age 75) deaths per year in the U.K.

- A 2007 Chief Scientist's Foresight Obesity Report found that obesity cost the U.K. 7 billion British pounds in 2002 (that's over 11.5 billion U.S. dollars).

- Food-related ill health costs the U.K. National Health System at least 6 billion pounds per year (that's almost 10 billion dollars).

In this report, the shift to a higher dietary percentage of refined sugar, refined salt, and processed foods were cited as the key concerns when it comes to people's health.

During the conference, experts cited that while each of us may see a lower cost at the grocery store, there are much bigger hidden costs in our own health-care bills, such as insurance; our taxes (which contribute to health care, food subsidies, and disability costs); and the great burden on the environment.

Often we look at one cost at the grocery store and forget all the hidden costs in our lives. For example, when you're eating healthfully, you often spend less on prescription drugs, trips to the doctor, beauty remedies (lotions, serums, anti-wrinkle creams, and the like), hair products, makeup, weight-loss aids, over-the-counter pain remedies, energy drinks, chiropractors, and other health expenses.

What you eat absolutely impacts your physical health, but there's a greater benefit: the way you feel. Most people who adopt healthier eating habits say they feel better. Their energy, moods, and memory improve. They tend to feel more motivated and productive at work and at home. The benefit of feeling better is priceless.

In *Interview with God,* edited by Reata Strickland, there is a wonderful quote: "they [humankind] lose their health to make money and then lose their money to restore their health."[14]

This is indeed what human beings tend to do. We think about the cost at the cash register and forget that we are a worthwhile investment. We often forget that our health is a product of what we think, what we eat, and how we live our lives. This is when we've disconnected from our life purpose as a whole and forgotten to love ourselves.

The greatest investment you can make for a happy, healthy life is loving yourself through your words, your thoughts, and your actions. A healthy body means a healthy mind: a healthy mind means more happiness and joy, and a healthy body means more energy and strength. Imagine yourself in a world where you and the people you share the planet with are happier, healthier, and stronger. How much support for each other and the planet could we provide when we start from a strong foundation of health?

You are worth the investment. Some people have told us that they don't feel that it's worth putting healthy food into a sick body. We want you to know that healthy food and thoughts are the way back to a healthy body. With every thought and every bite, you are training your body to move in some direction. You are worth the investment, no matter where you are starting from. It's okay to start with a small investment, as change builds over time. Your body responds to changes you make with love, no matter how small.

Part of your love story is believing that you are worthy of goodness in your life, even if it costs a little more. You may find, like we do, that you start to prioritize your values differently, like eating at home more than eating at restaurants and shifting your budget to higher-quality groceries instead. (Note that we have many tips for you to eat healthfully on a budget in Chapter 5.)

Taking Time for Your Health Is Taking Time for Yourself

In addition to not wanting to spend money on foods that best nourish their bodies, people often insist that they don't have enough time to prepare whole foods.

We completely understand! The three of us have been in a place where we've had to decide how to fit preparing food into busy schedules with work, families, paying the bills, running errands, business travel, and more.

Heather spent over 15 years working in the corporate world and, due to job offers and promotions, was in a constant learning curve to master a higher level of responsibility. In short, she was a self-described workaholic. When she learned that recovery from bulimia meant eating healthier foods and giving her body high-quality nutrients, she was working as an executive for 12 hours per day and most weekends. At the time her typical grocery shopping included all packaged and processed food, and mealtimes revolved around microwaves and fast-food windows. She had to completely overhaul her life, particularly the way she related to grocery shopping and preparing food, at one of the busiest and most stressful times in her career.

What happened was interesting. She got guidance from a natural-health coach, and started with a few easy recipes for soups and vegetables she'd never tried before and looked up how to prepare them. She asked for advice at the health-food store on how to choose produce. In fact, she had to ask for a lot of help, at home from her husband and at work from her employees and colleagues, which was very unfamiliar for her. She started working smarter so she could leave work earlier and stop working on the weekends, yet no one even noticed that she was working less. Her better health and state of mind allowed her to be more productive in less time. And she developed a love for cooking because it was the first time she was doing something so kind for herself. She was taking the time to heal, and to show herself that she mattered more than the self-imposed beliefs about all the work she had to do.

That year, Heather got promoted and her team was the most productive in the company. Not because she worked harder, but because she was so much healthier.

She had a healthy body and a stronger mind that was willing to set boundaries and create work/life balance, which she implemented in her team as well.

Heather's biggest discovery was that if you put yourself first, you can find ways to focus on what's important and to take good care of the people who rely on you as a leader or even a parent. Feeling good has a ripple effect with many benefits.

Ahlea and Louise have similar stories of learning how much they matter when it comes to making healthy food. As we write this book, Ahlea is in her first two years with her first baby. She is bringing him up with healthy, whole foods, which often means that they are made from scratch. And she's running a growing business. Like Heather, Ahlea has had to learn to ask for help, from her husband, friends, and family. She also makes gardening and preparing food part of the bonding process with her son. She brings him into the kitchen, where he stands in a toddler-safe learning tower to watch and participate in what she's doing.

One of Ahlea's greatest lessons in having a baby is that you have to accept where you are in this moment. Everyone has something or several things that compete for their time. Perhaps you feel as if you have so much to do and so little time. Remember, this is only a thought, and thoughts can be changed. If you have a goal to get healthy and want to prepare whole foods, start by accepting where you are, and then think about how you can incorporate small steps into your routine. Perhaps there are things you can let go of or people you can ask for help.

To that end, we cannot emphasize enough the importance of a "tribe." According to *The Blue Zones* by Dan Buettner, the world's longest-living populations all found, or were born into, a group of friends who supported their healthy habits and who helped them when they needed it.[15] Knowing that they could ask for help and receive it when needed was key to feeling safe and living longer. So if you're not sure of how to approach healthy eating, or you're having trouble finding the time, call on your friends, a support group, or your social network to get ideas and support. Maybe you have a friend who knows how to cook and would love to come to your kitchen and help you out!

Louise is brilliant at creating a tribe of like-minded people. She is always pulling people together to prepare food and have fun in the kitchen. Whenever she's learning something new, she brings in people who can teach her and her tribe helpful concepts, tips, and techniques. She's always willing to learn new things and "be the beginner," which is one of the keys to her health and longevity.

Since Louise is so busy with teaching and travel, she uses a calendar and schedules in time for what matters to her, which includes her time at the grocery store and in the kitchen preparing healthy food. This is a great tip: give your time in the kitchen and at the grocery store a slot on your calendar instead of leaving it on a long to-do list that might never get done. That is a great way to prioritize your self-care and make sure it happens.

Client Stories

Throughout this book, we'll share stories of how people healed from so-called incurable conditions naturally, so that you can see how lifestyle, nutrition, and beliefs play a powerful role in your health. First up is Mary, who came to see Ahlea for treatment of lupus.

Mary: Lupus

Lupus is an autoimmune disease that is considered "incurable" by mainstream medicine and typically consists of inflammation; swelling; and damage to the kidneys, heart, lungs, and joints.[16] Mary was in her 40s and had tried almost everything to treat the symptoms she was experiencing. Her doctor specifically told her that nutrition would have no effect on the lupus, but Mary's inner voice was questioning that. She felt that how she treated her body must have some impact on her health, but she wasn't sure where to start or what to do. That's when she decided to go see Ahlea.

Like many people with autoimmune conditions, Mary looked perfectly fine, so her family and friends often accused her of being a hypochondriac. The first thing Ahlea did was help Mary understand that her body was telling her something with love and wisdom. Because Ahlea can hear the stories the body is telling, she listened to Mary's body and shared the messages it wanted Mary to know. She also recommended ways in which Mary could talk to her family so that they would understand her situation and how she was working to resolve it.

Ahlea showed Mary how she was mineral deficient, which was contributing to her full-body aches and inflammation. Mary, a self-confessed fast-food and junk-food junkie, was resistant to changing her diet. So Ahlea encouraged her to start with just one change: giving up gluten. Gluten is protein found in grains that many people have difficulty digesting, so giving it up can often be the easiest way to reduce inflammation and joint pain and even lose weight.

Mary reluctantly agreed to give up gluten for a couple of weeks. She came back for her follow-up appointment very excited, as she had less joint pain and more ease of movement in her body. Pretty soon she was going for walks again because the pain was gone.

Mary was thrilled to realize that she was losing weight naturally and the lupus symptoms had dropped away. Like other clients with autoimmune conditions, Mary's body will speak to her with lupus symptoms if she starts to go too far off track, so she's learned how to adjust back to a healthy, loving lifestyle if that happens. Today, she truly understands how loving herself with a healthy diet and positive affirmations is the key to a happy life.

Empowering Yourself: Becoming Your Own Best Health Advocate

While the modern medical system does many things well, like saving lives in emergency situations, many of today's chronic lifestyle conditions, such as type 2 diabetes, obesity, and cardiovascular disease, respond better to nutrition than drugs.[17] Yet it's becoming a well-known fact that medical doctors are not taught nutrition in medical school. In 2010, researchers did a study of medical schools and found that only one quarter of the schools offered the recommended 25 hours of instruction in nutrition, and some made it optional or offered none at all.[18]

With so little emphasis placed on nutrition in medical school, your doctor may not be fully up to date on how nutrition can influence your health. The good news is that this gives you the opportunity to become a partner with your doctor. The Internet has brought many benefits, including online support groups and the ability to research just about anything you want. In fact, a 2012 study done by the Pew Internet Project found that 72 percent of Internet users had looked online for health information within the past year; of those with a serious health condition, 60 percent got information or support from family and friends, and 24 percent got information or support from others with the same condition.[19]

These days, we have many options to learn more about our health. Louise has always been an avid learner, and health and nutrition are two of her favorite topics. She is currently studying homeopathy and the healing power of spices. She attends classes and trusts that the right people will always come along with the right information. And they do!

Louise's passion for nutrition is one of the reasons she is so healthy, vibrant, and active at 88 years of age. Over a decade ago, Louise started working with Ahlea, and together, they have created a nutrition, exercise, and lifestyle routine that works for Louise's schedule, which includes a great deal of travel.

Here are some tips from Louise on being your own best health advocate:

— **Be willing to learn.** You don't have to have all the answers, just be willing to ask people or look the answer up.

— **Ask Life to provide you with the right people** to assist you in whatever you need help with.

— **Use this affirmation:** *Every hand that touches me is a healing hand.*

— **Choose a doctor who you feel supports your vision of health and well-being.** Choosing the right doctor for you goes beyond getting a referral from people you trust. Make sure this individual listens to your concerns and gives you the information you feel you need to make your best decisions. Does the doctor explain things in a way you can understand without talking down to you? Does he or she treat you as a partner in your own health? Do you feel comfortable asking follow-up questions? And above all else, are you comfortable with the steps your doctor is suggesting you take?

— **Create a team.** Your team could consist of a health expert you trust, along with knowledgeable friends or family members. Louise has created her own health team so that she has the support she needs to be at her best. Ahlea is the leader of that team and often will find others to come in as needed. Ahlea is also Louise's medical advocate and goes to doctors' appointments with her; in this way, Ahlea can partner with Louise and the doctor to be sure all medical advice is blended with a natural approach to health. This also gives Louise peace of mind that she doesn't have to know everything, because she has someone with her who knows how to speak with doctors and what is in the best interest of her specific health goals.

— **Keep a binder or online folder of your health tests.** Make sure to get copies of any medical tests your doctor or health provider does. Ask questions about the results, and make notes so that you understand them. This way, you can review your tests whenever you want and can take them to a new practitioner, if necessary.

— **Ask questions.** Prepare questions ahead of time and ask them when you see your doctor. If he or she advises something you are uncomfortable with or unclear about, ask more questions.

— **Get a second opinion.** If you are not sure about advice from your health practitioner, get a second and even third opinion.

— **Seek your own inner guidance.** This one is important. If a doctor tells you something that doesn't feel right to you, trust your inner guidance. Trust that you will find the answers you need. Louise, Ahlea, and Heather have all been in this situation more than once—take it from us, the most important thing you can do to become your own health advocate is to listen to your inner voice and trust its guidance.

You Can Heal Your Body: Moving Beyond Incurable Illness

You may already know that decades ago, Louise was diagnosed with cancer. At the time, she was scared, and yet she knew this was a huge opportunity to walk her talk. She already had a deep understanding of how her thoughts influenced her life and her health, and she suspected that Life was giving her a chance to prove it to herself.

One of the things you might not know about that time, though, is that in addition to working with her thoughts, Louise decided not to use a mainstream medical approach to treat the cancer. At that time, there was very little knowledge about natural treatments for cancer, but Louise's inner ding said to look to nutrition as a form of healing. One of the protocols she followed was eating two ounces of pureed asparagus three times per day. Because of her teaching and travel schedule, this often meant carrying her food. She looked around and found that film containers (back when cameras used film) were a perfect two-ounce size, so she cleaned them out and used them to carry her asparagus. (These days, there are lots of new and healthy options for carrying food for travel, and we'll share Louise's healing asparagus puree recipe in Chapter 10.)

What Louise noticed during that time was interesting. As she moved into a full-scale trust for her work—a trust in her thoughts, her commitment to nutrition, and in Life to take care of her—her clients and students got even better results. If you've ever met Louise, or just seen or heard her teach, you may understand this. When someone truly embodies what they teach, there is an almost magical quality that transcends what is being said. We learn more and change more because we can recognize and feel what is being taught. This is the beauty of investing time in yourself, loving yourself, and trusting Life to take care of you. When you do this, you change your own life, but you also become a beacon for others, just by being who you are.

When she was 12 years old, Ahlea was diagnosed with muscular dystrophy, which weakens the muscles and can result in the inability to walk or sit up. She was told she would require surgeries on all of her major joints. Ahlea knew in that moment that this diagnosis was not true for her—she was adamant that she would not visit that doctor again, nor would she be treated through mainstream medicine. Fortunately, Ahlea's parents had developed a deep respect for her intuition and alternative views on health after years of observing her within the family, with animals, and with her friends. They could see that she was determined to heal herself naturally, and they decided to support her and watch to see what happened.

From that point forward, Ahlea became deeply conscious of her body's needs, nutritionally, functionally, spiritually, and structurally. She learned everything she could about physical and emotional health and focused on loving thoughts and self-care. Decades later, she is strong, vibrant, and healthy, and she too embodies what she teaches. Over the years she has extended her childhood gift of seeing into bodies into her work, so she can hear the stories that unlock other people's ability to heal.

In the 16 years that Heather had bulimia, she had almost every scary, painful symptom you can imagine and had gone to countless doctors to find answers for them. The one thing she knew was that she did not want to be treated with gastro-intestinal-system surgery (for example, gallbladder removal, which one specialist insisted was the only thing that would work) or drugs—so, like Louise and Ahlea, her inner guidance turned away from mainstream medical approaches and found her healing in working with her thoughts, lifestyle, and nutrition.

Heather developed a strong belief that people could recover from anything. Some experts told her that she desperately needed to commit herself into a treatment center because she could die at any moment. There were times she was afraid she *was* about to die, and during those dark moments, she chose to believe in her health. What she learned was to be unafraid of symptoms, recognizing them as the body's way of giving clues for recovery. Today, her ability to see even the hidden symptoms in people's bodies and minds allows her to support her clients in healing naturally from addictions and chronic health conditions.

You see, we have each had conditions considered "incurable" by mainstream medicine. In each case, we followed our inner guidance, and we've gone on to work with many others to support them in doing the same.

Now, it's critically important to note that we are not saying to avoid medical doctors and medical treatments. We all work with medical doctors and we value them. We make sure our clients are working with their medical doctors as well, and we consider ourselves a part of their team.

What we are saying is that we truly believe there is no incurable illness. The word *incurable* means that something can't be cured by any outer means at the moment, so the answer lies in going within. We believe that your body is just asking you to come back to a loving relationship with yourself. That symptoms don't need to be scary; they can instead be a guidepost for when you are off track and need to make some adjustments in self-care. If you understand this, then you can allow your inner guidance to point you in the direction you want to take in your healing journey.

We also want you to feel comfortable researching and getting a second opinion about any diagnosis or drug you are asked to take, especially if your inner guidance is questioning it.

As we mentioned, Louise is studying homeopathy as we write this book, and one expert told her, "If you want to know your next health problem, look at the listed side effects of the pharmaceutical drug you are taking right now."

In 1998, *The Journal of the American Medical Association* published a study finding that *every year,* more than two million Americans become ill and 106,000 die from the toxic side effects of correctly prescribed pharmaceutical drugs.[20] This study only looked at pharmaceutical drugs *properly prescribed by doctors and properly taken by patients.* The study was not suggesting that people stop taking the drugs prescribed by their doctors, but instead, that the medical system should have better checks and balances in place to protect patients.

That's the thing with pharmaceutical drugs taken for long-term, chronic health conditions. Instead of having a clear picture of your relationship to yourself, where symptoms are your guideposts to readjust this relationship, it's like looking in a funhouse mirror—the picture is distorted by symptoms from the drugs' side effects, and you lose the ability to truly know how your body is doing.

The more you listen to your body, the more it will teach you what you need to know for your health and happiness. While you may not be certain of how to listen to your body at first, we will share some excellent techniques later in the book to help you discover how to listen to your body and understand the signals it's giving you.

When you learn to listen to your body and lovingly give it what it needs—and when you learn how to feed it with healing thoughts and food—your body responds with better health. Your body is always speaking to you with love.

Exercises to Love Yourself and Your Body

We have designed the following exercises to support you in creating a more loving relationship with yourself and your body.

1. Vision Exercise

Heather does a vision exercise with all of her clients because she finds that the first step to creating optimal health and lifestyle is to get clear about what we really want in life. Many of us operate based on what we think we "should" want or what others want from us. Or we find that we are unhappy and don't know how to change.

> "Whatever the mind of man can conceive and believe, it can achieve."
>
> — Napoleon Hill

Heather was still in her corporate job when she went to a seminar about writing visions. She was very skeptical since she had done similar exercises before, but she figured what the heck, and went ahead and wrote hers. Her vision included starting her own business and living on a tiny Caribbean island, two seemingly impossible goals. Because she was not sure what she wanted to do besides her current job, she just focused on the kind of work she loved and how it would feel. She included how she wanted to feel about herself and her relationships, as well as how she wanted to feel physically and emotionally from a health perspective.

Heather focused on her vision each morning in meditation and read it at night. After a few months, she stopped reading it at night and just focused on her morning visualization. The more she visualized her new life, the more comfortable and achievable it felt for her. At the same time, she wanted to be practical, so she and her husband, Joel, began discussing ways in which they could manage moving to the Caribbean. How could they make it work financially? Would Joel be able to work remotely at his corporate job?

What they found out was that the simple act of focusing on what they wanted to achieve allowed them to set some practical goals. First they made a budget to learn what they had to change to make their dream financially feasible. As they looked at their current spending, they realized that they could drastically reduce their expenses. They wrote up a detailed plan that included the following: (1) selling their current home and most of their possessions, (2) Heather becoming a writer and certified professional coach, and (3) Joel getting the go-ahead to work remotely. While each step had its challenges, their intense desire to create a simpler life in the Caribbean allowed them to stay focused and believe in themselves enough to make big requests that they might have been afraid to make previously. This is not to say that there weren't some very difficult decisions and fears along the way. And yet, the decisions and fears seemed small compared with their passion for creating their ideal life. Getting clear and committed about what they wanted seemed like the catalyst they needed to really change their lives.

Many people say that when you put your focus on something, you notice solutions you might never have seen otherwise. Heather and Joel felt that solutions seemed to pop up almost magically to make their transition much easier. A year later, the two of them were on a plane to Saint Martin. As they landed, Heather burst into tears. Joel asked her what was wrong, and she said, "I just realized that I've achieved most of my vision."

Heather had left her job and started her coaching business. Joel had gotten permission from his company to work from the island. And that was when Heather realized that writing a vision is not "woo-woo." Yes, it's a whole lot of belief and magic, but from a practical perspective, it's about getting clear about what you want and then creating a plan to get there.

♥

As a very simple example, you may know from work experience or even from having kids that clarity is very important when giving instructions. Would you tell your kids, "Don't come home too late" without telling them what time you want them to be home? Would you tell your employees, "Do a good job" without telling them what specific result you want them to achieve?

Your mind works the same way. The more clear you are about what you want, the easier it is to put the right messages and affirmations into your conscious mind, so that your subconscious can carry it out.

While you may have a focus on what you want to do (such as a career) as part of your vision, keep in mind that the most powerful part of doing this exercise is to identify how you want to *feel*. So although a vision for what you want to accomplish in your life or career is wonderful, there is a journey and steps to be taken from where you are now to accomplishing that goal.

On the other hand, once you are clear on how you want to feel, you can begin feeling that way today. And the great news is, since your body believes what your mind thinks, a juicy, positive feeling can bring all kinds of benefits to your body and your overall health.

There are two key benefits to writing your vision:

1. You get clear about what you truly want, so you can focus on what really matters.

2. You get clear on how you want to feel, so you can bring those feelings into your body and mind right away.

Let's get started!

Setting the Stage

- Go to a quiet room where you will have no distractions.

- Make sure your environment is one that will inspire peace and/or creativity—consider dimming the lights and lighting a candle or playing soft music.

Guidelines for Writing Your Vision

- Do this exercise in a way that feels best to you. Use your creativity and make it fun!

- Some people like to focus on their "ideal day" and identify what their dream day would look like. Others like to take a big-picture point of view and focus on what their ideal life would be like. Do what feels good to you—get as big picture or as detailed as you like. The main thing to remember is that you want to get a sense of what your ideal lifestyle feels and looks like. Bring as many of the five (or six!) senses into this experience as possible.

- Focus on what you're passionate about: What do you love? What makes your heart sing? The more strongly you feel for the things in your vision, the more likely you are to create them. This is about creating the life you love—the life of your dreams!

- Use as much detail as possible. That is, an ideal vision might focus on what your dream life is like from the time you wake up until the time you go to bed. A big-picture vision might focus on exactly how you feel as you go through your life, whom you're with, how you take care of yourself, where you live, and so on.

- Use language as if your vision is the present moment, and use positive language. Do not use "I will not" or "I don't have," but instead say, "I am," "I have," or "I choose."

- Include people you want in your life (specific people or characteristics of people you want to spend your time with).

- Include things you want to have in your life (the house of your dreams, your own business, or what have you).

- Include how you want to be or feel (such as *happy, healthy, energized, light, peaceful, joyful, charismatic, confident, smart, loving, forgiving, patient,* and so forth).

- Include what you want to do (such as *Travel to xyz countries, Be a leader, Work part-time and still make $X, Get married, Be fit, Eat healthy, Write a book,* and the like).

- Bring in as many of your senses as possible (what do you see, taste, touch, smell, feel?).

- Be as specific as you can about how your work and personal life flows together. You are inventing the *lifestyle* that is most ideal for you, not what you think is realistic.

- Avoid worrying about limitations (that is, "I have kids, so I can't live in a sunny place in the winter" or "My husband's job is here, so I can't go live in my dream city"). This is your time to dream about what *you* want, not what you think will work for everyone else.

- Are you dreaming big enough? Don't confine yourself to what you think is possible. You might not even know what is truly possible until you experience the power of getting clear about what you want and visualizing it coming true for you. Doing your mirror work and affirmations to support believing in your vision is another way to boost the power of this exercise.

Alternative Option: Vision Board

If you tend to have better success expressing yourself in visual ways, rather than in writing, you can do a vision board instead. Follow the same guidelines as you would in the written vision. Start with a blank poster board and add:

- Photos of yourself and of people you want in your life.

- Pictures of things you want in your life or that express the way you want to be or feel. Look in magazines, newspapers, or other sources.

- Words—use colored markers or something to write words that are meaningful to you.

- Add specific dates for when you want these things in your life. And remember, think big—don't get constrained by the how or worry about whether you can get it done by that date. This is your dream and you set the time frames!

Place your vision board on the wall by your desk or in your bedroom— anywhere you will see it often. Some people paste the pictures in a journal that they can carry around with them. Look at it every day, notice every detail, and believe in it!

If You Are Having Trouble with Your Vision, Consider These Questions

Is this the first time writing your vision? Don't know where to begin? Here are some questions to get you started:

- If money was no object and you could do whatever you wanted, what would it be?

- If you absolutely knew you could not fail, what would you do?

- If someone waved a magic wand and you could have whatever you want, what would it be?

- What are you passionate about?

- How do you want to feel?

- How can you love yourself more?

- What have you always wanted to do?

- What are your hobbies?

- What are your interests?

- Whom do you admire?

- What are you good at? (This is often something that feels easy because it comes naturally to you.)

- What are the qualities, characteristics, and attitudes of the people you want in your life?

- What do your ideal relationships look like?

- Where do you want to travel?

- Where do you really want to live (or what are aspects of your ideal place to live)?

- What is your day-to-day life like?

- How would others describe you?

- What is your ideal lifestyle (blend of work and play time)?

- How many days, ideally, would you like to work?

Then there's the "Keep It Simple" option: You may want your entire vision to simply be about how you want to feel, with no emphasis on anything else. In this vision, you'd focus on how you want to feel from the beginning to the end of the day, or how you want to feel throughout your life. You might focus on how you'll know you are feeling that way. (For instance, *I feel loving toward myself, and I know I'm feeling this way because I am kind to myself. I say yes when I truly want to say yes and no when I want to say no. I feel a sense of ease in how I do things, and I know this because I have very little stress in my life. I feel happy and calm as I go about my day.*)

<u>Your Vision Is Complete—Now What?</u>

— Once your vision is written or your vision board is completed, **keep it nearby.**

— **Read your words or view your vision board every morning and every night.**

— **Consider doing a morning and/or evening meditation** where you visualize everything in your vision being a part of your life today. If you aren't ready to meditate or visualize yet, simply read your vision while breathing deeply as you read. Do deep belly breaths, where you gently fill your lungs with air and feel your breath filling your abdomen. If you are tensing your abdomen, relax and let your breath expand it. Feel your breath filling your body with the words you're reading.

— **Act as if** you have everything in your vision right now. Since everything is energy, you are actually embracing this energy in the present to attract it in the future.

— **Really believe in it!** If you're having a difficult time with this, start by being open to believing it and as you accomplish that, move into really believing it.

— **Open your mind** to the limitless possibilities Life has to offer.

— **Take action.** Take steps that will bring your vision closer. Look for anything that will bring the feelings or people or things into your life, even if it's a small step.

— **Focus on inspiration.** Read books; attend seminars; watch programs; or listen to podcasts, radio shows, or other audio programs that inspire you!

— **Pay attention to events.** Start noticing when opportunities arise that will bring you closer to your vision—and take them!

— **Pay attention to your thoughts.** Catch yourself thinking thoughts that are negative and limiting and delete them! Replace them with positive affirmations or statements from your vision.

— **Eliminate doubt.** Look for proof that what you're doing is working, and write it down in your journal. Proof is anything big or small that shows you're moving toward your vision. It may be that you are actually feeling happier or calmer, or things may just get easier for you. Perhaps some magical things are happening in your life. Even if they feel very small compared to what's in your vision, they are still signs that Life loves you and is taking care of you. The more you notice signs each day, the less doubt and more belief you'll have. The stronger your belief, the easier it is to create the life you want.

— **Record and celebrate your results.** Keep notes in your journal about your progress. Notice the miracles that start to happen in your life, however small. Keep a record so that you can see how far you've come. Celebrate the miracles that happen. Sometimes you may even forget how you used to be—your journal will show you how much you have shifted by believing in your ability to create the life you love!

2. Affirmations

Here are some affirmations that will help you love yourself and your body more. Pick one to begin with; you can choose more when you feel ready. Say these affirmations as you look in the mirror. Practice them throughout the day, anytime you feel you need them.

Judgment and Compassion

We are going to start with Louise's affirmations on judgment and compassion because we find that those who judge others are often the most critical of themselves. Learning to stop judging is a great way to develop more compassion.

Often, when you think that something is wrong with yourself or someone else, it is really an expression of individuality. Every human being is unique and special, just as no two snowflakes are alike. We are meant to be different. When you can accept this, there is no comparison and no competition.

Affirm:

I am willing to release the feeling that I am unworthy.

I see myself and others with compassion and understanding.

The people in my life are really mirrors of me.
This allows me the opportunity to grow and change.

I have compassion for my parents' childhoods. I now know that I chose them because they were perfect for what I had to learn. I forgive them and set them and myself free.

There is no competition, no comparison,
for we are all different and meant to be that way.

I accept my uniqueness, and I accept the uniqueness of others.

Loving people fill my life, and I find myself easily expressing love to others.

I am worthy of the very best in life, and I now lovingly allow myself to accept it.

I radiate acceptance, and I am deeply loved by others.

My heart is open—I love myself, I love others, and others love me.

Loving Your Body

The subconscious mind has no sense of humor and does not know false from true. It only accepts what you say and think as fact, and this is the material from which it builds. As you say these affirmations, trust that you are planting seeds in the fertile soil of your subconscious mind. These affirmations can help you have a body you really love:

I love you dearly, body. I love every inch of you.

I have a happy, slender body.

It is my joy to love you to perfect health.

I love my beautiful shape.

The more I love my body, the healthier I feel.

My body is such a good friend; we have a great life together.

I love and appreciate my beautiful body just the way it is.

I rejoice that I have chosen this particular body because it is perfect for me.

I create my own security. I love and approve of myself.

It is safe to be me. I am wonderful just as I am. I choose joy and self-acceptance.

Health and Nourishment

We all have ideas and habits around the food we eat and the thoughts we think about health. If you put yourself in the position where you know you can create healthy habits around food and trust that you can be healed, the right information and support will come to you. If you believe something is too hard, takes too much time, or can't be done, your life and habits will reflect that. When you shift to believing it can be done, the how will show up.

Affirm:

Hi, body, thank you for being so healthy.

My health is easy and effortless.

I am healed and whole.

I am worthy of being healed.

My body knows how to heal itself.

Every day and in every way I am feeling healthier and healthier.

I love selecting foods that are nutritious and delicious.

My body loves the way I choose the perfect foods for every meal.

Planning healthy meals is a joy. I am worth it.

When I feed myself healthy foods, I nourish my body and mind for the day ahead.

<u>Troubleshooting: If You're Having
Trouble Believing Your Affirmations</u>

Many people ask how affirmations about loving themselves or their body work if they don't believe it when they say it. First of all, be patient and kind with yourself. You are digging up years of negative conditioning, and it sometimes takes time and practice to plant new seeds in fresh, fertile soil.

One step you can take is to simply say, *I am open to loving and accepting myself.* When you begin there, you may find that being open to this belief allows you to move into actually believing it with time and consistency in your mirror work.

Another great way to start seeing how your thoughts can change your life is to depersonalize the whole experience. Louise suggests that you consider starting by believing that you will get a green light or a great parking spot. Since these have nothing to do with you personally, you don't have to work through so much old conditioning.

Give yourself 30 days to practice focusing on getting green lights on your way to work or to the grocery store. Or focus on believing that you will find a great parking space. As your belief grows, notice how Life brings you these things. This is proof that positive thinking works, and it may help to give you confidence in how affirmations and mirror work can change your life and health in other ways.

In the next chapter, we'll teach you more about how your body works, so you can create a strong foundation for health.

♥ ♥

Chapter 3

Step #3: Know How Your Body Really Works— the Foundation for Health

If we asked you *why* you eat, how would you answer?

From an intellectual perspective, it's easy to understand that human beings eat to satisfy hunger and fuel the body. Some of you might even say that you eat to be healthy. What you may not realize is that our food choices are more complicated than you think. We make over 200 decisions each day about food based on emotions, habits, environment, whom we're with, and food chemistry (the food additives designed to get you to eat more).[1]

> "I digest life and assimilate all new experiences peacefully and joyously."
>
> — Louise

While that may seem overwhelming, we're going to keep it very simple here. Because there is only one emotion, one habit, and one environment to cultivate: *loving yourself.* When you practice loving yourself, you set the stage for making the best food choices. In this chapter, we are going to share how your body works, so you can love yourself with food that is the most nourishing for you.

Where We Got Lost, and How to Find Ourselves Again

Both experts and laypeople agree that eating a healthier diet is a great way to feel our best. So why don't more people do it?

If we were to go back in time, before people moved into cities, before the Industrial Revolution and back to when people lived off the land, we'd find that our ancestors ate food that came from nature. Our agricultural-era ancestors had a connection to nature and ate what they grew. They learned to cook and prepare foods from scratch because that is all they had access to.

In her book *Food in History,* Reay Tannahill explains that the Industrial Revolution changed "the face of the earth." The population grew dramatically in Europe (from 180 million to 390 million people) in the 1800s, people moved into cities, and a food crisis began.[2] During this time, the focus of society was building machines, and people worked in factories instead of on the land. With less time and access to land, and a subsequent food shortage, machines were employed to manufacture food. Canning, freezing, and transportation efforts grew as food was imported across cities, countries, and the world.

To stretch food and lower costs, the first food shenanigans began. Local retailers would stretch cocoa powder by adding brick dust. Everything from mustard husks to sweepings from the store floor were added to stretch black pepper. Ash leaves were mixed into tea. And as late as 1969, an Italian manufacturer was charged with making a "Parmesan cheese" out of plastic umbrella–handle shavings![3] Tannahill calls this the period of food "adulteration," and while there were many complaints and government policies enacted around it, the crisis to feed a growing population was the larger concern.

While the British government thought it was doing a great job feeding the poor, they realized they were wrong when 41 percent of the men examined for war duty between 1917 and 1918 were deemed unfit due to health deficiencies.[4] Right around this point, the new science of nutrition was uncovering the need for vitamins and minerals, but the challenge of feeding a growing population and keeping them healthy became its own battleground, one that still exists today.

It's no surprise that there would be so much confusion about what to eat and how to nourish our bodies. At one time, nature's food was all people had. Today, we still have those options, but we also have what social scientist Claude Fischler calls UFOs, or "unidentified food objects."[5] We no longer know what's in our food.

Fischler's views were aptly summed up in an article by Ashley Braun: "What happened with food in the West is that food became disenchanted. . . . When we grab food without thinking, without ritual, there is a loss of meaning. . . . When food is commodified and processed, it retreats into a black box. We are what we eat and if we don't know what we eat . . ."[6]

We believe that the disconnection from real, all-natural, nourishing food is creating a focus on eating for taste and convenience, rather than health. For many of you who *do* eat for health, we know it can be confusing to know how to eat with all the mixed messages today.

The good news is that in the next two chapters, we are going to provide you with two simple yet important concepts that will empower you to make the best choices for your own health. In this chapter, we're going to share how your digestive system works, so you can see how miraculously your body was created to support your wellness. And then in Chapter 4, we'll teach you how to listen to your body, so you can follow your own inner guidance when things feel confusing.

We invite you to take a moment right now to put one hand on the center of your chest and the other on your abdomen. Take three deep breaths. Tell yourself how much you love yourself, and then ask if you believe you deserve to feel your best. Whatever comes up, tell yourself: *I am willing to release the patterns in me that created these conditions. I am worth healing. I am worth the time it takes to learn how to nourish myself. I love you, body.*

Most of us didn't learn to nourish ourselves well. We learned about food from advertisements, our families, and our friends. We ate what was convenient. Very likely, we were never taught how our bodies worked and what they truly needed to feel calm and balanced.

One of the most important things you can be aware of when it comes to the thoughts you think and the food you eat is that this is what you are feeding yourself. If you are focused on thoughts that make you feel bad and foods that do not nurture your body, you are denying yourself love and feeding yourself misery. You deserve to feed yourself love and let go of the misery. Misery is not the path to good health or happiness.

There are many studies that show that acts of love, such as reducing stress, getting exercise, and improving sleep, can positively affect your digestion. A healthy diet positively affects your digestion, too—and a little-known bonus is that it positively affects your brain, including your moods, memory, and willpower! (We will focus on your gut-brain connection later in this chapter.)

We would like to give you the important highlights for how your digestive system works. We'll keep this as simple as possible and then share some amazing ways that the brain and digestive system communicate with one another.

Digestion: Your Body's Miraculous Way of Nourishing You

Your digestive system is the only system in the body that can function without the help of the brain; the gut has its own enteric nervous system, which is often referred to as a "second brain."[7] It's one of the most important systems you can learn about, because it is through the digestive system that you get all the nutrients your body needs to look and feel your best.

The digestive system, also called the gastrointestinal tract (GI tract), is essentially a 25- to 35-foot muscular tube running from your mouth to your anus.[8] Its job is to break down the food you eat into the building blocks for energy, healing, growth, good moods, and every function your body performs. Yet between one-third and one-half of all adults have digestive illness, and it seems to be a growing epidemic among children as well.[9]

Symptoms Related to Digestive Challenges

While you may recognize some of the wide range of symptoms related to faulty digestion, others may surprise you. They include[10]:

- Abdominal pain
- Arthritis
- Autoimmune issues
- Back pain
- Bacterial and fungal infections
- Balance and gait (walking) problems
- Bloating
- Constipation
- Crohn's disease
- Diarrhea
- Dysbiosis (a microbial imbalance in the body that often causes digestive symptoms, fatigue, and mood issues)
- Fatigue
- Flatulence
- Food allergies or sensitivity
- Gastroesophageal reflux disease (GERD), heartburn, or acid reflux

- Headaches or migraines

- Indigestion

- Infertility

- Irritable bowel syndrome (IBS)

- Leaky gut syndrome

- Memory and learning issues

- Mood issues or disorders (depression, irritability, and the like)

- Premenstrual syndrome (PMS)

- Skin problems

- Sleep problems

- Ulcerative colitis

Changing Your Lifestyle Can Improve Your Digestion

The best thing about your digestion is that the more loving your choices, the healthier it can be! Aside from your genes, the most common contributors to digestive challenges are lifestyle related. As we learned from Bruce Lipton's work earlier in the book, genes are only a blueprint, and positive changes in your beliefs and perceptions can change your genes. The science of epigenetics is also uncovering more research showing that better nutrition can "switch off" negative gene expressions as well.[11]

Here are some of the major contributors to digestive challenges[12]:

- Alcohol abuse

- Chronic stress

- Cigarette smoking

- Dehydration

- Environmental and food toxins

- Genetic predispositions

- Infections

- Lack of exercise

- Low stomach acid

- Poor nutrition

- Prescription and over-the-counter medications

We believe that when you start by making loving choices in how you think and live your life, you are setting the stage for your best health.

The Brain: Where It All Begins

While many people will tell you that digestion begins in the mouth, it really begins before the act of eating. Digestion actually starts in your brain: when you think about, see, or smell food, your brain sends signals to your digestive tract causing your mouth to water, your stomach to contract, and your pancreas to secrete enzymes.[13] Your body is now primed for digestion.

Your brain is also very involved with choosing the foods you eat. When you choose real food that grows in nature, you're giving your body something that it understands. (We will talk more about food choices and willpower later in this chapter, and then in Chapter 5, we'll give you an abundance of information on choosing delicious whole foods that can help nourish your body and boost your willpower. We will even include menus and recipes to make your choices that much easier in Part II!)

It's helpful to know how important your brain is when it comes to your digestion. The body believes what the brain thinks, so if you visualize your meal digesting well and nourishing your body, you will also prime your body for better health. There are affirmations and meditations at the end of this chapter that will support you in doing this.

Let's take a closer look at each part of the digestive system. On the next page, we have included a handy illustration that you may want to refer to as we move along.

THE DIGESTIVE SYSTEM

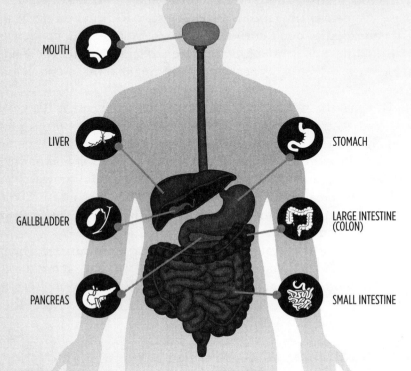

MOUTH

LIVER

GALLBLADDER

PANCREAS

STOMACH

LARGE INTESTINE (COLON)

SMALL INTESTINE

MOUTH
As you chew, your mouth secretes saliva, which contains amylase, an enzyme to help initiate the breakdown of carbohydrates. Chewing well is a great way to prime your body for better digestion.

LIVER
The liver filters almost all the blood in your body, creates bile to break down fats, breaks down hormones, processes all nutrients, including vitamins and minerals and neutralizes toxins.

STOMACH
Your stomach secretes hydrochloric acid (to break down food), intrinsic factor (starts digestion of vitamin B12) and the digestive enzymes, pepsin and lipase.

GALLBLADDER
Your gallbladder stores and releases bile to help you digest fats.

PANCREAS
The pancreas regulates blood sugar and secretes pancreatic enzymes to break down carbohydrates, protein and fats.

LARGE INTESTINE (COLON)
Good bacteria in your colon keep bad bacteria under control and help with peristalsis. Nutrients are extracted from the chyme and the remaining waste (feces) is stored in the rectum.

SMALL INTESTINE
The small intestine is responsible for digestion and absorption. Microscopic finger-like structures, called villi, produce enzymes to break down food and absorb nutrients.

The Mouth

Once you've made the decision to eat something, it goes in your mouth. Note that chewing your food well and getting it into a mash is one way to love your stomach, because you deliver the food in a way the stomach can best do its job. When you inhale your food or don't chew well enough, you create a challenge for your stomach by sending it chunks of food that are too large. If you experience indigestion, gas, bloating, belching, or heartburn, you might want to take a look at how well you are chewing.

While you may have heard from a variety of experts that it's best to chew between 15 and 40 times before swallowing, the important thing to focus on is chewing enough so that you can swallow your food easily. Over time, as you eat mindfully, you will learn what amount of chewing works best for your digestion.

As you chew, your mouth secretes saliva, which contains amylase, an enzyme to help initiate the breakdown of carbohydrates. Saliva also cleanses your mouth and teeth and signals your parotid glands (in the jaw behind your ears) to secrete hormones that tell your thymus to prime the immune system.[14]

Keep in mind that the health of your teeth and gums matter when it comes to healthy digestion. When you have healthy teeth, you have more surface area to chew better. Additionally, when you choose healthier foods, your teeth tend to be healthier.[15]

Health Alert: Silver Mercury Fillings and Choosing a Holistic Dentist

We recommend that you work with a good holistic dentist who understands how the health of your mouth works in harmony with the health of the rest of your body. This type of dentist can assist you in choosing approaches for healthy gums and teeth—and if you need fillings, crowns, or other dental work, they will help you choose materials that are most compatible with your body.

If you do happen to have mercury (silver) fillings, like so many people do today, and you are having health challenges, a holistic dentist can talk to you about the benefits of removing those fillings. Mainstream dentistry did not know in the past that mercury fillings could adversely affect people's health. While the great mercury debate has waged for years, more studies have begun to reveal what holistic dentists and practitioners have known for some time: mercury fillings in mothers can affect the health of newborns[16]; they may also contribute to autoimmune illness, chronic fatigue, and other health conditions.[17] The debate came to a head in

October 2013 with the International Mercury Treaty, an international agreement to phase out the use of mercury fillings and mercury-containing products worldwide by the year 2020.[18]

To find a holistic dentist, here are some steps you can take:

— **Ask your health-minded friends, family, or practitioners** for a recommendation.

— **Use the Internet.** Do a search for holistic dentists and check health-minded social-media groups, forums, and review sites for information on the quality of practitioners in your area. There are also online directories where you can seek out a holistic dentist, including: Mercury Safe Dentistry, the International Academy of Oral Medicine & Toxicology, the International Academy of Biological Dentistry & Medicine, the Holistic Dental Association, the American Academy of Craniofacial Pain, and dentists recommended by the Weston A. Price Foundation.

— **Meet with the dentist** and see if they are willing to work with you and listen to your goals and concerns. Do they answer your questions? Are they considering your whole health (not just your mouth)? Do they treat you like a partner in your health?

— **Look at their methods and recommendations.** Truly holistic dentists do not use amalgam (mercury) fillings, do not promote the use of fluoride, seek out other alternatives before choosing to put on crowns, and tend to prefer implants as opposed to root canals. Holistic dentists use digital x-rays or dye staining to reduce your exposure to radiation. If dental surgery is required, they tend to suggest natural therapies to support it, such as vitamin C therapy, lymphatic massage, and a cleansing diet. Often, they will provide natural or homeopathic remedies for pain as well.

— **Above all else, follow your inner guidance.** Make sure you feel comfortable with the dentist and the approaches that are recommended to you. Heather had an experience where a new holistic dentist suggested she get a very invasive surgery to correct her bite so that she could chew her food better and improve her digestion, but that didn't feel right to her. Another specialist said that since her digestion had already improved with her positive nutrition and lifestyle changes, her bite was probably not the root cause of her history of digestive challenges. Instead, he gave her the option of doing nothing if she wanted, respecting the adaptability of the human body. After researching the pros and cons of invasive dental surgery,

Heather decided to follow her inner guidance, sticking with the dentist who was willing to work with her on natural approaches instead of surgery.

You may have chosen differently than Heather did. It's not about the choice itself, but about listening to your inner wisdom. By all means, do your research and get a second or third opinion with matters relating to your health, but always trust what your inner voice is telling you, too.

Down the Esophagus to the Stomach

When you swallow, your food goes through your esophagus, which is like a tube. If food is too large or too dry, it can get stuck along the way. At the bottom of the esophagus is a protective flap (the cardiac or esophageal sphincter), which protects it from stomach acid and opens during peristalsis, the wavelike motion that propels food into your stomach.[19]

Common challenges that can occur during this point of digestion are difficulty swallowing and acid reflux, or heartburn. These symptoms have a variety of causes, including hiatal hernia, which is when an organ, typically the stomach, protrudes up through the opening of the diaphragm.[20] (We provide some solutions for acid reflux in Chapter 6. We also have some exercises you can do at the end of this chapter to support your entire digestive process.)

Next up is your stomach, located on the left side of your upper abdomen, below your heart. Your stomach secretes hydrochloric acid, which helps break down food into a blended, souplike consistency (called *chyme*) and kills bacteria in the food. It also secretes intrinsic factor (which starts the digestion of vitamin B_{12}) and the digestive enzymes pepsin (to break protein into amino acids) and lipase (for fat digestion). Finally, your stomach produces a mucus barrier to protect itself from the stomach acid.

Some common health challenges associated with the stomach stem largely from too little stomach acid. Surprisingly, ulcers can be the result of too little stomach acid, as opposed to too much. (In Chapter 6 we'll show you how to do a stomach-acid test, as well as provide tips for supporting your digestion.) For a variety of reasons, including poor diet and aging, the body may produce too little stomach acid and too little intrinsic factor. Without enough intrinsic factor, your body cannot digest and assimilate vitamin B_{12}. Symptoms tend to be depression, memory issues, dementia, low energy, tingling extremities, nervous-system conditions, and more (see "Vitamin B_{12}: The 'Master Key,'" on the following page).

One way to lovingly support your digestion is to reduce stress, particularly during meals. Stress basically shuts down digestion and lengthens the time food stays in your stomach, which can set the body up for gut challenges. Typically, food will stay in your stomach between two and four hours, then empty into your small intestine through the pyloric valve.

Vitamin B$_{12}$: The "Master Key"

While all nutrients are important, there are some that stand out because of the sheer number of systems they support in the body. One of these is vitamin B$_{12}$ (also called cobolamin). B$_{12}$ gets its master-key status from researchers because it plays a functional role in a long list of organ systems and can be used to correct problems caused by other issues, even if a person's B$_{12}$ levels are adequate.[21]

Some medical professionals are calling B$_{12}$ deficiency a silent epidemic because even low-normal levels can cause symptoms. A Tufts University study of B$_{12}$ levels in participants between the ages of 26 and 83 showed that nearly 40 percent of participants were "low normal," 16 percent had a near deficiency, and 9 percent were deficient.[22]

While low B$_{12}$ and B$_{12}$ deficiency can happen at any age, it's most common among the elderly, vegans, and vegetarians. It is estimated that over 80 percent of long-term vegans and over 50 percent of long-term vegetarians who don't supplement with B$_{12}$ are deficient.[23]

People with eating disorders, anemia, autoimmune disorders, infertility, diabetes, or a history of alcoholism—or those with gut issues such as IBS, Crohn's, or low stomach acid, or those who regularly use antacids—could be at risk for low or deficient levels of B$_{12}$.[24]

Some symptoms of B$_{12}$ deficiency are[25]:

- Abnormal sensations (tremor, tingling, tremor, muscle spasms)
- Chronic fatigue
- Deep vein thrombosis
- Diarrhea or constipation
- Digestive pain (poor digestion, full or bloated feeling)
- Generalized weakness (weak arms or legs, difficulty walking)
- Heart attacks, coronary artery disease, or congestive heart failure
- Incontinence

- Infertility
- Loss of appetite, weight loss, or anorexia
- Memory issues and dementia
- Mood issues (depression, irritability, apathy, paranoia)
- Osteoporosis
- Palpitations
- Paralysis
- Premature gray hair
- Pulmonary embolism
- Shortness of breath
- Strokes or transient ischemic attacks (TIA, or "mini-strokes")
- Tinnitus
- Vision changes or damage to the optic nerve
- Vitiligo

If you think you have a B_{12} deficiency, talk to your health practitioner. Keep in mind that doctors may not recognize the value of B_{12} testing, so you might need to work with a naturopathic doctor. The urinary methylmalonic acid (MMA) is the best test to get, if you do decide to get tested. Keep in mind that some people with certain genetic mutations that adversely affect methylation (a key body function that keeps all systems running smoothly) could have tests showing false normal or false high B_{12} levels due to something called "methyl trapping." The bottom line is that if you feel you have vitamin B_{12} deficiency, work with a health practitioner who can guide you through testing, interpreting test results against your symptoms, and supplementation options.

If you do need supplementation, you'll likely want to look into the active forms of B_{12}: methylcobalamin and adenosylcobalamin (also called dibencozide). These forms are the most bioavailable and can be obtained in sublingual form or shots (at the time of this writing, adenosylcobalamin is no longer available in shot form, but it may return to market in the future).

Because dosage is different for everyone (some people need to start low and slow, others need higher doses), we recommend that you work with a knowledgeable practitioner to identify the type and dosage of B_{12} that is right for you.

The Small Intestine: The Body's Factory

Once the stomach delivers partially digested food to the small intestine, it enters the duodenum, the first 12 inches of approximately 20 feet of small intestine. The small intestine is like a factory, responsible for digestion and absorption. Microscopic fingerlike structures called villi are like factory workers, producing enzymes to further break down food, absorbing nutrients that are needed and blocking those that aren't.[26]

The wall of the small intestine acts as a gatekeeper, letting through water and needed nutrients and keeping out harmful substances. Poor diet, medications, and bacterial or fungal overgrowth can compromise the lining, causing leaky gut. Symptoms of leaky gut are varied but can include food sensitivities, allergies, headaches or migraines, arthritis, eczema, hives, and chronic fatigue.[27]

Pancreas, Liver, and Gallbladder: Three Key Players Supporting the Small Intestine

While 90 percent of digestion is taking place in your small intestine, three most valuable players fill very important roles:

— Your **pancreas** is located toward the back of your abdomen, partly behind your stomach and partly connected to the duodenum of your small intestine. As food moves from your stomach to your small intestine, the pancreas secretes bicarbonate of soda (like baking soda) to neutralize the acid before it enters the small intestine. From there, it secretes pancreatic enzymes: protease (breaks down proteins), amylase (breaks down carbohydrates), and lipase (breaks down fats). If your pancreatic enzymes are too low, nutritional deficiencies can result, like B_{12} deficiency. The pancreas also regulates blood sugar by secreting the hormones glucagon and insulin. Diabetes could result if this system is out of balance.

Symptoms that could indicate challenges with your pancreas are: pain radiating to your back, nausea, vomiting, fever, increased heart rate, loss of appetite, bloating, or foul-smelling or fatty stools (which have an oily appearance and may float).[28,29]

— Your **liver** weighs about three pounds and sits on the right side of your upper abdomen, under your diaphragm. It is the largest glandular organ, and arguably the hardest working in your digestive system, performing over 500 known functions to support your health.

The liver, which is Ahlea's favorite organ, plays the following roles: filters almost all of the blood in the body; creates bile to break down fats; breaks down hormones; processes all nutrients, including vitamins and minerals; and neutralizes toxins. This workhorse loves us so much that it makes 13,000 chemicals and 2,000 enzyme systems, and it can lose 70 percent of its function and still show no signs of disease.[30]

The liver will neutralize the toxins it can, and whatever it can't neutralize will be stored in the lower lobe of the liver and other tissues in the body. This is why we recommend regular liver cleansing (we'll share some tips on how to support your liver in Chapter 6).

Signs of issues with your liver could include: addiction to substances like nicotine, alcohol, or food you're allergic to; changes to your skin (such as a yellowish hue or itchiness and inflammation), urine (changing to a dark color), or stool (becoming pale, bloody, or tar colored); fatigue; weakness; or abdominal pain (cramping, gas, and pressure).[31]

— On the underside of the liver is your **gallbladder**, a small pear-shaped organ that stores and releases bile to help you digest fats. The most common symptoms indicating that your gallbladder needs love are: gallstones, pain after eating (particularly processed fats or fried food), mild symptoms of abdominal pain that may radiate to your right upper back or shoulder, a lingering bitter taste in your mouth, constantly running nose, painful feet, sore tongue, rectal itching, or peeling skin on the palms of your hands.[32]

The Large Intestine (Colon): The Catcher

Your large intestine is three to five feet long and runs up the right side of your lower abdomen, across the front and down the left side. Water, fiber, and bacteria are delivered from your small intestine to your large intestine, where 80 percent of the water is extracted and delivered back to your bloodstream and stool is produced.

Your colon is full of good bacteria (flora), which keep bad bacteria under control and help with peristalsis, the motion that keeps chyme, the partially digested food, moving through your colon. Nutrients are extracted from the chyme and the remaining waste (feces) is stored in the rectum. When enough feces has collected in the rectum, your sphincters relax and you have a bowel movement. (See the next box to learn more about what a healthy stool looks like, symptoms of constipation, and the metaphysical meaning of poop.)

Challenges can arise with colon health if chyme moves too quickly through the colon, causing diarrhea, or if stool sits too long in the colon, causing constipation. Diarrhea and constipation could actually be considered two sides of the same coin because if one is chronically constipated and compacted stool builds up in the colon, only watery stool may be able to pass through, appearing as diarrhea. Other challenges associated with the colon are: bacterial overgrowth, diverticulitis, IBS, Crohn's disease, ulcerative colitis, inflammable bowel disease (IBD), hemorrhoids, and parasites.[33]

The Scoop on Poop

About 80 percent of people experience constipation at some time in their lives.[34] What some people or health professionals think of as "normal" when it comes to bowel movements varies widely, from three times per day to three times per week.

The fact of the matter is that what goes in, must come out. If you've experienced constipation, how do you feel? While constipation may not cause symptoms in some people, it's not uncommon to have symptoms such as: bloating, abdominal pain or cramps, foul-smelling gas, irritability, fatigue or lethargy, inability to pass gas, rectal bleeding, or changes in appetite or vomiting.[35]

The reality is that you live in your body, and you know when you are not feeling comfortable or something doesn't feel right. (We encourage you to trust yourself when it comes to how you feel, and you'll learn more about how to do this in Chapter 4.)

Luckily, there are also some signs you can look for if you are not sure what a healthy bowel movement should look like. Take a look at the following lists and chart to learn more.[36, 37, 38]

Signs of healthy poop:

- Brown in color

- Well formed, like a banana with a tip at the end

- Consistency like toothpaste and well hydrated

- Slips out easily with no straining or discomfort

Signs of unhealthy poop:

- Stool that is pencil thin, loose like pea soup, hard, lumpy, or in balls

- Soft, foul-smelling stool that sticks to the sides of the toilet

- Whitish mucus in the stool

- Having to strain or experiencing discomfort

- A feeling of incomplete evacuation

- Pale, yellow, green, black, or red in color

- Feeling like you have to manually manipulate your abdomen to push stool out

- Feeling like you have a blockage in your colon

- Feeling like you have to extract stool with fingers

- Undigested food in stool

Note: in the illustration on the next page, type 4 is what a healthy stool looks like. The Bristol Stool Scale was developed as a tool to assess gastrointestinal health. It can be a helpful way to identify how quickly stool is moving through your colon and, therefore, if you are tending toward constipation or diarrhea. The first two stool types would indicate constipation; types 3 and 4 indicate more normal transit time, with type 4 being the easiest stool to pass; and types 5 through 7 leaning more toward diarrhea. While this scale is not definitive proof of your digestive health, it can provide insightful feedback for nutrition and lifestyle choices.[39, 40]

Your poop is just one sign of the relative health of your digestive system. Typical suggestions to improve the health of your stool and your digestive system harken back to the basics of health: eat more fiber, drink plenty of water, get enough sleep, exercise, and reduce stress. Surely, we can all agree that these are great guidelines, along with paying attention to your thoughts and doing mirror work! At the same time, there are other aspects that can create challenges to your digestive health, as you've seen thus far. The exercises at the end of this chapter, along with those in the rest of the book, will give you plenty of ways to improve your digestive health, including the health of your stool.

The Metaphysical Meaning of Poop

When Louise was asked to share the metaphysical meaning of poop, she said:

> Bowels or poop are an indication of how we live our lives. All of life is: taking life in, assimilating what is good for us, and releasing and letting go of that which we no longer need.

BRISTOL STOOL FORM SCALE
WHAT DOES HEALTHY POOP LOOK LIKE?

TYPE 1 — Separate hard lumps, like nuts (hard to pass).

TYPE 2 — Sausage shaped but lumpy.

TYPE 3 — Like a sausage but with cracks on the surface.

IDEAL → **TYPE 4** — Like a sausage or snake, smooth and soft.

TYPE 5 — Soft blobs with clear-cut edges.

TYPE 6 — Fluffy pieces with ragged edges, a mushy stool.

TYPE 7 — Watery, no solid pieces. Entirely liquid.

When intake, assimilation, and elimination are all in Divine right order in my body, I feel great. There is nothing that feels like a really good poop. Then we flush and it's on its way, never to return! This is nature's way. I do not know of anyone who tries to go into the sewer to retrieve their poop.

If only we could treat all of our life experiences the same way. Intake, assimilation, elimination, and *flush!* How often do we dig into the garbage of our past, try to bring back a situation so we can rehash it, go over it again—worry some more—and look for a different solution, when it no longer exists in our life?

When I find myself doing this, I say to myself, "*Flush,* Louise!" and I bring myself back to the *now.* Now is where the action is.

Working with Your Body's Loving Army

It's worth noting that 70 percent of your immune system is located in your gut. This makes sense when you realize how many toxins work their way through the digestive system. Your miraculous body has been designed to keep you healthy and strong!

Your gut-associated lymphoid tissue (GALT) is like a loving army that protects your body. When Ahlea works with clients with low immunity, she can actually hear that their GALT feels like "unequipped, lonely soldiers." A healthy diet and lifestyle is one way you can make the job of the GALT and your entire digestive system much easier. Imagine how much energy would be left over for you if they could take a rest from working so hard!

From your digestive organs to the 100 trillion bacteria that live in your gut, your body was designed to work in perfect harmony. Over the years, modern lifestyles have become busier, with more stress, increased exposure to toxins, less sleep, and a diet full of fast and convenient processed food.

We don't go wrong when we live in the modern world. We go wrong when we let the speed, convenience, and fears of the modern world disconnect us from our bodies. For example, if you want a break, but you feel you must push on and "get through" a difficult week out of fear of some consequence, it requires disconnecting from your body's cry for rest.

The truth is, we live in human bodies that have needs, and we inhabit a world that often asks us to put aside those needs and keep going. After a while, we fear that if we listen to our bodies, we will have some adverse financial, social, health, career, or relationship situation. Too often, we live based on what we fear could happen.

Most of us have not been taught to listen to our bodies and inner wisdom, so we don't trust it. While we will talk more about this later in the book, we wanted to make an important point now: when you stop listening to your body or your inner voice, you move from harmony to disharmony. It's harder to make loving choices for yourself when you don't even know what your body is asking for. When it comes to your food choices, it becomes easier to follow the more obvious signals, like cravings, the need for speed (fast, processed food), or disconnecting from the sensory experience of food (eating while multitasking).

These behaviors set the stage for eating a nutrient-poor diet, eating too quickly, overeating, and a vicious cycle of cravings. What's happening inside your body is even worse: your organs don't know what to do with the chemicals in processed foods; your body can become depleted through lack of real, usable nutrients; and other symptoms, like fatigue, joint pain, irritability, depression, and weight gain, become your body's only way to reach out to you.

Going deeper into your digestive system, your gut bacteria—once a health team working together to get you everything you need for good health—are waging a battle with "food-like" chemicals that they don't know how to deal with. The good guys begin to die off, allowing the bad guys to overtake your system, creating a state of dysbiosis (the absence of harmony). These bad bacteria adore sugar because it helps them grow even bigger and stronger. They love a "messy room" to play in, and as they start partying in your system, you may begin to feel out of control, like you have no willpower and just can't figure out what to eat or how to heal.

Have you ever de-cluttered your office and felt like you could work better, or cleaned a room and felt happier? If you are feeling confused about how to move forward in your life, or you feel that you can't stick to healthy habits, cleaning up your diet is a great place to start because it essentially cleans up your digestive system and helps good gut bacteria thrive.

Digestive Health: Starving Bodies, Full of Food

There are three important steps in the digestive process for good health:

1. Food must be broken down into nutrients.

2. Nutrients must be absorbed and assimilated.

3. Waste must be eliminated.

When your diet consists largely of processed foods, you set your body up to have difficulty with all three steps in the digestive process. Over time, the body

BE KIND TO YOURSELF:
DITCH THOSE HARMFUL SOFT DRINKS & ENERGY DRINKS!
While research shows that most people know soda is bad for them, sales data shows that people are drinking it anyway

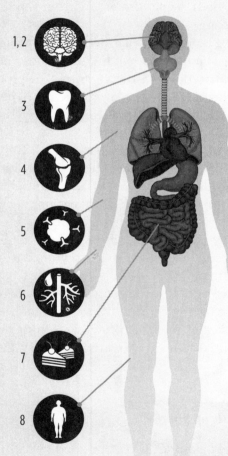

1. BRAIN & MENTAL HEALTH
A study on adolescents found that energy drink consumption was linked to poor mental health, depression and substance abuse.

2. MOODS & MEMORY
Artificial sweeteners contribute to panic, anxiety and irritability. Consumption of energy drinks has been linked to insomnia.

3. TEETH
High levels or acid and sugar in sodas and energy drinks promote tooth decay.

4. BONES
The phosphoric acid in sugar may contribute to lower bone density.

5. CELL DAMAGE
Soda contains the preservatives sodium benzoate or potassium benzoate, which are responsible for cell damage and contributing to asthma and allergic conditions.

6. BLOOD SUGAR
Rapid boost and then crash of blood sugar adversely affects moods, appetite and willpower.

7. CRAVINGS
Artificial sweeteners in soda can promote loss of taste for healthy foods and increased cravings for junk food.

8. WEIGHT GAIN
"If everything else in their diet is equal, a person who has a can of Coke a day adds an extra 14.5 pounds per year, just from the calories alone," says Dr. Christopher Ochner, assistant professor of pediatrics and adolescent medicine at the Icahn School of Medicine at Mount Sinai. Yale University researchers found that people ate more food on the days they drank more soda. Studies show regular soda consumption can lead to:
34% increase in risk for metabolic syndrome
26% greater risk of developing type 2 diabetes
75% higher risk of gout in women

As an act of self-love, one step you can take is to replace your soda or energy drink with options that will better nourish your body and mind. **Chapter 6** has ideas for boosting energy naturally and our recipes section has some ideas for replacing soda drinks with healthier options.

How Soda & Energy Drinks Affect Your Health

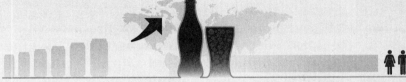

Energy drink sales are on the rise: estimated at **$20 billion** in 2013 in the US alone.

Nearly **50%** of Americans drink **2.6 cups of soda** per day on average and even with some declines in soda drinking due to a link with obesity, sales are expected to increase by 17% by the end of the decade.

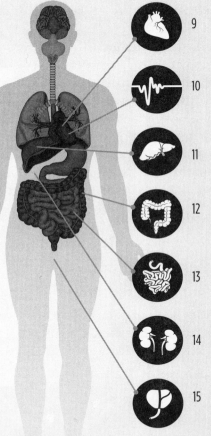

9. HEART
Dehydration and caffeine consumption from soda and energy drinks were found to increase heart rate and blood pressure. Energy drinks are not heart healthy. Consumption is associated with: palpitations, rapid heart rate and raised blood pressure, seizure and even death. Diet soda has been linked to high cholesterol.

10. STROKE
Consumption of soda has been linked with an increased risk of stroke.

11. LIVER
Researchers found that increased consumption of soda was linked to an increase in non-alcoholic fatty liver disease.

12. DIGESTIVE SYSTEM
Carbonated drinks and high fructose corn syrup contribute to gas in the digestive tract, like bloating, belching, abdominal pain and flatulence.

13. INTESTINES
Artificial sweeteners in diet cola can reduce good gut bacteria.

14. KIDNEYS
A Harvard study found that diet soda consumption had adverse effects on kidney function, particularly when drinking more than 2 sodas per day.

15. REPRODUCTIVE SYSTEM
BPA (bisphenol A), an endocrine system disruptor responsible for reproductive problems, can leach from soda cans into the soda people drink.

SOURCES

National Institutes of Health. "Gas in the Digestive Tract." National Digestive Diseases Information Clearinghouse. Web. 24 Apr. 2014 / Bray, George A, Nielsen, Samara Joy, Popkin, Barry M. "Consumption of high-fructose corn syrup in beverages may play a role in the epidemic of obesity." The American Journal of Clinical Nutrition. (2004): vol. 79 no. 4. 537-543. Web. 24 Apr. 2014 / Rudavsky, Shari. "Study: Diet soda doesn't help you lose weight." USA Today, July 10, 2013. Web. 24 Apr. 2014 / University of Waterloo. "Energy drinks linked to teen health risks." ScienceDaily. ScienceDaily, 6 March 2014. Web. 24 Apr. 2014 / Ellis, Marie. "Energy drinks alter heart function, study shows." Medical News Today. MediLexicon, Intl., 2 Dec. 2013. Web. 24 Apr. 2014 / Bernstein, et al. "Soda consumption and the risk of stroke in men and women." The American Journal of Clinical Nutrition. (2012). Web. 24 Apr. 2014 / Saad, Lydia. "Nearly Half of Americans Drink Soda Daily." Gallup Wellbeing. Gallup, 23 July, 2012. Web. 24 Apr. 2014 / Team, Trefis. "The Coke And Bull Story: Why Soda Sales For The Company Could Improve. Forbes. 24 February 2014. Web. 24 Apr. 2014 / Oaklander, Mandy. "7 Side Effects of Drinking Diet Soda." Yahoo Shine. Prevention Magazine, 17 September 2012. Web. 24 Apr. 2014 / Harvard School of Public Health. "Soft Drinks and Disease." Harvard School of Public Health. Web. 24 Apr. 2014 / Shaw, Gina. "Soda and Osteoporosis: Is There a Connection?" Osteoporosis Health Center. WebMD. 2007. Web. 24 Apr 2014 / Abid, Ali, et al. "Soft drink consumption is associated with fatty liver disease independent of metabolic syndrome." Journal of Hepatology 51 (2009) 918–924. PDF file.

can become deficient in the nutrients it needs to stay strong, energized, and happy. Muscles can lose tone, caffeine or energy drinks may be needed to get through the day, and you may experience cravings and mood swings. Over time, this could progress to aches and pains, lack of sleep, constant stress or "frayed nerves," and weight gain.

Did you know that cravings and overeating are signals that your body may in fact be starving? Now you can see how weight gain may actually be related to nutrient deficiency. However, keep in mind that weight alone is not an indicator of digestive health.

Now let's say you are eating a healthy diet, but you still have trouble with the second and third steps of digestion—this is a sign that you may have a compromised digestive system. The fact that you are already eating a healthy diet is a beautiful way to love yourself, and you may want to continue by focusing on improving absorption, assimilation, and elimination. Make sure to read the client stories in this chapter to learn how others have healed their digestion. This may give you the encouragement you need to continue the healthy habits you have started!

Symptoms that you may have problems with the second and third steps (and may have dysbiosis or malabsorption) are:

- Abdominal pain and cramps

- Constant cravings (especially for sugar or carbohydrates)

- Constant hunger

- Constipation

- Diagnosis of parasites, fungal overgrowth, or bacterial overgrowth (candida, small intestine bacterial overgrowth [SIBO], *Clostridium difficile,* and the like)

- Diarrhea

- Eating disorders

- Fatigue

- Feeling simultaneously hungry and full

- Gas, including that which feels trapped and painful

- IBS

- Joint pain

- Low blood sugar or hypoglycemia

- Mood issues (such as depression, anxiety, apathy, or irritability)

- Skin problems (such as acne, eczema, psoriasis, or rashes)

- Stool changes (see "The Scoop on Poop," and particularly the Bristol Stool Scale, earlier in the chapter to discover why the type of bowel movement you have can be an indicator of digestive health)

- Ulcers

No matter where you are in your digestive health journey, we will have some solutions for you in Chapters 5 and 6. For now, please take a look at the "Be Kind to Yourself" section earlier in the chapter to see how soda affects your body. Soda is full of chemicals that your digestive system does not understand. You'll clearly see what happens to your body when you ingest harmful chemicals in processed foods and beverages.

Methylation: A Biochemical Process That's Key to Your Health

You can see that your digestion is a very important process for keeping your mind and body healthy and strong. Another lesser-known yet critical function of your body is methylation. According to Dr. Mark Hyman, methylation is a biochemical process that occurs billions of times every second, affects just about every system in the human body, and is essential for health and longevity.[41]

We've already learned about Bruce Lipton's work in epigenetics, which proves that environment and perception can change your genes. Some doctors refer to epigenetics as "a second chance that allows the body to make changes to its genes," and this second chance is made possible through methylation.[42]

Methylation is a set of processes that work hand in hand to give your system what it needs for optimal brain and body health. You can understand why when you see that methylation is involved in important processes such as: gene expression; building energy, mood, and stress chemicals in the brain; digestion; detoxification; nervous system function; mobilization of fat and cholesterol; hormone control and production; allergic response; cellular function; homocysteine regulation; and the production and repair of proteins (including collagen and elastin).[43]

According to Dr. Hyman and other experts, problems with methylation can contribute to a wide and seemingly unrelated set of health issues, including: birth defects (such as spina bifida and Down syndrome), miscarriage, diabetes, osteoporosis, gut dysbiosis, fibromyalgia, cancer, depression and other mood disorders, and addictions.[44, 45]

One of the more talked about methylation defects is called MTHFR, which stands for *methylenetetrahydrofolate reductase*. MTHFR is estimated to affect more than 40 percent of the population, but there are several other defects that also play a role in methylation problems.[46] If you or a loved one has a chronic health condition, auto-immune disease, an addiction, or autism, or if you find that you aren't improving despite many efforts, we recommend getting tested for methylation defects. Women wishing to conceive a child may also want to be tested. The best way to do so is to work with a doctor who is familiar with MTHFR and related methylation-pathway challenges. Your doctor can recommend a methylation-pathway blood test or may direct you to a saliva test that you can get yourself by mail from 23andme.com.

The test you receive from 23andMe is a genetic one that provides information about your ancestry and other DNA, including your methylation genes. It's helpful to work with a doctor or qualified health practitioner to interpret your results because 23andMe provides them to you as "raw health data," which means you receive a bunch of letters and numbers (such as "rs4477212"). The raw data is very difficult for laypeople to do anything with, so companies like LiveWello (LiveWello.com) have developed online technology applications to take the 23andMe raw data and put it into a more organized report.

While many people are choosing to go this route for genetic testing, the data you receive can still be confusing. If you have a health background or are a skilled researcher, you can learn a lot about your own genetic health with a combination of the 23andMe saliva test and the LiveWello report. However, it takes a knowledge-able practitioner to interpret the data and help identify a natural health, nutrition, and lifestyle protocol based on your genetic blueprint and the symptoms you are experiencing. (To find a list of doctors around the world who understand MTHFR and related methylation challenges, go to Dr. Ben Lynch's website, MTHFR.net, and select "find a doctor.")

Remember, your genes are just blueprints—they do not dictate whether or not you can create a state of good health!

Diet, Thoughts, and Lifestyle Can Positively Affect Methylation

Methylation is an interesting and fairly new hot topic in health and medical circles. Much of the conversation is around gene defects and how to resolve gene ex-pressions, or symptoms. What's fascinating is that for most people with methylation problems, the prescription is to "heal the gut." A healthy diet is one of the most critical ways to support methylation. And many people with methylation issues have digestive issues as well.

It may not surprise you to hear the additional recommendations for improving methylation: getting plenty of sleep, reducing stress, exercising . . . all the "basics" that we've heard over the years, regardless of the latest trends.

Now, there are vitamin and mineral supplement recommendations as well, but very few prescription medications are available. We are happy to see this because the focus on optimizing methylation may encourage mainstream medicine to embrace nutrition and lifestyle recommendations that have shown success, rather than pharmaceutical drugs. While we would not be surprised if pharmaceutical companies start to create drugs to improve methylation, we are excited to see more scientists and medical professionals teaching their patients how diet and lifestyle can improve their health dramatically. Although it's currently rare to find medical doctors who work with patients to correct diseases associated with methylation defects, we are seeing more emerge. These doctors are excited about the successes their patients are having with all-natural supplements, nutrition, and lifestyle changes like stress reduction.

We are even seeing scientists talk about Bruce Lipton's work and taking a more positive mental outlook to improve methylation.[47]

Besides Genes, Here's What Impacts Methylation

Methylation is important for everyone to understand because it can be adversely affected for reasons besides a genetic expression. For example, the following also contribute to methylation issues[48]:

- Poor diet
- Poor gut health (low stomach acid, malabsorption of food/nutrients)
- Smoking
- Alcohol abuse
- Medications (birth control pills; acid blockers; high-blood-pressure medication; and medications for cancer, arthritis, and autoimmune issues)
- Conditions like cancer, kidney issues, and low thyroid

- Pregnancy

- Toxins (in food, water, and the environment)

- Stress (chronic stress can even affect the genes of future generations)[49]

Methylation is yet one more reason to make your health your greatest love story! Science is continuing to give us more evidence that healthy food and healthy thoughts are the keys to wellness.

Why Now? Processed Food Has a Negative Effect on Methylation

Now that you understand how a poor diet can negatively affect methylation, there's one more interesting piece to this puzzle. Since 1998, the U.S. government has mandated that folic acid (synthetic folate or vitamin B_9) be added to flour and other processed cereal and grain products. The government chose to regulate this because folate deficiencies in pregnant women led to babies being born with neural tube defects, such as spina bifida.[50] While statistics for neural tube defects began to fall, other methylation issues cropped up that seemed unrelated because no one knew about MTHFR at the time. If someone is one of the over 40 percent of people who have MTHFR, they likely cannot break down folic acid.

In some recent studies done on women who took folic acid (synthetic folate) and ate folic acid–enriched foods (processed flour and grain products), unmetabolized folic acid was found in 78 percent of the participants.[51]

Unmetabolized folic acid causes the following symptoms[52]:

- Low immunity

- Anemia, memory problems, and cognitive impairment from B_{12} deficiency that is masked by folate levels that are too high

- Higher incidence and development of certain cancers

- Neural tube defects *(Yes, the folic acid that was added to processed grain products can actually contribute to neural tube defects in babies with the MTHFR gene defect. This is problematic for pregnant women who don't know they have MTHFR and are prescribed a folic acid supplement during pregnancy.)*

The U.S. Food and Drug Administration (FDA) has guidelines for how much folic acid is safe to consume in processed foods, but it's not likely that the average person knows what these levels are, or that they are aware of exactly how much they're eating as they go through the day. Additionally, taking a B-complex vitamin supplement, a multivitamin, or any supplement with "folic acid" just adds to the problem when someone has MTHFR.

We suggest that you avoid folic acid in food and supplements, and instead focus on getting folate from healthy greens (romaine lettuce, parsley, collard greens, spinach, mustard greens, and turnip greens), asparagus, lentils, cauliflower, and beets.[53] Some people may need to supplement due to pregnancy or gut issues; in that case, using the active form of folate, called methylfolate, is better than folic acid. People with MTHFR are able to process methylfolate. You can look for methylfolate supplements like: L-5-MTHF (important to avoid racemic R forms), Quatrefolic (glucosamine form), Metafolin (calcium form), L-Methylfolate, and 6(S)-5-Methylfolate.[54]

We highly recommend that you research carefully and/or work with a knowledgeable practitioner before starting a methylation protocol. When your body starts methylating again, you may have symptoms or need to make adjustments, and it will help to have guidance for how to modify your protocol.

Diet, Thoughts, and Lifestyle Can Positively Affect Digestion

In her classic bestseller *You Can Heal Your Life,* Louise asked an important question about stomach problems and digesting: "What or who can't you stomach? What gets you in the gut?" For decades, Louise has taught that there is a connection between your digestion and how you digest life.

Think for a moment. Do you like your life? Do you trust it? As long as you're afraid of life, you're not digesting it. If you find yourself worrying about the future or upset about the past, if you are constantly working a long to-do list without any time to relax, if you feel like no one is there for you, or if you fill your time with work—even work you love—with no time to relax and have fun, you are likely not digesting life.

The first time that Heather went to the health-food store with Louise, they were approaching the elevator with their shopping cart. There were only a few bags in the cart, so Heather asked, "Do you want to leave the cart and we'll carry the bags?" Louise looked at her and said with a smile, "Let's take the cart. I'm not into suffering." At that moment, Heather realized how much of a habit she'd made of "shouldering" things—this went well beyond grocery bags to how she approached her life. Thanks to one simple, yet profound, statement by Louise, Heather realized that she could choose the easier path, rather than the one that required a great deal of strength and energy . . . or suffering.

Where can you make life easier on yourself? Where are you choosing to carry heavy bags, rather than taking the shopping cart and floating along?

Breathe deeply into your body several times and ask yourself the following: *Am I feeling safe? Is life safe for me? Am I giving myself what I need? Am I saying yes to please others when I want to say no? Where am I denying myself?* Sit with these thoughts for a few minutes and write down what you learn.

Remember the vision exercise at the end of Chapter 2? That is a great way to focus on creating a balanced lifestyle, with more of what you truly want in your life, while letting go of what you want less of. We have also provided affirmations at the end of this chapter, and we encourage you to continue doing mirror work so that you can learn to deeply love yourself and trust Life to take care of you. This step alone will go a long way to healing your digestion.

The Body-Mind Connection: Digestive Health and Your Brain

Have you ever had a gut feeling? Or felt butterflies in your stomach? If so, then you have experienced the gut-brain connection. Some experts once believed that issues in the brain should be handled separately from the gut, but more research is showing that if you want to improve your moods, memory, and brain function, look to the health of your gut.

There's a good reason why. Let's start as early as conception, when a baby is in the embryo stage. During this stage, a clump of embryonic tissue separates, and one becomes the brain (the central nervous system, which is the brain and spinal cord) and the other becomes the gut (your digestive system and its enteric nervous system).[55] Connecting your brain and gut is the vagus nerve—like a telephone line, it carries messages from the brain to the gut and vice versa. It's also how the bacteria in your gut speak to your brain.

Michael Gershon, professor and chair of pathology and cell biology at Columbia University, has done groundbreaking work on how the gut's brain, or enteric nervous system (ENS), works. Here are a few key facts[56, 57]:

- The enteric nervous system is embedded in your entire digestive tract from mouth to anus.

- It relies on, and in many cases creates, more than 30 neurotransmitters that are *identical* to those in the brain. (Serotonin is one of these.)

- Approximately 70 to 80 percent of your immune system is located in your gut. This makes sense because your digestive system has a big job. It takes in food, water, and bacteria from the outside world and transforms it into nutrients to grow, repair, and maintain the human body. This is the true definition of the old adage "You are what you eat."

- Approximately 90 percent of the body's serotonin is located in your gut. Serotonin helps regulate mood, sleep, and learning, and can influence your happiness and self-esteem. Serotonin also plays a critical role in digestion by helping to secrete enzymes that help you digest food.

- Your gut sends signals to your brain that directly affect feelings of sadness or stress, even influencing learning, memory, and your ability to make decisions. In turn, your brain's emotions affect your digestive tract. Anger, anxiety, sadness, joy, and other emotions can trigger symptoms in your gut.

Today, more studies are showing that food affects mood and that gut health has a big impact on disease, including osteoporosis, autism, depression, and auto-immune conditions.

Here are three studies that further highlight the gut-brain connection:

1. What you put in your stomach can change your mood. A study by Belgian scientists found that eating fat has the power to lift our emotional state and make us feel happier.[58] This is why people go for comfort food when they're upset.

2. Chronic stress can create gut-to-brain cravings. Studies on mice showed that under chronic social stress (like trauma from abuse or bullying), mice would go for high-fat, high-calorie foods and gain more weight than their less stressed counterparts.[59] Additionally, researchers found that it was the gut telling the brain what to eat and not the other way around. Under stress, the brain produces ghrelin, a hormone that stimulates hunger in the brain. Ghrelin makes food more exciting to the brain, especially when it is high in fat and calories.

3. Your diet influences your gut bacteria, and your gut bacteria influence your brain. According to neuroscientists, the good bacteria in the gut, which they call "the gut microbiome," act as auxiliary DNA. Essentially, what you eat controls the makeup of your gut bacteria, and these bacteria can change how your genes function. In other words, if you are eating a diet that promotes healthy gut bacteria, they in turn can influence a healthy body, regardless of your genetic predispositions.[60]

Another important takeaway from the studies in neuroscience is that your gut bacteria are constantly speaking to your brain. The gut microbiome influences how the brain is wired from infancy to adulthood, along with moods, the ability to learn, memory, and how to deal with stress. When the gut microbiome is healthy, it sends happy signals to the brain; when it's unhealthy, it can send signals of anxiety. Because of this signaling, neuroscientists are starting to investigate how to manage gut bacteria to treat mood and stress-related disorders, such as depression, IBS, and IBD.[61]

In other words, what you eat matters. What you digest or absorb matters. Your gut is responsible for how you feel, how you act, what you focus on, whether you sleep or not, your overall health, and your overall enjoyment of life. When you take care of your gut, you take care of your whole body-mind.

Reaching Your Goals: How Your Gut Impacts Your Willpower

For years, Louise has been teaching that everything is thoughts and food. She has always intuitively known about the gut-brain connection because she experienced it herself when she changed her diet. When people come to her and say, "I'm having a hard time sticking to my affirmations. They don't seem to work for me, so what can I do?" Louise's reply is, "What did you have for breakfast?" (You can imagine the look of surprise on their face!)

What happens next is a very interesting discussion about how changing the person's diet can support them to be at their best. It can support how they think, how they feel, how focused they are, and how happy they are. And guess what else it affects? Their willpower.

If you want to stick to something or reach a goal, your gut has a bigger role than you think.

Willpower is one of the most studied topics in social science because experts believe that in addition to intelligence, it is one of the most important attributes for success in life. Willpower is defined as self-control or your ability to overcome temptations that might keep you from achieving your goals.

A 2011 Stress in America survey showed that 27 percent of respondents felt like a lack of willpower was the most significant barrier keeping them from making positive changes.[62] A separate study involving over one million participants asked about the human virtues they felt they had, and willpower came in dead last.[63]

In the book *Willpower: Rediscovering the Greatest Human Strength,* research psychologist Roy F. Baumeister investigated how willpower could be strengthened. What he found is that willpower is not this elusive quality that only the lucky have. In fact, it's something everyone has, but it needs to be fed and, like a muscle, needs to be exercised.

Willpower needs to be fed because it—surprisingly—relies on blood sugar. If your blood sugar is low, you have less willpower; if it is stable, you have more willpower. Imagine the implications for dieters who are depriving themselves of food, even if they are getting hunger signals from their body. Blood sugar drops when you're hungry, so if you eat when you're hungry and raise your blood sugar back to normal, you are more likely to have stronger willpower.[64] Baumeister stresses that what you eat matters, though. If you eat sugary foods that spike your blood sugar, you're not creating sustained willpower; in fact, it's more "boom and bust." Just like your blood sugar can crash after a spike, your willpower can, too.

Now keep in mind that if you have malabsorption or gut dysbiosis, you may experience blood-sugar challenges even though you're eating a healthy diet or at regular intervals during the day. As you heal your digestion, you will likely find that you also feel a greater strength of willpower emerging.

Of course, blood sugar is not the only factor when it comes to willpower. Baumeister notes that willpower is like a muscle and must be exercised to develop strength, but the challenge is that you use the same "muscle" to make decisions. So if you're making a lot of decisions about whether to give in to temptation or not, you're likely to fatigue the muscle and lose willpower.

German researchers found that people spend at least four hours per day resisting temptations in order to achieve their goals. The most commonly resisted temptation was the desire to eat. After that, it was the temptation to sleep, the urge to take a break for fun, and the desire to surf the web.[65] When the participants in this study tried to resist temptation, they succeeded only half the time. For this reason, Baumeister and his colleagues found that the most successful people structured their lives to avoid having too many temptations. One example is having only healthy food in the house—with no junk food around, these people had fewer temptations to overcome and could conserve their willpower muscle for when they really needed it.

Food and Weight: How to Move Into Slim Mode

In Chapter 2, we talked about how weight is not the main indicator of health, yet we know that many people strive to reach a healthy weight. One thing you have learned in this chapter is that a body starved of real, whole foods can suffer from cravings and overeating that lead to weight gain. And denying yourself food when you're hungry, especially in restrictive diets, can blow your willpower and set up a vicious cycle.

So how does one become naturally slim? The first step is to love and accept yourself and your body, just the way you are, as you you've already learned. Another important step is to eat the foods your body actually needs to function properly. In other words, making choices about health is a combination of listening to your body and choosing real, whole foods that will support its needs.

When you count calories and follow rules, you are listening to other people, not to your body. You're not taking into account special situations your body may be in that require more food on one day and less on another. Calorie counting and weighing food can also set up a vicious cycle of judging yourself if you eat more than what you were "supposed" to eat.

When Heather was recovering from bulimia, she had to learn to trust her body and her appetite. Before her recovery, she would meticulously count calories and follow all the rules about staying fit and thin. These rules made her feel like she was in prison, always checking to make sure that she was doing things right. Once she recovered, she began to listen to her body. At first, because of malabsorption and digestive issues, her body was very hungry. She had blood-sugar issues, so she ate more than she had in the past. In fact, her appetite was so voracious that it concerned her. She felt like once she started eating, there was no "shutoff valve" to let her know when to stop. However, she knew that she was making healthy food choices, and she decided to trust her body and see what happened. She knew that if she didn't learn to trust her body, she'd never know what it was capable of. Affirmations and mirror work were key for her as she learned to trust the process.

It took about two years for Heather's appetite to come back to normal. After more than a decade and a half of bulimia, her gut needed to heal, her blood sugar needed to stabilize, and the hormones that signaled appetite and satisfaction needed to balance out. During this time, she gained some weight; however, because she had researched the healing process, she knew that this was a normal part of how the metabolism heals.

In her book *The Schwarzbein Principle II,* Dr. Diana Schwarzbein explains that when you have damaged your metabolism, you will likely gain weight as you heal your body. She explains that as you eat healthier food, your metabolism will heal, and you can more easily reach your ideal body composition.[66] No longer bound by calories and rules, Heather began to feel free to allow her body and her natural appetite to guide her.

When women have babies, they often feel pressured to lose weight right away. This kind of thinking can actually damage the metabolism. From conception to birth, women's bodies go through a lot of changes, affecting every system of the body. When a baby is born, moms tend to get less sleep and are focusing on caring for this precious being around the clock.

In Chinese medicine, one of the key concepts in digestion and healthy weight is *qi* (pronounced "chee"), which means energy. All bodies are different in the need for qi, and some women's bodies may have a good reason for losing weight more slowly after birth: to conserve qi and allow for better health in the long run.

Knowing this, Ahlea focused on eating healthfully and building energy after the birth of her baby. Instead of giving in to the external pressures of society for weight loss, she did her affirmations and focused on how miraculous her body was at producing milk to feed her baby and staying healthy after many late-night feedings. Her weight loss happened naturally, which allowed her to appreciate her body, rather than feel uncomfortable in it.

The key here is that the body is both mysterious and miraculous. When you love it and make loving choices, it responds in the time it needs to create sustainable, lasting good health and a naturally slim body. Take exercise, for example. When you start to exercise, there is a period of time when your body is building muscle before it releases the excess fat. During this time, you can feel as if your clothes are tight and you're gaining weight. If this creates fear, you might take drastic measures or stop exercising altogether, missing the moment that your body balances out and is more lean than ever.

Remember, *never use your body as a focal point for self-hatred.* Instead, look upon yourself with love. Louise teaches that being overweight represents a need for protection—an overweight person seeks protection from hurts, slights, criticism, abuse, sexuality or sexual advances, and life in general. Louise had observed in her own life that when she would feel insecure and not at ease, she would put on a few pounds. Then, the excess weight would go away when the threat was gone. She realized that fighting fat was a waste of time and energy, and she watched over decades as people tried and failed at different trendy diets.

The exercises at the end of this chapter will give you better solutions to focus on. Loving yourself, feeling safe, trusting your body, and trusting the process of life will enable you to make loving choices for your body.

Client Stories

Ahlea's ability to listen to the body and organs has allowed her to see, hear, and feel what is happening in her clients' bodies when they are not making loving choices in their food, thoughts, and lifestyle. Some of the most common patterns she sees are:

- The liver gets sucked up into the diaphragm and becomes dry as it struggles to do its job. When the liver is dry, it creates a dryness in the duodenum (the first 12 inches of the small intestine), which puts an extra burden on the digestive process.

- Sphincters (the rings of muscle that work to open or close a passage in the digestive system, such as the stomach or anus) tend to hold on to things, losing their natural ability to allow digestive material to flow easily through the body (for example, things like acid reflux can occur when the lower esophageal sphincter loses its ability to function properly).

- Feces becomes hard, dry, and impacted in the colon, which can contribute to challenges like constipation and bacterial overgrowth.

As Ahlea works on her clients' bodies and teaches them to make loving choices, the body responds. She's noted that after about ten sessions, her clients' organs begin to heal and thrive. The body is miraculous, and Ahlea has seen how beautifully organs respond when they are listened to with love and treated in loving ways

The following stories will show you how the digestive system responds to loving food, thoughts, and lifestyle changes.

Carter: Depression, Mood Disorder, and Chronic Fatigue

Carter, a man in his 70s, came to see Ahlea for depression, mood swings, and chronic fatigue. He was in relatively good health otherwise, but wanted to feel better and age healthfully. Carter's diet was actually quite healthy, so Ahlea listened to his organs, found out what his body needed, and focused on supplementing his nutrition with herbs and an exercise routine that would support his body energetically and structurally.

Carter was enthusiastic about making changes, and he had great progress, feeling happier and more energized, and developing more physical strength and muscle tone. People commented that he looked healthier than they'd ever seen him look. There were still some challenging mood swings he wanted to smooth out, though.

Since Ahlea and Heather consult with one another on many cases, they felt it would be a good idea to have Carter's methylation pathways tested. Not only does this help with mood issues, but they felt they could design a protocol for healthy longevity as well. Through genetic testing, they found that Carter had MTHFR. With some dietary changes and a protocol of vitamins, minerals, and herbs, Carter was able to smooth out his mood swings. His friends and family noticed changes very quickly and were very excited about his progress.

Carter is a good example of how a genetic condition that is expressing in symptoms can be shifted with good nutrition, improved lifestyle, and supplementation.

Becky: Bipolar Disorder

Becky, a woman in her early 50s, came to Heather to address a recent diagnosis of bipolar disorder, which is a major affective disorder with severe ups and downs in mood, energy, and daily activity.

Becky was on three different medications and following a vegan diet. An admitted workaholic, she had very little time to prepare food, so her diet included a lot of bread and junk food. In addition to her mood symptoms, she experienced bloating, excessive gas, constipation, terrible PMS, cravings, binge eating, and low energy. Becky felt hopeless because she thought that something was wrong with her brain, and she'd have to live with bipolar symptoms forever.

Heather told Becky about Dr. Natasha Campbell-McBride's research showing that people who suffer from issues such as bipolar disorder, depression, ADHD, schizophrenia, and obsessive-compulsive disorder all have digestive problems. Heather also shared recent research about the links between bipolar disorder, mineral deficiency, and methylation. This immediately resonated with Becky, and she became inspired to make some changes in her life.

The first step Heather took with Becky was to change her lifestyle, starting with a more reasonable work schedule, better sleep, affirmations, and more self-care. This gave Becky more time and energy to take action with her new eating habits. Heather helped Becky slowly incorporate a healthier diet and supplements to enhance methylation so that Becky's digestion, moods, and nervous system could heal.

One of the keys was making sure that Becky kept her blood-sugar levels stable and supplemented with vitamin B_{12} and zinc, since she was not getting these nutrients from her vegan diet. Over time, Becky was willing to add some animal protein, and she noticed bigger improvements in her health and mood stability.

Within three months, Becky was feeling better. She began taking more time for herself and working less. Since she was still on medication, she included her doctor in every change she was considering. The good news is that he had heard about how genetic mutations could be behind Becky's condition and was very supportive. Over the next year, Becky was able to make big changes in her diet and get off her medications. She felt so much better that she was committed to treating her body with love and following the methylation protocol that helped her recover.

As someone who travels a lot, Becky still has challenges sticking to her healthy diet and remembering her supplements when on the road—but she is gentle on herself, because she knows she's still learning and trusts that she will get better with practice.

Cara: Cushing's Disease and Eating Disorder

Cara, a woman in her 30s, came to Ahlea with Cushing's disease and bulimia. Cushing's disease is a condition that creates too much cortisol, the stress hormone. This excess cortisol contributes to extreme pain and symptoms such as acne, upper-body obesity, easy bruising, weak muscles, and thinning bones.[67]

Cara was full of pain throughout her body, including her joints and digestive system. The only food she felt safe keeping down was yogurt and diet soda. As Ahlea listened to Cara's body, she could hear the fear in her organs. She also saw that Cara's body was carrying resentment toward her husband.

Ahlea realized that this woman needed to start by feeling safe digesting life, so she gave her affirmations for mirror work. She also worked with Cara to design an initial nutritional program that Cara would feel safe following, to get some important nutrients into her body. Cara did agree to give up diet soda as a first step and replace it with water with fresh-squeezed lemon and a couple of high-quality green drinks each day.

Over time, Cara began to gain strength and energy, and her pain started to dissolve. As she felt stronger, she was ready to face the resentment she was carrying about her husband. Ahlea supported Cara in making lifestyle changes and communicating her needs to her husband.

As of the writing of this book, Cara is making wonderful progress and feeling better than ever as she continues her health journey with Ahlea. Part of this includes a methylation protocol to support the next level of Cara's recovery.

Mindy: Weight Loss and Metabolic Healing

Mindy, a CEO in her 50s, came to Ahlea to lose weight and gain energy. She was a very driven woman who worked hard and ran a large corporation. She was used to taking action and getting things done.

As Ahlea listened to Mindy's body, she heard her organs and tissues crying out for rest. Ahlea could tell that Mindy's metabolism was damaged from over-work, over-responsibility, and a lack of rest and repair. Ahlea recognized that Mindy's body was not going to cooperate with more action. At this point, Ahlea had quite a challenge. Her protocol for Mindy was one of rest, but she knew that Mindy favored action, believing that hard work and a vigorous exercise routine was the path to weight loss.

Ahlea asked Mindy if she was willing to trust that her body needed rest. Mindy wasn't sure, but she agreed to follow Ahlea's recommended protocol: to lie down and rest for their entire session.

Ahlea had Mindy lie on a yoga mat, and she did some energy work on Mindy's organs. While Mindy remained skeptical, she kept coming back and agreeing to just rest. After a month, Mindy had lost ten pounds and looked fresher and younger. She was so excited about the changes in her body and mind that she was willing to move forward with the rest of Ahlea's suggested protocol.

Mindy began to approach her lifestyle and her body with more kindness, realizing that rest, relaxation, and fun were important parts of a balanced, healthy life.

*Exercises to Get to Know Your Body
and Create the Foundation for Health*

1. Tips for Improving How You Digest Life

Good digestion starts with how you digest life. When you are afraid of life or don't trust it, you tend to focus on things that reinforce that belief. Remember, it's only a thought, and a thought can be changed!

We have created a list of tips that you can follow to be kind to yourself, love yourself more, and learn to feel safe. Pick one thing that feels good to you from the list below and practice it each day.

— **Continue your mirror work and affirmations** (see the next section).

— **Kiss your hand and say, "I love you."**

— **Hug yourself.**

— **Tell your body how much you love it**—when you look in the mirror, as you walk around during the day, as you exercise, or anytime you think of your body. Tell your body how grateful you are for how it supports you, how strong your legs are as they carry you from place to place. Pick something to appreciate, and tell your body how much you love it.

— **Eat mindfully and stop multitasking.** When you sit down to a meal, turn off the TV and stay away from your phone and computer. Sit in a quiet place, and focus only on your food and the sensory experience you are having. Give love to the food and your body as you eat. Truly enjoy your food! If you're stressed, take time to breathe deeply and relax before eating, so that your body calms down and can digest your food.

— **Fill your environment with things that connect you with the feeling of love.** Write affirmations and post them on your computer, on the refrigerator, on your bathroom mirror, or in your car. Have keepsakes that you love in places where you want to be reminded to be kind to yourself.

— **Choose to stop engaging with media that is violent or reinforces negative thoughts.** Turn off the news, stop reading women's magazines that focus on weight and perfection, and choose movies and TV shows that make you feel uplifted.

— **Spend more time with friends who support you in making loving changes in your life,** and spend less time with friends who are not supportive of your new habits.

— **Practice trusting Life to take care of you.** If you are afraid of something, repeat: *All is well. Everything is working out for my highest good. Out of this situation, only good will come. I am safe.* Say this as often as you need to in order to feel more comfortable and safe.

— **Keep in mind that you are responsible only for yourself.** Some people take responsibility for the stress, health conditions, and upset emotions experienced by their spouse, kids, extended family, friends, clients, co-workers, and anyone they care about. If you take in the stress and upset from others, it can have a negative effect on your own stress levels and health. You are essentially taking responsibility for their stress. Practice loving them instead of taking on their stress and burdens. You can do this by sending them a loving affirmation, such as, *I lovingly release this energy. They are free and I am free. All is well in my heart now.* Allow yourself to release the energetic stress and trust that the energy of love is the most healing of all.

— **Ask Life for help.** If you are feeling stressed or upset, notice whether you're pushing to accomplish something. Move from pushing to allowing. Ask Life to help you make it happen, and focus on allowing it to be easy.

— **Keep a gratitude journal.** Since what you focus on expands, write down all of the wonderful things that happened in your day, as well as the things you are grateful for. Remember, one can have gratitude for seemingly small things, too, like a cat purring, a dog wagging its tail, a child's smile, clean bedsheets, the healthy meal you had, a good book, and so on. If you do this each day, you can capture all the proof that Life loves you, which can help eliminate doubt. Also, you get to choose what you focus on, and gratitude is a very healing emotion that is so good for your body.

— **Feed yourself love instead of misery.** Throughout your day, ask what you're feeding yourself. If you notice that you're feeding yourself misery, shift into feeding yourself love with nourishing foods and positive, loving thoughts.

— **Move from suffering to simplicity.** Instead of choosing the harder approach, ask yourself how you can make things easier on yourself. Make it a game to find out how you can keep things simple and easy. Remember, there's no need to suffer!

2. Affirmations

Have you been doing your mirror work consistently? This one loving act can set the stage for so many of your health goals. Here are two affirmation treatments to practice in the mirror, during meals as well as throughout the day. You can also use them as meditations.

"Accepting My Physical Perfection" Treatment

I am vibrantly healthy, happy, healed, and whole from the top of my head to my big toes. Every part of my body is in a state of perfection. My hands and arms embrace all of life with great joy. My nerves, muscles, and bones express comfort and ease. My mind and body are flexible and flowing. I have the freedom to move in any direction I choose. From inner to outer, my body is a joy to live in. My inner child is nourished, loved, and happy. I forgive everyone and everything I have forgotten to forgive. I see only perfection in my body and in my world. Life loves me, and I love life. And so it is!

"Healthy Body, Healthy Mind, Healthy Digestion" Treatment and Meditation

Close your eyes, take a deep breath, and quiet the chatter of your mind. Take another deep breath and tune in to your body. As you breathe, breathe love into your body and let it surround you.

Imagine yourself looking into your eyes with love. And now imagine having a conversation with yourself . . . allow yourself to let go, and affirm:

I am willing to let go. I release all tension. I release all fear. I release all anger. I release all guilt. I release all sadness and let go of old limitations. I let go, and I am at peace. I am at peace with myself and the process of life, and I am safe.

Now, see yourself talking to your body:

My body is a glorious place to live. I rejoice that I have chosen this particular body because it is perfect for me in this lifetime. It is the perfect size, shape, and color. It serves me so well. I marvel at the miracle that is my body. I choose the healing thoughts that create and maintain my healthy body and make me feel even better.

I cooperate with my body's nutritional needs and feed it delicious, healing foods. I drink clean, clear water and allow it to flow through my body, washing away all impurities.

I deserve to be healed, and my healthy cells grow stronger every day. I am safe. My body knows how to heal itself, and I trust Life to support my healing in every way. When I need support, I attract the right people to help me heal. Every hand that touches my body is a healing hand, including mine. Every day and in every way, I am growing healthier and healthier.

I love and appreciate my beautiful body!

My digestion starts with my mouth. I love my mouth. I nourish myself by taking in new ideas. I prepare new concepts and healthy foods for digestion and assimilation. I learn to choose new foods that are delicious and supportive of my body. I have a good taste for life and for healthy food. I choose to eat slowly, savor my food, and chew well so that I can digest with ease. This is how much I love my body. I love and appreciate my beautiful mouth!

I love my stomach. It is with joy that I digest the experiences of life and the healthy, delicious food I eat. Life agrees with me, and I choose nourishing foods that agree with my body. I easily assimilate the food I eat at every meal. I chose the thoughts and the food that glorify my being. I trust Life to feed me that which I need. I am good enough as I am, and I am worth taking the time to digest my food. I assimilate this thought and make it true for me. I love and appreciate my beautiful stomach!

I love my liver. I let go of everything I no longer need, and I joyfully release all irritation, criticism, and condemnation. My liver knows how to cleanse and heal my body. Everything in my life is in Divine right order. Everything that happens is for my highest good and greatest joy. I find love everywhere in my life. I love and appreciate my beautiful liver!

I love my intestines. I am an open channel for good to flow in and through me—freely, generously, and joyfully. I create new habits of choosing foods that assimilate well in my body, keeping me energized, healthy, nourished, and strong. I willingly release all thoughts and things that clutter and clog. All is normal, harmonious, and perfect in my life. I live only in the ever-present now. I choose the thoughts that keep me open and receptive to the flow of life. I have perfect intake, assimilation, and elimination. I love and appreciate my beautiful intestines!

Next, see yourself sitting down to a meal. It could be any meal of the day.

I am so grateful to have this wonderful food. I choose the best food for my body, and I bless this food with love. I love selecting foods that are nutritious and delicious. Planning healthy meals is a joy, and I can easily make anything taste good. My body loves the way I choose the perfect foods for myself. Mealtimes are happy times, and my body heals and strengthens with every bite I take.

I am one with Life, and Life loves me and supports me. Therefore, I claim for myself perfect, vibrant health at all times. My body knows how to be healthy, and I cooperate by feeding it healthy foods and beverages, and exercising in ways that are enjoyable to me.

I listen with love to the thoughts I think about my health. I open myself to the wisdom within, knowing that Life will bring me everything I need to know to create new, healthy habits. I trust my body to guide me, knowing that whatever I need comes to me in the perfect time, space, and sequence for me.

The world I live in is safe. It is full of delicious, healthy options I can choose as I create new habits for my health. I choose to love myself with each thought I think and with the food I eat.

This is a new day. I am a new me. I think differently, speak differently, and act differently. My new world is a reflection of my new thinking. It is a joy and a delight to plant new seeds for my best health.

I have within me all the ingredients for good health. I now allow the success formula for wellness to flow through me and manifest in my world. I only need to do one thing at a time. I trust Life to guide me to each new step when I am ready. I am safe making changes at my own pace. My pathway is a series of stepping-stones to ever greater health, energy, and joy. All is well in my world.

I am not my parents, nor do I choose to re-create their illnesses. I am my own unique self; and I move through life healthy, happy, and whole. This is the truth of my being, and I accept it as so. All is well in my body.

I am open and receptive to all the healing energies in the Universe. I know that every cell in my body is intelligent and knows how to heal itself. My body is always working toward perfect health. I now release any and all impediments to my perfect healing.

I learn about nutrition and feed my body nourishing, wholesome, healing food. I watch my thinking and only think healthy thoughts. I release, wipe out, and elimi-nate all thoughts of hatred, jealousy, anger, fear, self-pity, shame, and guilt. I love my body. I send love to each and every organ, bone, muscle, and part of my body. I flood the cells of my body with love. I accept healing and good health here and now.

These affirmation treatments and meditations are incredibly helpful for loving and accepting yourself more and more each day. As you go about your day, make sure to pay attention to your thoughts, the choices you make, and any physical or emotional symptoms you have. These are indicators of your overall well-being and as you become aware of them, the idea is to make loving adjustments rather than judging yourself.

Natural Beings, Natural Foods

By now, you know that your body has two critical processes that rely on whole foods: digestion and methylation. So it bears repeating that if something doesn't grow, don't eat it! We are natural beings, and we run on natural foods. You have now seen why our food history is pockmarked with goals that have nothing to do with fueling our natural bodies and everything to do with figuring out how to feed a growing population. And you are likely very aware that many of us have come to rely on food that is fast, so we can get about our daily lives.

We invite you to take a deep breath in this moment. Put one hand in the center of your chest and the other on your abdomen. Breathe deeply for three breaths. Remind yourself that you are worth good health. You are worth investing time to relearn what we humans have forgotten in the past few centuries. You don't have to do it all in one day. In this moment, all you need to do is tell yourself how much you love yourself and how much you love your body. Tell yourself you only need to take one baby step at a time, that you are safe, and that all is well in your world.

In the next chapter, you'll learn how to listen to your body's messages so that you can deepen your intuition and take loving action in support of your best health.

♥ ♥

Chapter 4

Step #4:
Listen to Your Body—
a Powerful, Yet Little-Known
Health Secret

Long before it was fashionable to discuss the mind-body connection, Louise published her book *Heal Your Body,* in which she talked about health conditions and the probable thought patterns behind them. In the ensuing years, more and more scientific evidence has cropped up to prove the mind-body connection, yet it still seems so mysterious to many people.

You probably were not taught to listen to your body or even your feelings. In fact, if you go back to your childhood, you may remember being told that you were wrong about things you felt. Perhaps you were told not to feel something: "Don't be sad," or "You're not hurt." Maybe you were told that you were "too sensitive." If you had the typical upbringing, you likely got the message that concrete evidence, science, and proof were more important than how you felt or what you thought you knew.

> **"I listen with love to my body's messages."**
>
> — Louise

Dreams, instincts, intuition, and extrasensory perception (ESP) used to be relegated to the "woo-woo" or considered "airy-fairy"; and knowing in advance that something would happen was called a "coincidence." Yet studies show that more than 50 percent of U.S. adults believe in ESP and psychic or spiritual healing, even though science does not confirm its existence.[1]

We know from Chapter 3 that we get "gut feelings" all the time for a very good reason—a reason science didn't know about until the 1950s. And our bodies give us many other clues about what is right or not right for us, if only we'll listen. Gavin de Becker, author of *The Gift of Fear,* explains intuition as the brain looking at something and processing it so quickly that conclusions are drawn without the person understanding how or why. Whatever the reason—intuition, ESP, your inner voice, or the "inner ding" as Louise calls it—this is something we all have.

De Becker also points out that the root of the word *intuition (tuere)* means "to protect" or watch over.[2] Life loves and protects us at all times. Listening to our inner guidance is a beautiful way to trust that Life always takes care of us, and it's a way that we can take loving care of our bodies.

The Still, Small Voice Inside

Intuition operates in mysterious ways. Did you ever have a time when you just "knew" something? Perhaps you were thinking of a friend just before she called out of the blue. Or you had a dream that later came true. Maybe you got "a feeling" about something or made a seemingly innocent decision, and it ended up saving your life. That's the power of intuition.

Michael Lomonaco was head chef at New York City's Windows on the World, at the top of the World Trade Center. On September 11, 2001, he had a noon appointment to get his glasses repaired, but for some reason, he decided to see if he could go in before work instead.[3] The first plane hit the World Trade Center while he was in the lobby, so he was able to get out safely. Had he gone right to work, he may not have survived.

While many stories of intuition involve dramatic life-or-death events, it's also at the heart of countless day-to-day decisions that guide people's lives. For example, Oprah Winfrey, who continues to make the *Forbes* most powerful celebrities list, says that while she listens to proposals, data, and reports, all of her successful decisions have been made by intuition or from the heart. As she says, "When you don't know what to do, do nothing. Get quiet so you can hear the still, small voice—your inner GPS guiding you to true North."[4]

This still, small voice is what Louise has relied on throughout much of her life. When asked if she always heard her inner ding, she said no, it was something she actually had to practice. In fact, when Louise was first learning to listen to her intuition, she used a pendulum, which is a weight (oftentimes a crystal) suspended on a string or chain, to help her access her subconscious mind. (When first using a pendulum, you learn how it moves when the answer is yes or no, and then you can ask questions. The idea is that your subconscious will affect the way the pendulum moves. If you're not sure how to trust your intuition, using this tool can help you see the guidance you're receiving.)

Louise started out using her pendulum to make simple decisions, like what food on a restaurant menu would be most healthful for her body. Over time, she continued to play with using the pendulum and realized she could get the same feeling without it. She said that there were times when it appeared that her inner ding was wrong at first glance, yet in the long run, it was that "wrong" choice that acted as the pathway to the choice that was right for her. She ultimately learned to trust her inner ding deeply, and even more so, trusted Life to guide her to the right thing at the right time.

Ahlea always knew how to listen and see into people. While she was sometimes punished for saying the things she knew (which no one had told her, and no one believed she could know), she continued to believe in her inner guidance. This is not a typical path for children, so it was clear that this gift Ahlea had was very strong in her life. As a teenager, she went to work in the radiology department of a hospital, where she got to test and confirm her ability to see into bodies by reading x-rays and observing how patient cases progressed. She went on to further learn about what she was seeing in bodies by studying anatomy and physiology and doing an anatomy lab with the cadaver of a deceased person who had chosen to donate his body to science. In this way, she could have the full sense of what human bodies need and what influences good health.

Heather had some connection to intuition growing up, too. Yet although she was mildly aware that she was using it to be successful in her job, where she often had to predict which products and processes would become popular in global companies in the future, she had largely abandoned listening to her own body. Instead, she was focused on doing her job well in a fast-paced company, which often meant not listening to her body and just pushing forward to get things done. There were times she had a "bad gut feeling" about something, and even described it as such to her boss as they contemplated acquiring a company—but while she was proven correct a year later, these feelings had little credence in the corporate environment.

Everything changed when Heather started working with a life and business coach. Her coach would ask Heather to describe the feeling she was having and then find out where she was feeling that emotion in her body. For at least a month, all Heather could feel was pain in her abdomen. This was in her initial stages of recovery from bulimia, and she felt like this "feel into your feelings" thing was hard to trust because all she felt was the same pain in her gut, over and over again.

With continued practice, though, Heather became aware that there were emotions behind that pain. They were scary for her to look at because they were about her job and how it was not right for her. Listening would mean a major upheaval in her life, including leaving the corporate world, selling her house, and building a new life somewhere else with her husband. It was much later that Heather realized she got a lot of intuition in her gut that almost had a "sick" feeling in it. However, once she understood it was just information, the sick feeling would leave immediately. She realized how long she had made herself sick by not listening all those years.

As Heather discovered, physical symptoms are the body's way of talking to you. This is especially true if you're ignoring other signals in your life and continuing on a path that is not right for you. As you learned in Chapter 2, when you are not making loving choices for yourself, your body will often speak to you in symptoms. Remember, your body knows how to heal and it wants to heal—it just needs your loving care to support the process.

Certain people, called physical sensors, can be so sensitive energetically that they pick up on symptoms that other people are having and feel them in their own bodies. Other people are emotional sensors, or empaths, and feel the emotions of others very strongly. The first thing to do if you are (or think you may be) one of these people is to stop, take deep breaths, and ask your body if this symptom or feeling is yours or if it belongs to someone else. If you feel that it belongs to someone else, ask what it has to tell you. Once you know it's not yours, it will typically start to dissolve.

People who are energetically sensitive in these ways often tell stories of being "sickly" children until they realized that the symptoms and/or emotions were intuitive messages and learned to work with their sensitivity. One very effective technique is to say, "Thank you, body, for giving me this message. It belongs to someone else. I lovingly release it from my body, and I send loving energy to them and to myself."

If you find that the symptom is in fact yours, the simple act of listening to that symptom and giving it your love can make a huge difference. Ahlea has her clients put their hand on their body where the symptom is, ask it what it needs, and then just listen. While you may not hear anything in the beginning, the body responds to the fact that you are listening. As you tell your body how much you love it and that it's safe with you, your body hears that and relaxes. You may feel the intensity of that symptom come down a bit. For example, if you have a great deal of pain, you may feel the pain soften. Some have felt it completely dissolve.

When Ahlea was 16 years old, she got an intuitive message to stay home from her after-school job. While she was not sure why she was getting this message, she listened and stayed home. That day, her horse got stuck in a fence and would have died had she not been there. As she released him from the fence, she massaged his body where he had hurt his neck, feeling where the tissue had tightened up and giving it loving energy. Her horse began to breathe deeply, and she could feel the tissue releasing under her fingers.

Ahlea has noticed that the tissues and organs in our bodies release in just the same way when we stop, breathe deeply, listen, and respond with loving energy. If you have any troubling symptoms, practice doing this and see what happens.

Listening for What Your Body or Your Life Wants

Intuition, or your inner voice, is there to support you in moving toward your highest good. While symptoms are just one way your body speaks to you, there are many other ways your body or your life could speak to you. Additionally, each person is different when it comes to how they get these signals.

Here are some ways your inner guidance may signal you:

— **Feelings.** Some people refer to them as "gut feelings," or getting a "bad vibe" or a "good vibe." You may not know what the feeling exactly is, though: it could be very vague, like something that just feels bad, uncomfortable, or "not right"; or wonderful, uplifting, or "right."

— **Emotions.** Similar to feelings are emotions, yet to some, they have subtle differences. You may experience an emotion that seems to come out of the blue. Perhaps you have thought of something or someone right before that emotion came up. Or maybe you walked into a place and felt the emotion. While emotions, like symptoms, feel as if they're really yours, remember to check to see how this emotion is speaking to you. It may be telling you that something is or is not aligned to your greater good.

Years ago, for instance, Heather was walking along and suddenly felt depressed. Her first thought was, *I haven't been depressed in years, so why am I feeling this way?* As she tuned in, she realized that it was not her emotion—it had come from a woman she'd just passed, who was sitting on the porch and talking on the phone. Heather sensed some things about this woman and her life and sent her the energy of love. The depression immediately went away. At that point, Heather began to think about all the years she had depression, wondering what really belonged to her and what she was picking up from others. As you can see, if we don't learn to tell the difference, we can be caught up in or hold on to emotions that are not our own.

— **ESP.** Extrasensory perception is a category of intuitive abilities that includes telepathy (the ability to read people's thoughts), clairvoyance (the ability to see what is happening somewhere else), precognition (the ability to predict the future), retrocognition (the ability to see things that happened in the past), psychometry (the ability to touch something and pick up information), and mediumship (the ability to channel spirits).[5]

— **Symptoms.** This could be any physical sensation, such as tingling, chills, fatigue, energy, pain, "pit in the stomach," aches, lightness, and so forth. One of the easier ways to notice this is to see how you feel when you're with different types of people. Notice if you feel normal (that is, as you usually do), energized (or uplifted), or drained. If you consistently feel drained with certain people, look more closely at how you feel about them—you may find that they are not right for you. Some teachers refer to these people as "energy vampires." We like to think of them as not being aligned to what you need in your life.

— **Thoughts.** Sometimes you may think of something and it's actually your intuition guiding you. An example of this is when Heather first started recovering from bulimia, she would notice that she'd think of food when she wasn't feeling physically hungry. She judged this as old, disordered eating behavior, as if she "could not stop thinking about food." Within a week of watching her thoughts around this, she realized that within 30 minutes of having a thought about food, her blood sugar dropped so drastically that she was in blood-sugar emergency. At that point, her body was so hungry that it felt like no amount of food could solve the hunger. Overeating can be very common as a way to get the body back into comfortable balance when blood sugar has gotten too low.

What was happening is that Heather's digestive system hadn't healed enough for her body to get the right signals of hunger at the right times. A bloating in her small intestine sent a signal of fullness when her stomach was actually hungry. What she realized is that her body was compensating for her digestive issues by using her thoughts to send the "time to eat!" signal. She began to eat when she'd think of food, and this worked beautifully until her digestive system healed.

See, our bodies love us! When we judge the signals we're getting as "wrong" or "bad," we lose the opportunity to allow our bodies to guide us to better health.

— **Words.** Louise has always been incredible at listening to the words people use and understanding how they play out in their thoughts and beliefs. She has seen the relationship between how they speak and how things happen in their lives.

Listening to the words you use, along with the words other people use, is another way you may get an intuitive hit on what is working or not working for you. For example, do you find yourself saying things like "This is so hard," "I can't stand this," "The body starts breaking down at the age of 40," or "They'll never accept me"? If you're saying things like this, it may be time to look at your belief systems and see how you can change them so that you can love yourself more. In Chapter 3, you learned that the inability to digest life can create health challenges. So remember to use loving words—your body is listening. Listening to your words, using affirmations, and doing mirror work can help shift the thoughts you think and the words you use into more loving ones.

— **Dreams.** For some people, signals come in dreams. Sigmund Freud, the father of psychoanalysis, believed that dreams tapped into the unconscious mind. According to some researchers, he may have been right. In one study, amnesiacs with no conscious memory of their past would have memories of their past when they dreamed. Studies like this have led scientists to believe that when dreaming, we are accessing parts of our brain that we don't often use in our waking lives.[6]

If you're unsure of what steps to take in your life, ask yourself before bed to have a dream about the next best step you can take. Another great way to work with your dreams is to write them down when you wake up and ask yourself what meaning they have for you. There are many books on dream interpretations that you can use if you want to learn more. At the same time, make sure you practice paying attention to these interpretations so that you can learn the language of your dreams.

— **Patterns.** Some people get signals through recurring events: Perhaps someone tells you about a book they love, then two more people tell you about it. This kind of pattern could be a signal to check out the book. Or maybe you keep having the same experience over and over again, but in different situations. For example, one of Heather's clients had a pattern of being the expert or helper in every relationship. She had very few equal relationships because all of her friendships and even her significant other seemed to rely on her for her strength, knowledge, and support. When she came to Heather, she was exhausted with adrenal fatigue and felt that no one would ever be there for her.

Notice the patterns that keep happening in your life, whether they're circumstances that occur, things people keep telling you, or situations you keep finding yourself in. These are signals that can help you take action in your life.

If you get any of these signals, or even others that are not mentioned here (remember, everyone is unique and special in how these signals show up!), get curious about them. Ask what they want you to know. You are starting a conversation, and learning a new language that no one has ever taught you. The more you listen, the more you'll understand what your body and your life are telling you.

Over time, you'll learn to trust these signals and may come to find that life feels a lot easier. Think of a car with no dashboard—no speedometer, no gas or temperature gauges. How would you know how fast you're going, when you need gas, or when the car is overheating? Know that you have an inner dashboard that you can learn to read as easily as you read the dashboard in your car! It may take time, and that's okay. You are on a beautiful journey of discovery with your body, so allow it to unfold at its own pace. (The exercises at the end of this chapter will give you some ideas for how to teach yourself the language of your body as you go.)

How to Listen to Your Body and Inner Voice

We want to stress how important the simple act of listening—being aware of the signals guiding you in your life—is. You don't have to know what to do about those signals right away. Trust that Life will continue to show you the way. Even if you only get one little step at a time, that is all you need! You don't have to figure everything out all at once, especially if you trust Life to show you the next step as you're ready for it.

When you're learning to listen to your body, it's important to get still and quiet. As you first start to listen, the signals you get may be very quiet, like a whisper, or very vague, like a slight feeling or symptom. The more you tune in to that signal, though, the more clear it will get.

As you begin to practice, here are some tips that may make listening to your intuition much more successful:

— **Focus on being present and aware.** Pay attention to what is happening in the moment and drop any thoughts about the past or the future. The more you're aware of this moment, the easier it is to tap into how you are feeling. Think of it as taking a moment to put your radar up and scan the environment, noticing exactly what is happening, and then noticing how you are feeling. This is the best way to develop your intuition. And there's a bonus: being in the present moment reduces the stress of mind chatter and worry about the past or the future while you're doing something else in this moment. Multitasking is stressful, and many people are on autopilot while they are moving through life because they are constantly focused on the past or the future instead of being in this moment now.

— **Develop a relationship with yourself—think of it as dating yourself.** Think about going on a first date: You don't know much about the other person, what they like or dislike, how they behave, or whether you will "click" with them. You are just getting to know them and might feel a little uncomfortable. It's likely that you are really listening to what they say and watching their body language.

Sometimes thinking of this process as a first date is helpful because if you don't yet have rapport with yourself, it can take time to get comfortable and get to know how your body responds as you communicate with it. By the second or third "date," you'll feel more comfortable. Maybe communication is a little easier. You may have started to recognize the signals or language your inner voice speaks.

— **Get quiet and still.** You might want to begin by setting aside some time in your day so that you can get quiet and still. Choose a space where you won't be disturbed for a period of time. You can use this time in any way that supports you. At first, you may want to spend time in meditation, clearing your mind of all chatter and focusing on not thinking at all. As you reduce mind chatter, you can invite your inner wisdom to speak to you in whatever way it chooses.

Another option is to do Ahlea's listening meditation at the end of this chapter. This allows you to focus your attention on your body in specific ways and tune in to any symptoms or signals that come up, learning what they have to tell you.

Or you can ask yourself a question and remain quiet, seeing what shows up. If you don't hear anything right away, that's okay! Just tell yourself that you are open to hearing an answer in the right time and space. As you stay open, you may find that an answer comes to you at another time during the day, in a dream you have, or in something another person says. Life works in magical and mysterious ways, and if you trust that answers will come, they will!

Remember, simply asking and being open to an answer in the perfect time and space is all that is necessary. You may be guided to do your own entirely different process during your quiet time, so go with whatever feels most supportive as you learn to listen to your inner guidance.

— **Tune in to your body during the day.** It can be great practice to check in with your body as you do various things throughout your day. For example, on your commute to work; in a meeting; as you're making a decision; when you're with friends, family, or pets; or as you plan your schedule. Tune in to your body to see how you feel during these activities. Look for signals that may be telling you what is right or not right for you. Be willing to take more time for a decision if you aren't feeling right about it and want to sit quietly to learn more. Tuning in to your body allows you to get very present and aware in the situation, which can heighten your intuition.

— **Keep an open, judgment-free mind.** Because everyone's intuition works in different ways, it's crucial that you stay open and avoid judging the signals that you get. It's best not to judge the importance of a signal, whether it's big or small, clear or vague, or the way it shows up. Stay open and curious as you learn the language of your inner wisdom.

— **Keep a journal.** Journals are wonderful because you can record your experiments and the results. Have fun with this! Write down what you learn about yourself and document the language of your inner voice. With time and practice, this language or the signals you get may change, and journaling can help you pay attention to how things progress. It can also help you to remove doubt by focusing on the successes you have with your intuition, particularly as time goes by. Sometimes it's with the passage of time that we can look back and see the true wisdom of our intuition.

— **Start small and build.** Start listening to your inner guidance in ways that feel easy for you. These are very simple steps that will tell your body that you're listening and that it matters. Here are some examples:

- When you have to go to the bathroom, go! Most people put off urinating or having a bowel movement until they have the "time." Instead, go when you feel you have to go.

- When you're thirsty, get a drink of water. Thirst is another signal that people tend to put off until they have time. Even if you have to stop what you're doing, get up and get a drink.

- Ask your body when it's ready to stop working for the day. Many people push on, even when they've put in a full day of work and are starting to feel like they want to stop. Notice what happens when you listen and stop working or when you push on. Some people report that their neck and/or shoulders start to ache if they push beyond their limit. Tune in and see what the right balance is for you, and then notice what happens when you follow that inner guidance!

- Notice what other people are saying or doing; listen to their words and watch how they behave. If you do this with curiosity and not with judgment, you may pick up some helpful inner guidance.

- Recognize what feels like "truth" to you. When Louise first started attending the Church of Religious Science, the information was completely new to her, yet she had a feeling that what she was hearing was true for her. When you feel that something is true, it's probably true for you, regardless of what others think. There will always be people who argue about what is true. The key is what you feel—practice listening to your own feelings about what is true *for you.*

— **Practice, practice, practice.** The more you tune in to your inner guidance and the more you follow it, the easier it is to understand how your body and life speak to you. The signals tend to get clearer and it becomes easier to trust your inner guidance. This practice goes a long way in trusting Life.

What Could Get in the Way of Listening to Your Body or to Life

There are many things that could get in the way of listening to your inner guidance. First and foremost being that we aren't taught to listen. On top of that, we live in a world that currently values science, evidence, and things that can be immediately observed . . . things that other people can see as well. Intuition does not work that way. It's subtle, it speaks its own language, and it is different for everyone.

And if you really think about it, many companies today are making products that are not healthful for our human bodies. If we were all running around listening to our inner guidance, these companies would be out of business in no time. For example, how would the fashion, cosmetics, and weight-loss industries survive if we all loved our bodies and were happy with our size and the way we looked? How would pharmaceutical companies survive if we started looking at symptoms as signals and shifted to more loving thoughts and actions, thereby getting healthier on our own? These are the very companies that put out ads that teach us not to love or trust ourselves, but rather to look outside ourselves.

The good news is that we can begin to listen more, to accept who and where we are right now and pay attention to the signals that allow us to move into what supports our overall well-being.

There are other reasons we may not be able to hear our inner voice very well. Some examples are:

— **Pain.** When you have physical pain, that may be the loudest "voice" that draws your attention, making it seem difficult to listen to your body or hear your inner guidance. Just like Heather's story of always going to the pain in her lower abdomen when her coach asked her to feel into the emotion in her body, you may find that you can't find anything underneath the pain at first. Continue to listen to your body. You may find that the pain lessens, or you may be able to feel emotions underneath the pain. Loving your body by listening to and loving that area of pain is the perfect way to start learning its language. Put your hands on that area of your body or visualize it and surround it with love.

— **Being too busy or not taking time for yourself.** If you overschedule yourself with work or friends or family, leaving little time to be still, you are less likely to take the time to listen to yourself. Taking this time is important, especially at first. When you're overbooked, you have little time to place awareness on your body, to meditate, or to develop a rapport with your inner guidance. Giving yourself time to get to know how your intuition works is one way you can love yourself more. It's also a beautiful way to get some much-deserved rest and replenishment.

— **Addiction.** One of the outcomes people have when addicted to alcohol, drugs, sex, food, negative thinking, or any other pattern is that it numbs them from feeling. This is a very big subject and beyond the scope of our book, but we want you to know that listening to your inner guidance and focusing on loving yourself is one of the key steps you can take in recovering from an addiction, even if it feels challenging at first.

— **Sugar and junk food.** In Chapter 5, you will learn more about how sugar and junk food mess with your brain and body. From addiction to brain fog, fatigue, and reduced willpower, sugar can rob you of energy, attention, and focus, making it challenging to hear your inner voice. As you begin to eat foods that work for your body, you will get even more clear messages from your intuition.

— **Fear.** One type of fear is worrying that once you start listening, there will be so much emotion that it be too much for you to take. We have never seen this to be the case in all of our work with clients and students. Instead, what we see is that when you look inside with love, your body responds to that love. In his book *Change Your Thoughts—Change Your Life: Living the Wisdom of the Tao,* Dr. Wayne Dyer said: "I know that we humans are like the rest of the natural world and that sadness, fear, frustration, or any troubling feeling cannot last. Nature doesn't create a storm that never ends. Within misfortune, good fortune hides."

Another type of fear is that you might not like the answer because it could mean you have to overhaul your life in ways that make you uncomfortable (such as leaving a bad marriage). Even if something feels scary for you, it's important to remember that your inner guidance wants what is in your highest good. Typically, if you ignore one signal, another arises and another, getting louder or stronger each time until you listen. If you become aware of a step you're afraid to take, consider working with a practitioner or seeking support from a friend who can be there for you. Ignoring your inner voice won't make it go away. Listening, on the other hand, can put you on a more glorious path.

Yet another type of fear is when something happens that makes you question following your inner voice. Perhaps your inner guidance told you to talk to someone and they were rude to you, or told you to eat a certain way and you began to gain weight. Or maybe you followed your intuition about a business deal and it fell through. What we see oftentimes is that these results occur when you still have a lot of doubt. It's almost like you're on the fence. You trust your inner guidance, but a big part of you (maybe in the back of your mind) doesn't believe it will work. Life has a way of showing us what we believe. So if you follow your inner guidance and things go wrong, there are two possibilities: (1) that the "wrong" result is actually a blessing in disguise that is setting the wheels in motion for the right thing to show up, or (2) you still have doubt, and Life wants you to examine that doubt so you can learn to trust more.

No matter which situation you are in, you are being offered an opportunity to listen again. Ask yourself if you have doubt. If you don't, practice trusting (or being open to trusting) that Life has an important plan for you and it's all working out for your greatest good. This is the perfect time to say one of Louise's favorite affirmations: *All is well. Everything is working out for my highest good. Out of this situation, only good will come. I am safe.* Louise says that she has said this affirmation hundreds of times on some days, and it's always helped her trust Life.

As long as you don't judge the current situation too quickly, you may find that there are great lessons and blessings for you there.

— **Negative media programming.** This can include ads on television or the radio, in magazines, or online; or it could be movies, books, TV shows, gaming, or any type of experience that serves to separate you from love. In particular, we recommend that you reduce or avoid media that makes you feel like you are not good enough or programs that have a great deal of violence, mean behavior, or other negativity that leaves you feeling sad or unsafe. One way to assess this is to check in with your inner body and just see how you are feeling, then check in again after engaging with an ad, TV show, movie, game, or other media. Notice how you feel. If you feel bad, sad, or like the world is a terrible place, we recommend you choose something that contributes to feeling good instead. What you focus on continues to grow—so if you focus on media programming that makes you feel bad, you'll continue to reinforce those messages in your life.

— **The discovery that the result isn't perfect.** Perhaps you didn't get the exact result you wanted when you followed your intuition. You may automatically think that it's faulty, but this could not be further from the truth! Life brings you things in the right time and space.

For example, Heather's client Beth was offered a job with a salary lower than what she wanted. While it required Beth and her family to move across the country and her husband to relocate his business, Beth's inner voice said to take it anyway. Within two months, her boss felt she was doing such a good job that she gave her a raise. While the salary was still not exactly what Beth wanted, she realized how great she felt being so valued in the new company. She loved the work and colleagues, and she had better work/life balance. Had she questioned her intuition and focused only on salary, she feels she would have missed out on her dream job.

— **Concern that others don't see visible results.** Sometimes when you're following your intuition, you may question it because the results aren't visible. This happened with Heather's client Jordan. Jordan's wife died when he was in his late 20s, and his grief caused him to question everything in his life. He began to listen to his inner voice and realized that he was not doing work he loved. While in the grieving process, he left his job and started studying Reiki (a Japanese healing method for relaxation and stress reduction) and taking yoga teacher training. His family and friends began to worry, feeling that he was getting too much into woo-woo practices and not being serious anymore. But over the next two years, Jordan felt happier than he had ever felt before. He missed his wife, but at the same time, he was grateful that he found himself through the process of his grief. He did question why other people didn't notice how much better his life was, though, as they continued to judge him and think he was "doing nothing." The people in his life could only seem to ask him when he was going back to a real job.

Four years after his wife's death, Jordan had a successful business in the healing arts. He had gotten a great deal of media attention for his work and became well known for helping other people overcome grief and loss. He finally realized that, had he listened to everyone else three years earlier rather than sticking to his intuition, he would have given up too early and possibly returned to a corporate lifestyle that didn't work for him.

Sometimes results happen from the inside out. In the wintertime, when we think a tree looks dead, there are actually amazing things happening inside. In a process that even scientists call magical, the cells inside the tree transform so that they can live and thrive through the winter. If we just looked at the tree, we might think nothing was happening and then become surprised in springtime when it blooms again. Like Jordan, if you trust your inner guidance and trust how *you* feel, it doesn't matter what others see on the outside.

— **Worry about disappointing others or "shirking" responsibility.** What if your inner guidance tells you to do something that disappoints someone, or you have to leave in the middle of an important work meeting? Ahlea had this happen to her several years ago. She was working with a client when she got a strong intuitive hit to go home. She had a paying client in the middle of a session—but since Ahlea trusted her intuition, she apologized to her client and went right home. When she arrived, she found that her small dog had gotten into a box of raisins and was eating them. Raisins are toxic to dogs and can cause kidney failure. Ahlea was able to save her dog because she listened to her inner voice. Her client was perfectly fine with being rescheduled, especially given that Ahlea's intuitive gift was one of the big reasons she was working with her!

While we recognize that it could be difficult to decide what to do when your inner voice conflicts with responsibilities you've committed to, we recommend that you learn to love yourself enough to listen and follow your inner guidance anyway. Just as Ahlea did, you'll learn how to talk to people about why you need to renegotiate a commitment. The more comfortable you are with making loving choices for yourself, the easier it will be to renegotiate with others.

— Lack of support from family and friends. It's not uncommon to make changes in your life that your friends and family don't understand. Earlier in the book, we talked about how humans tend to resist change for a variety of reasons. When you change, your spouse, family, or friends may also feel resistant to the changes you are making. They may worry that you're going to change so much that your relationship with them will change, too. Or they may feel jealous or miss the "old you." If you begin to listen to your inner guidance and your friends or family put you down for doing so, recognize that this is their fear—it's about them, not you.

Part of listening to yourself means having the courage to commit to yourself; that is, what *your* heart wants. In the beginning, you may not fully trust your inner guidance, so it is easier to fall off track when family or friends become naysayers. Instead of agreeing with them and abandoning your inner voice, see if you can instead become curious and open to experimentation. Dip your toe in the water. Take a step in the direction of listening to your inner voice and see what happens. Keep in mind that if you have a lot of doubt, you can create a self-fulfilling prophecy. Instead, keep an open mind and have fun experimenting. You can even start by choosing to listen to your inner voice about something that is less important to you so that you don't have a lot at stake, like Louise did with her pendulum at restaurants. The more you see how your intuition guides you, the more you will trust it.

Remember, instead of taking what your friends and family say personally, recognize that naysayers often have their own very personal reasons for not supporting others. These reasons do not have to take you off track for developing a strong inner guidance system.

Exercises for Learning to Listen to Your Body

Psychologists and relationship experts teach people that one of the keys to better relationships is to make sure the other person feels heard. This is because it's more common that people listen to each other through a filter of their own experiences and emotions, without fully hearing the person speaking.[7]

The thing is, no one else can understand you the way you understand yourself. No one lives in your skin and in your experience the way you do. And no one else knows how to love you the way you know how to love yourself. This is why it's very important to listen to your inner voice. You are the only expert on the planet on *you*. On your deepest hopes, dreams, and desires. Since we are most often taught to follow rules and care about others before ourselves, it's very common to not know what we want.

Chances are, you've listened to others for too long. The more you listen to your inner voice, the more you can give yourself the love, kindness, and understanding that only you know you need. The more you commit to giving yourself what you need, the easier it becomes to ask others for it, too.

And the more your needs are met, the more you begin to trust life. This whole process starts with you loving yourself enough to listen. And then loving yourself even more by taking action on what you feel guided to do. Knowing that you have this inner guidance system that you can trust makes it easier to remember that you are loved, protected, and watched over by Life. That is the gift of your intuition.

The exercises below will help you learn how to listen to your body, which is truly the key to trusting yourself and your life.

1. Affirmations

The following affirmations are a great way to let your body know that you are listening. Use these for mirror work and throughout the day:

I listen with love to my body's messages.

My body is a glorious place to live, and it always guides me to my highest good.

I trust my body to guide me.

Life loves me. I am safe trusting my body.

I appreciate my body's wisdom.

I am at peace with my inner guidance. No person, place, or thing has any power over me, for I am the only thinker in my mind.

I know how to love myself.

I am safe. I willingly and lovingly release old concepts and ideas.

I am an open channel for the good to flow in and through me—freely, generously, and joyfully.

I choose the thoughts that glorify my being.

I know what is true for me.

I am a unique individual, and I respect my individuality.

My inner wisdom is my own unique approach to life.

It is safe to listen to my body and my intuition.

Life loves me. My body loves me. I am always guided and protected.

Life supplies everything I need.

I am guided to what is in my highest good in the right time and space.

I nourish myself by taking in new ideas.

I recognize my own true worth.

*The point of power is in the present moment. The more
present I am, the more I tune in to my intuition.*

Hi, body, we can change. I want to hear you—let's be friends. I want to love you.

2. Listening Meditation

There are few things as satisfying as really feeling heard or felt. When our best friend or partner truly listens to us, knows us, gets us, and loves us, it nourishes us on such a deep level.

The following meditation was designed to take you on a journey through your body, deeply listening along the way. In Ahlea's healing practice, she often sees or hears what people's bodies are trying to tell them. The biggest pattern she sees is that people's bodies feel unheard and even frustrated. Think about how you feel when you're in a conversation and feel unheard or shut off—it's not uncommon to feel hurt, angry, or unacknowledged. Your body feels this way when you don't listen to what it wants to tell you.

Remember, listening effectively occurs when a person is in a state of loving nonjudgment. As you listen to yourself in this state, notice how nourishing it feels. There is no need to fix, change, or figure anything out. You are simply being with your body in a state of love.

As you take time to do this meditation, think about what it's like to spend time with a loved one, perhaps your partner, child, or dear friend. If they were having trouble, you'd want to listen to them, support them, and soothe them with a compassionate heart. You deserve to do the same for yourself.

Sit or lie comfortably in a quiet location and turn off any distractions, like your cell phone. Close your eyes and settle into your body, taking deep breaths and letting go of what happened today with each exhale.

Come into the present moment and gently wiggle your hips, making adjustments to relax your body more deeply. Feel yourself relaxing more with every breath.

Now bring your attention to your right baby toe. With all of your attention, focus on your toe and really feel it. Wiggle it a bit to get even more sensation into your toe. Notice how it feels: feel the skin, bones, and muscles.

Move to your left baby toe with the same attention, and then bring your awareness to all of your toes on each foot. Feel the life and energy in your toes and as you wiggle them, feel how responsive they are.

Bring your awareness to both of your feet. Feel the power of your feet and arches, all the bones and muscles, your ankles. As you feel this, thank your feet and toes for all that they do for you. Is there anything they want you to know? Listen for a moment and notice if you get any signals.

Now feel this attention and appreciation move up your ankles and into your legs. Feel the muscles and bones in your calves, shins, knees, and thighs. Feel the warmth and circulation of your blood. Now move your attention to your hips, where your leg bones attach to your pelvis. Take a moment to feel your feet and legs together. Relax them and give them love and gratitude for carrying you through life. Is there anything your legs want to tell you? Listen for any signal that comes.

Move your focus from your legs to your pelvis, lower abdomen, and buttocks. Notice the bones and how they support you. Feel the energy of love surrounding and nourishing this area of your body, bathing your sex organs and nourishing your intestines. Feel the powerful protection from the bones and muscles in your lower body and lower back. You may feel a difference in the energy of the bones, muscles, tissue, and organs. Bathe them in your love and ask them what they want you to know. Remember, you are not here to fix, change, or figure anything out, just to listen with love.

Now bring your attention to your abdominal area, just before your chest. Feel the strong bones of your spinal cord, up the back of your body. Feel the soft tissue, muscle, and digestive organs. Place your hands on your abdomen, near your belly button, and surround it with love, feeling your breath moving your hand up and down. As you touch your abdomen, thank it and feel the warmth of that love spread. Let your body know you are ready to digest life with ease. Ask your abdomen and chest what it wants you to know.

Now bring your hands to your chest and connect to your heart. Feel your heart pumping with love and strength, bathing your body with nourishing blood. Acknowledge your heart with love and ask what it wants you to know.

As you move your attention upward, feel your shoulders, arms, hands, neck, throat, jaw, face, ears, eyes, and right up to the top of your head. Relax this whole area. Relax your shoulders, arms, hands, neck, jaw, and mouth. Relax your scalp, forehead, and ears. Relax your mind. Allow any tightness or burdens to release as you exhale. Bring in love and relaxation as you inhale, and feel it spreading throughout this area of your body. Now ask, "What do you want me to know?"

As you bring your awareness to your whole body, every part, inside and out, tell your body, "I want to know you more. I want to love you more. I am ready to listen. I'm doing my best to listen. It's okay if it takes time. Thank you, body, you are a masterpiece. I know you love me and are always protecting me. I know you know how to heal. Is there anything else you want me to know right now? Thank you, body. I love you, body."

This meditation is a beautiful daily practice that nourishes your whole body with love. Yet you can also do this with just one part of it if you want to go deeply into that area. The more you practice listening, the more your body will share its messages with you. Remember, every story your body has to tell you is part of your love story. Your body always keeps you safe and guides you. Together, you know what true love is, and together, you heal. The more you listen, the more you can nourish yourself lovingly in all ways.

In the next chapter, we will provide a variety of guidelines on how to choose and prepare healthy foods. We will give you some easy and fast options, along with tips for fitting healthy eating into your life. And we will keep reminding you to take time for yourself.

There is something magical that happens when you take time for yourself. You don't lose in other areas of your life—you actually gain. You will find out how much Life loves you and wants you to have a healthy, nurturing, nourishing existence. If you allow it, Life will show you how to do this at your own pace, and how it can be more rewarding than you'd ever expect.

♥ ♥

Chapter 5

Step #5:
Emphasize Food
and Thoughts That
Heal Your Body and Mind

Food is one of the most controversial topics, along with religion and politics, isn't it? Everyone from the government to nutritionists to doctors have been arguing about it for decades. And food trends change so often that it's hard to keep up with what's "good for you" and what isn't.

This book is not about food trends. This book is about honoring nature and natural foods, and then listening to your body to see what works best for you. The one thing that everyone can agree upon is that eating whole foods from nature is one of the healthiest things you can do.

As you have already learned, packaged and fast foods have changed what and how we eat a great deal. We've moved farther and

> "Everything is thoughts and food. If you have good nutrition, it serves your brain. If you start to shift and change the food you eat, then it's easier to grasp on to new, positive thoughts and make better choices in your life. Start with this affirmation: *I love myself, therefore, I lovingly feed my body nourishing foods and beverages and my body lovingly responds with vibrant health and energy.*"
>
> — Louise

farther away from nature, and this has created a disconnection—both a disconnection from what is natural, and a disconnection from one another. In this chapter, we are going to bring you back to connecting with your body, as well as introduce you to some foods to emphasize and avoid for your best health.

Learn from Our Ancestors and Our Bodies

In ancient times, the way people made sure food was okay to eat was through taste and a form of conscious eating. We all know about the little bumps on the tongue called taste buds that signal whether we like a food or not. For our ancestors, though, taste buds were a very important tool for detecting the safety of foods. Plants that have poisonous compounds tend to produce a bitter taste, and since humans have about 30 genes for bitter taste receptors, the taste buds were a great way to identify if a plant was poisonous.[1]

Today, our ability to taste is not as advanced as it was in ancient times. In some cases, this is because our survival is not dependent upon detecting poisons in food, and in other cases, we have simply disconnected from the experience of mindful or conscious eating.

While early humans may have paid attention to their reaction to foods for survival, they were also getting a sense of what worked for them, personally. As they tasted, experimented, and watched for reactions, it's easy to surmise that they'd get a sense for the foods that worked best for their bodies. In this way, they would have a better sense of the foods that would be most energizing and healing for them.

One of the biggest questions we get is: "With all the conflicting nutritional guidelines, how do I know what diet to follow?" This especially comes up when we meet with clients who have autoimmune conditions and other chronic health issues. As you've already learned, your genetics and your gut bacteria make you very different from everyone else when it comes to the ideal nutritional program for you. What we've found, however, is that there are three important things you can do to identify your ideal diet:

1. Seek guidance from experts. You can do this by reading books or doing other research, joining online support groups, or working with a health practitioner who specializes in healing nutritional protocols. We are excited about all of the great health books and websites these days that focus on healing the body with nutrition. However, do keep in mind that experts are sharing guidelines from their own research and experience, which understandably includes generalizations that may not pertain to your specific situation. There is no book or website in the world that can account for all the differences in each unique individual—nevertheless, there are often excellent clues that can point you in the right direction. Social-media groups and forums can also provide a way to discuss unique situations with others who can provide further aha's.

2. Listen to your inner guidance. Your body will give you signs and even put you in situations that allow you to learn how it works best, if only you'll trust it! As you ask your body what it needs and listen for the answers, Life will bring you the signals and situations you need to find out what's best for your health.

Heather remembers that when she first started listening to her body, she was also traveling quite often. She noticed that she felt better when she traveled and started to investigate why. This was when she realized that certain foods she was only eating at home were contributing to her abdominal pain. Once she eliminated those foods, she felt better. She was allowing her digestive system to rest and heal while she worked on the root cause of her abdominal pain. Eventually, she was able to add those foods back in.

One of the easiest ways to listen to your body is to keep a food diary. This tool allows you to write down the foods you're eating, along with any symptoms, emotions, and signals you have that day. Over the course of the next two weeks, you can see a relationship between the food you eat and your energy, moods, and physical symptoms. (You can learn more about keeping a food diary in the exercises at the end of this chapter.)

3. Eat mindfully. This is where you can benefit from the habits of our tribal ancestors. As you eat, make it a sensory experience: Look at the food, smell it, and taste it. Chew it well and feel it in your mouth. Give yourself a chance to sink into every bite with no multitasking. This not only allows you to really taste the food you're eating, but it also allows you to tune in and identify if the food is working for you. Is it truly satisfying you? Go beyond your taste buds and notice if you're experiencing a deep, grounding feeling. Does your body feel nourished and satisfied?

When Heather first recovered from bulimia, she was struck by the difference between whole and processed foods. She recalled eating processed, microwavable mashed potatoes (made with real potatoes, but with chemical additives and microwaved in its plastic container), aware that they had satisfied her taste buds but created no deep level of satisfaction in her body. The constant ravenous hunger in a binge was often her body asking for real, nourishing fuel that the processed food could not provide.

When you're only eating for your taste buds and not listening to your body while eating, you may not even realize the signals your body can give you. Heather was able to successfully stop binge eating because she noticed the signals of physical satisfaction from real food. Once she genuinely listened and identified that feeling, it was easier to choose foods that gave her body that deep fulfillment, and her appetite came back to normal.

Go deep into your body and feel beyond your taste buds. The more you are mindful of the full experience of eating, the more sensuous and deeply satisfying it is. This is one of the greatest ways to reduce binge eating and cravings. Over time, you'll choose foods that your body needs because you will have a new level of rapport with your body.

Everyone needs food. Food is life. We come from food. Vikas Khanna, chef and author of *Return to the Rivers,* described the Dalai Lama as saying, "We are not isolated as humans. We are all connected. And food is one thing which connects us all." From nature to the farmer to the harvest and then the ritual of cooking, there is "a long thread that connects all of us in the universe."[2]

When you reconnect with your body and the experience of nourishing it with natural, whole foods, there is an almost magical thing that happens: you begin to feel more connected to nature and to others.

No-No's: What to Avoid for Your Best Health

If you're ready to achieve better health, there are some foods we invite you to avoid. An easy way to start changing your diet is to eliminate just one of these No-No's and work your way through the list at the pace that works for you.

Before getting into the foods to avoid, we'd like to share some observations with you. First and foremost, food affects behavior—it can ground you and help you feel calm and centered, or it can send you on a roller-coaster ride of symptoms or mood challenges. One of the easiest ways to see this very quickly is with sugar because it absorbs so quickly into the bloodstream.

While studies on sugar and behavior vary, enough scientific evidence has been found to show that sugar adversely affects willpower, decision making, addictions, and cravings. Additionally, researchers have found that rats fed a high-sugar diet show a decreased memory, learning, and ability to process emotions.[3]

Instead of listening to what the researchers say, however, we invite you to listen to your own body. Tracking your food intake, moods/emotions, energy, and physical symptoms is the best way to understand how food affects you personally, so you can be empowered to eat in a way that supports your well-being. It can also be eye-opening to observe people around you as you go through your day. When you're first learning to listen to your own body, it can sometimes seem easier to spot changes in others than in yourself. Have fun with this!

For example, Louise and Heather once went to a Weston A. Price conference where the focus was on healthy, traditional whole foods. There was another event taking place at the convention center, and they both allowed children. Louise suggested that Heather watch the kids at both events to see what she observed. As Heather observed the children at the Weston A. Price event, she noticed that they were relatively quiet, calm, and well behaved; when they were in the seminar rooms, they did not make noise or act out. On the other hand, the kids at the other event were running in circles, screeching loudly, and seemed "wired."

Louise had seen this before at another nutritional seminar, where the children who were eating whole foods and no sugar were quieter and seemed more content. They played, but their play was more focused and less hyper.

Ahlea saw this type of thing firsthand in her own home when her ten-year-old nephew, Christopher, came to visit. Her brother and sister-in-law had been eating a Standard American Diet, which typically contains a lot of sugar. The first thing Ahlea noticed was that Christopher's body emitted a metallic smell as he slept at night, which she recognized as being related to toxins in the body.

Since he was used to eating processed foods and sugar, Christopher was not enthusiastic at first about the healthy whole foods in Ahlea's home, but as he ate meals containing them, he realized he liked the taste. Ahlea gently asked her nephew to notice how he was feeling as he was eating these meals, and after a few days, he told her that he felt a lot better. He confided that the teachers at school felt he had ADHD (attention deficit/hyperactivity disorder) and were recommending drugs to keep him calm and focused. What he realized now was that he felt more calm and focused than he had at home. As Ahlea talked with him, he began to realize the food he ate made a huge difference, which was exciting to him. Perhaps he didn't have ADHD after all!

When Christopher returned home, he ate pretty well for about a week, and then Halloween came. Eating Halloween candy put him on a three-day bender where he felt wound up, hyper, and anxious. He and his parents spoke with Ahlea and realized that the sugar and junk food had contributed to his symptoms. This was a big "aha moment" for the family. They began to focus on whole foods so that Christopher would feel better, and were relieved that he wouldn't have to go on drugs after all.

Most people have no idea how much food is contributing to their well-being or lack thereof. The No-No's that follow consist of foods that contribute to adverse mood, energy, and health symptoms. If you avoid them, like Christopher, you'll start to feel much healthier.

1. Sugar and Other Sweeteners

— **Sugar.** Of the 85,451 unique commercially available foods that were on the market between 2005 and 2009, 75 percent of them contained added sweeteners.[4] Sugar has many names and many forms, and Americans consume too much of it: 156 pounds of sugar per year, according to the U.S. Department of Agriculture (USDA).[5] That is 16 pounds over the 140 pounds of sugar that experts consider a "pharmacologic dose," which causes obesity and disease.

The refined white table sugar that most of us are familiar with is made of sucrose and considered a source of "empty calories." Sucrose is a disaccharide, which means that it's made up of two simple sugar molecules: fructose and glucose. Glucose causes a spike in blood sugar, and if your liver has to process too much fructose, it can cause a buildup of fat. In addition, sugar not only feeds bad bacteria and pathogens in the gut, it also provides no nutrients, while using up valuable nutrients in the digestive process at the same time.[6] In fact, most experts agree that we can achieve better health by reducing or eliminating it altogether.

Dr. Nancy Appleton, author of the classic book *Lick the Sugar Habit,* recently wrote a list of nearly 150 reasons to avoid sugar, and we're including just a few of them here. Sugar[7]:

- Suppresses the immune system and contributes to bacterial infection.
- Can cause hyperactivity, anxiety, irritability, and difficulty concentrating in adults and children.
- Contributes to premature aging, constipation, blood-sugar problems, food allergies, and obesity.
- Can contribute to multiple sclerosis, Alzheimer's disease, alcoholism, cancer, hemorrhoids, periodontal disease, osteoporosis, varicose veins, and diabetes.
- May cause cataracts and weaken vision.
- Can damage organs such as the kidneys, liver, small intestine, and pancreas.

When you're reading labels at the grocery store, look for these additional names for sugar (sucrose): beet sugar, brown sugar, cane sugar, confectioners' sugar, invert sugar, powdered sugar, raw sugar, saccharose, table sugar, and turbinado sugar.[8]

— **High-fructose corn syrup (HFCS).** HFCS is much cheaper than sugar, and is best avoided because it's often found in very nutrient-deficient processed food. Nevertheless, Americans consume about 60 pounds per person per year of it.[9] Note that HFCS is not the same as sugar, nor is it even close to natural, no matter what corn manufacturers would like you to believe. This manufactured food is a blend of fructose and glucose with no chemical bond (sugar does at least have a chemical bond between the fructose and glucose). This means that it absorbs in the body much faster than sugar does, causing insulin spikes and contributing to metabolic issues, obesity, increased appetite, diabetes, heart disease, cancer, energy depletion, inflammation, accelerated aging, and dementia.[10]

— **Artificial sweeteners.** In an America that spends $66.5 billion on the weight-loss industry, it's no surprise that food manufacturers would jump on the bandwagon with calorie-free sweeteners.

The FDA has approved five artificial sweeteners[11]:

- Saccharin (Sugar Twin, Sweet'N Low)
- Acesulfame-K (Sunett, Sweet One, DiabetiSweet)
- Aspartame (AminoSweet, NutraSweet, Equal)
- Neotame (NutraSweet's new and "improved" artificial sweetener)
- Sucralose (Splenda, Nevella, SucraPlus)

Be aware that FDA approval does *not* mean that these sweeteners are good for you! In Chapter 3, you learned exactly why the weight-loss industry does more harm than good, and the same is true for artificial sweeteners. They pretend to save you calories while giving you a sweet taste, but the reality is that they contribute to a whole host of undesirable health issues, such as[12, 13]:

- Increased cravings for sugar, sweets, and carbohydrates
- Weight gain
- Food addiction
- Loss of taste for healthy, natural foods due to overstimulation of sweet-taste receptors
- Decrease in good gut bacteria
- Possible migraine trigger

- Skin rashes

- Mood changes—panic, anxiety, irritability, nervousness

- Bladder issues

- Stomach pain

- Intestinal cramps

- Diarrhea

- Swelling

- Accumulation of formaldehyde in the brain (attributed to aspartame)

- Multiple sclerosis

- Fibromyalgia

- Lupus

- Dizziness

- Pregnancy complications

The main thing to keep in mind with artificial sweeteners is that they are chemicals that the body does not understand, which can lead to adverse effects on your health and your moods. These sweeteners are designed to trick the body, and good health is not about tricking the body. A positive relationship with your body means that it works in harmony with you to feel your best. It's about balance. Your appetite does not need to be fooled to keep you slim and healthy.

Remember, if your health is your greatest love story, it's not about deceit and manipulation—what relationship has ever been safe, calm, happy, and healthy under those conditions? A good relationship with your body is the same as a good relationship with a loved one: when you nourish it and meet its needs, everything falls into place. Loving your body is about meetings its nutritional needs. Once you do this, everything will fall into place. From your brain to your taste buds to your body, everything will be in harmony. This is how you create and sustain a naturally slim, healthy body.

2. Excitotoxins

Excitotoxins are molecules that are so stimulating to the nervous system that they can excite neurons to death. In his book *Excitotoxins: The Taste That Kills,*

Dr. Russell L. Blaylock outlines how they contribute to health problems such as hormone imbalance, obesity, amyotrophic lateral sclerosis (ALS, or Lou Gehrig's disease), Parkinson's disease, Alzheimer's disease, free radical damage, and inflammation.[14]

Examples of extitotoxins found abundantly in our food supply are glutamate, aspartate, and cysteine. The following two are increasingly used in foods, however, so we wanted to highlight them:

— **Monosodium glutamate (MSG).** While MSG is often linked to Chinese food, this excitotoxin is added to many processed foods, such as chips, packaged meals, and soups. It is often disguised with the following terms: *natural flavoring, spices, vegetable protein, hydrolyzed vegetable protein, soy protein isolate, glutamic acid, enzymes, protein fortified,* and *yeast extract.*[15] MSG is even used in some high-end restaurants because it excites the taste buds and makes food taste better. Even so, many people notice that they don't feel well after eating foods with MSG.

— **Aspartame.** In addition to being an artificial sweetener, aspartame is also an excitotoxin, giving you more reason to avoid it altogether.

3. Genetically Modified Organisms (GMOs)

GMOs are plants or animals that have been genetically altered with DNA from other plants, animals, bacteria, or viruses.[16] Scientists are on both sides of the fence as to whether GMOs are safe for the planet or not, and there are many issues embedded in the GMO controversy. Let's start with genetically engineered seeds.

In 1980, the U.S. Supreme Court ruled that genetically engineered life-forms could be patented.[17] Keep in mind that when something can be patented, companies can use it to create and control products on the market. This brings us to Monsanto, the foremost producer of genetically modified crops. It makes Roundup Ready seeds, which are genetically modified to withstand the use of Roundup, a wildly popular broad-spectrum chemical herbicide mostly made up of glyphosate.[18]

Since the beginning of farming, farmers have been saving seeds from past crops to plant new crops the following year. Now that companies like Monsanto have patented genetically engineered seeds, however, they can stop farmers from saving seeds. Instead, farmers have to purchase new seeds each year from Monsanto, removing their ability to work with nature as they always have.

In addition, as is nature's way, the wind pollinates plants. This means that farmers who choose not to grow GMO plants are at the mercy of the wind pollinating their non-GMO crops, resulting in an unintended genetically modified crop. Organic farmers and health-conscious scientists and consumers are very concerned that cross-pollination will result in genetic contamination and the end of organic food options.

Are GMO foods dangerous to the planet and our health? Amidst much controversy, studies are showing that GMO foods are not living up to their promise of higher crop yields and are in fact showing adverse effects. In addition[19]:

- There is concern about genetic changes producing toxic or allergenic properties in food—toxins from GMO corn has been found in the blood of pregnant women and their babies.

- Crop contamination—studies found that GMO corn has contaminated indigenous non-GMO corn in Mexico.

- Other living things may be harmed—the larvae of some monarch butterflies have been destroyed by GMO corn.

- While GMOs promised to boost the food supply by creating pest-resistant plants, there is no evidence of increased crop yield. Instead, an unintended consequence has emerged: the growth of herbicide-resistant pests, causing concern about infestation by a new breed of superbugs.

- Twenty-six countries have either fully or partially banned GMOs, including: Switzerland, Australia, Austria, China, India, France, Germany, Hungary, Luxembourg, Greece, Bulgaria, Poland, Italy, Mexico, and Russia. Additionally, about 60 other countries have some form of GMO restrictions.

- These foods are the most likely to be GMO (unless they are organic): corn, canola, cottonseed, papaya, soybeans, and sugar beets.

We are lovers of nature and believe that when you support it, it comes into balance; when you go away from nature, there are unintended consequences. For this reason, we feel that GMO foods and Monsanto's practices are bordering on the criminal and we urge you to avoid them. While there is no law to force food manufacturers to label GMO food, you can look for non-GMO labels on prepared and packaged health foods and choose organic whenever possible.

You can get a shopping guide and learn more about how to choose wisely at the Non-GMO Shopping Guide website: NonGMOShoppingGuide.com.

Pesticides: Are They Really Necessary?

Nature is amazing. It is phenomenal at creating balance, if only we would trust it and learn its wisdom. In Chapter 3, you learned how the food industry has inserted modern machinery and chemicals into the food supply, often resulting in food that is lower in nutrients.

The same has happened over thousands of years of farming. The fruit and vegetables our ancestors grew was lower in starch and sugar and higher in phyto-nutrients (which are important chemicals that we will describe in the next section). However, over time, farming practices have favored sweeter, starchier fruits and vegetables—and a focus on breeding them has resulted in produce that is lower in nutrients. In other words, it takes more food to give us the nutrition we need than it did for our ancestors.

Louise and Heather visited Cowhorn, a biodynamic vineyard near Ashland, Oregon, years ago. Biodynamic farming practices go way beyond organic and use no pesticides or toxic chemical methods to produce their wine. The farmers at Cowhorn explained that they cut the weeds in the fields and use them to fertilize the vines.

This lost art of using weeds is actually quite smart: For hundreds of years, weeds such as dandelions have been used for their medicinal value. In addition, weeds have a special ability to pull in concentrated minerals from the soil, which makes them excellent sources for fertilizer![20] This native fertilizer is extra special because the plants all live in harmony in the same land. Organic gardeners and permaculture enthusiasts often make weed teas as a mineral-rich compost in their own home gardens.

The Cowhorn farmers found that as they honored nature with their biodynamic farming practices, the end result of their wine-making process yielded what they call "happy yeast." In their research at other conventional wineries, they noticed that the yeast had an unpleasant odor and the final product had to be doctored up in order to make the wine palatable for bottling; that is, the sick yeast had to be fixed up in final production.

At this biodynamic farm, the yeast didn't need doctoring because it was happy and healthy right from the start. Customers with wine sensitivities told them that they could drink Cowhorn wine without any allergic reaction.

Phytonutrients: Nature's Secret Nutrient-Packed Natural Protector

In her book *Eating on the Wild Side,* author Jo Robinson explains that phytonutrients are nature's nutrient-packed plant protector. Phytonutrients are antioxidants, which nourish the body and scavenge the free radicals that can cause cell damage and aging. So phytonutrients help protect and keep us alive, and they do the same for the plant!

Phytonutrients protect plants from insects and disease. When plants are sprayed with pesticides—or genetically engineered to be "pesticide ready," as Monsanto does—their need to create phytonutrients to protect themselves has been eliminated. What's left are plants lower in phytonutrients and higher in toxins from the pesticide.

Modern practices sometimes get so enamored with science that they forget nature. Yet when human beings turn away from nature, we lose the ability to benefit from the already-encoded balance it provides. Imagine the result if we honored nature in our modern practices—what seems to take more time and effort up front would lead to faster, higher-quality results in the end, just like Cowhorn winery's happy yeast. Honoring nature can lead to a happier, healthier planet, as well as happier, healthier people.

Now, the good news is you can still find plants that are richer in phytonutrients. Here are some examples of great high-antioxidant choices[21]:

- Arugula

- Dandelion

- Green onions

- Lettuce—be sure to choose really green lettuce (not iceberg!) like romaine and any lettuce that is tinged red (such as red leaf lettuce)

- Kale

- Black, red, and dark red grapes

- Blueberries

- Artichokes

- Parsley

- Herbs and spices (see more on these in the Yes-Yes section of this chapter)

4. Gluten

Gluten, a protein found in grains like wheat, rye, barley, and oats, is difficult for the small intestine to digest and can cause autoimmune responses in some people. About 1 in 133 Americans have celiac disease, an autoimmune digestive disease in which gluten damages the villi of the small intestine, and which can include over 300 symptoms.[22] Additionally, the National Institutes of Health estimate that up to 10 percent of people may suffer from gluten intolerance.

Symptoms of gluten intolerance include[23]:

- Acid reflux
- Brain fog
- Chronic fatigue
- Depression
- Gas, bloating, constipation, diarrhea, or IBS
- Headaches or migraines
- Joint aches and pains
- Skin conditions, like eczema and acne

According to Dr. Natasha Campbell-McBride, author of *Gut and Psychology Syndrome,* improperly digested gluten can turn into substances that act like opiates in the body, causing a reaction similar to heroin and blocking parts of the brain.[24] This is particularly an issue for people with a damaged digestive tract or conditions like schizophrenia, autism, postpartum depression, epilepsy, Down syndrome, and some autoimmune issues, according to Campbell-McBride.

A great way to identify if gluten is a problem for you is to eliminate it from your diet for two weeks and see if you feel better. Many people find it challenging to remove gluten because it's in so many foods today, like bread, crackers, and cereal. However, most of these ready-made foods create nutritional challenges, so if you are experiencing chronic symptoms, it is worth doing an elimination diet for a period of time. Often, once your symptoms resolve and your gut heals, you can add them back in. (We will provide options for you to replace bread and other grains in Chapter 10.)

Bread: The Staff of Life?

Bread is often referred to as the "staff of life" because historically it has been an on-the-go, inexpensive staple for warding off hunger. However, the bread of our ancestors was very different from the prepared bread we eat today.

First, the wheat of yesterday has evolved to a very different species in our modern times. In the quest to make dough rise for a fluffier, longer-lasting loaf, wheat was bred over the years to have more gluten and gliadins and fewer minerals.[25]

Furthermore, over time the milling and processing of grains continued to remove important nutrients in the flour. And because wheat had a brown color that people disliked, bleach (which is not friendly to the good bacteria in your gut!) was used in countries like the U.S. to give it a pleasing white color. These practices alone reduced the overall nutrition and healthfulness of bread.

To add insult to digestive injury, the preparation of bread has changed dramatically as well. Our ancestors fermented the flour (much like a sourdough process), which predigested the grains, broke down the difficult-to-digest antinutrients, and added healthy bacteria. These days, this step is skipped, making bread more difficult for the digestive system, especially if the gut is damaged in some way, which is very common today.

While many people are opting to remove bread (at least bread containing gluten) from their diets as they heal from chronic health conditions, you could consider exploring organic, gluten-free sourdough. Bread prepared properly and eaten sparingly can be a nice treat, and you can learn to prepare sourdough bread at home or find a baker who uses traditional methods.

Many artisanal bread makers are emerging today to meet consumer demand—look for one who uses organic, gluten-free grains and sprouted flour for the easiest-to-digest bread.

5. Trans Fats, Olestra, and Refined Fats and Oils

You can think of trans fats and olestra as artificial fats—in essence, just as dastardly as artificial sweeteners.

Olestra is a fat substitute introduced during the "fat free" craze that was later found to cause gastrointestinal upset, loose bowels, and nutrient deficiencies. A 2010 article in *Time* magazine called olestra one of "The 50 Worst Inventions."[26] It was banned in Europe and Canada, but is still used in the U.S.

Trans fats, also called partially hydrogenated fats and trans-fatty acids, were introduced into manufactured foods to make oils more solid at room temperature, increase shelf life, and improve other product characteristics.[27] Dr. Mary Enig, a nutritional biochemist and expert on fats, has reported that they contribute to cancer, challenges with hunger and satiety (cravings), and obesity.[28]

Examples of trans fats are: margarine, vegetable shortening (like Crisco), and anything with the terms *hydrogenated* or *partially hydrogenated* in the label. Often this includes foods such as: French fries, pie crusts, pancake and cake mixes, battered and fried foods, cookies, ice cream, nondairy creamers, microwave popcorn, biscuits, and pizza dough.

Be aware that food-labeling laws allow companies to say "0 trans fats" on any food with less than 0.5 grams of trans fat per serving. Since food manufacturers can manipulate the number of "servings" in a package, they can hide trans fats this way.[29] The more you avoid processed foods, the more you will avoid trans fats.

We recommend that you avoid refined fats and oils as well. Refined oils have been heated and treated, creating dangerous free radicals and removing antioxidants. They also have toxic preservatives like BHA and BHT (see the "Processed Food and Food Additives" section later in the chapter) added in to keep them from going rancid.[30]

Another oil to avoid is canola oil. Nutrition experts Sally Fallon and Dr. Mary Enig wrote an article called "The Great Con-ola," in which they explained that this much-used oil is not as healthy as we've been led to believe. Canola oil is derived from the genetically engineered rapeseed, which has toxic properties (such as erucic acid, hemagglutinins, and cyanide-containing glycocides) known to cause: mad cow disease, blindness, nervous disorders, clumping of blood cells, and depression of the immune system.[31]

As you learned in Chapter 3, healthy, unrefined fats and oils have the ability to lift your mood and satisfy your body, thereby reducing cravings and satiating your appetite. We will talk about some wonderful fats and oils in the Yes-Yes section of this chapter.

6. Soy

Soy was once so widely touted as a health food that it ended up in just about every processed snack food, protein bar, and packaged health food that you can imagine.

Soy is one of the most highly genetically modified crops after corn, so if you do eat it, be sure that it's organic or non-GMO. Second of all, it's important to know that soy is high in phytoestrogens, so it can mimic estrogen in the body and reduce testosterone.[32]

Soy also contains some antinutrients like protease inhibitors, goitrogens, phytates, and lectins, which may interfere with your digestion, inhibit the thyroid, and steal minerals from your body.[33] These properties can be significantly reduced if you ferment the soy, which tends to make it easier on your digestive system and much healthier.

- *Examples of unfermented soy foods are:* tofu, edamame, soy nuts, soy milk, soy lecithin, and many vegetarian meat and cheese substitutes.

- *Examples of fermented soy foods are:* soy sauce, tamari, tempeh, natto, and miso.

We have included soy in the No-No's section because we feel that there are some very good reasons to limit or avoid unfermented soy. As the debate about the pros and cons of soy rages on in the health industry, we invite you to listen to your own inner guidance, and if you do eat soy, listen to your body. Trust that your body loves you and will always guide you to what works best for your specific needs.

7. Factory-Farmed Animal Protein (Meat, Poultry, Eggs, and Dairy)

While we'd like to think that any animal we eat was well treated, had plenty of room to roam the land, and ate its native diet, this couldn't be further from the truth when it comes to conventional animal protein from factory farms.

It's not surprising that many kindhearted people choose to become vegetarian or vegan because of the cruel and inhumane practices that happen on factory farms. Animals are crowded together so that they can't move properly, they don't get much time outside (if any at all), and they eat cheap feed that is not their native diet. Just like when we eat chemically altered food of low to no nutritional quality, animals fed this way develop health problems.

Let's take factory-farmed cows, for example. They eat grass for the first six months of their lives while nursing and then are fed GMO corn and grain, which their digestive systems are not designed to deal with (they're supposed to eat grass).[34] The result is a cow that gets very fat, very fast. To speed their growth, they are often injected with hormones. And because these cows are jammed together indoors with the wrong diet, they sometimes develop diseases and need antibiotics. Just imagine what that means when humans eat this meat from hormone- and antibiotic-injected, unhealthy animals. It doesn't take a scientist to recognize that eating the meat of unhealthy animals does not do much good for us. Yet most people do not realize that conventional animal protein—red meat, poultry, eggs, or dairy—from animals who are not treated or fed well can contribute to adverse health effects.

In the book *Heat* by Bill Buford, we learn from award-winning chefs and butchers just how different the meat of grain- and corn-fed cows is: "They eat *mush*. They taste of *mush* . . . the meat behaves like *mush*: it disintegrates in days."[35]

While some people have become used to eating grain- and corn-fed animals and claim that they prefer the taste, we invite you to learn to work with organic and pasture/grass-fed and finished meats and poultry instead. Choose farmers who treat their animals well and allow them to roam free, eating their native diets. This ensures a better quality of animal protein that passes its good health on to you!

A Special Note about Dairy

Depending on the source, it's estimated that up to 90 percent of people have trouble digesting dairy products because of the inability to digest lactose, the main sugar found in milk.[36] Because lactose intolerance (due to absence of the lactase enzyme in the gut) is so pervasive, scientists feel that it's not a disease, but is in fact quite normal. They say that it's actually abnormal for people to tolerate milk as adults, and those who can likely have a gene mutation called "lactase persistence."[37]

Additionally, many people are allergic to milk and dairy products because of allergies to the two main proteins: casein and whey. Whether due to an allergy or intolerance to lactose, casein, or whey, symptoms could include: lethargy, brain fog, itchy rashes, hives, acne, abdominal pain and cramping, cravings, nervousness, swelling, trouble swallowing, and trouble concentrating.[38]

Removing dairy foods such as milk and cheese from your diet is recommended by many nutritional experts; Ahlea and Heather have both recommended this to their clients with excellent results. In particular, children with autism, ADD/ADHD, and other gut- or mood-related disorders tend to improve when dairy is removed.

The one exception is raw, organic butter or ghee (clarified butter) from pasture-fed cows because it contains virtually no lactose or casein.[39] Additionally, some people do well with homemade yogurt or dairy kefir made with raw, organic, and grass-fed dairy. These days, you can find raw, organic, pasture-fed cheese at health-food stores. If you want to experiment with raw milk, you can find out more by going to the Campaign for Real Milk website at: RealMilk.com.

What about Vegetarian or Vegan Cheese?

We have not found any fake cheeses that have truly healthy ingredients. Most have soy, canola oil, or some other refined oil (see more in the "Trans Fats, Olestra, and Refined Fats and Oils" section earlier in the chapter), annatto, and natural flavors or yeast/brewer's yeast, which could be sources of excitotoxins.

Remember, it's important to listen to your body when it comes to the food you eat. This is especially true for dairy or dairy substitutes.

8. Farmed Fish

Another food controversy is farmed fish versus wild fish. Wild fish swim in the open, eating their natural diets (like algae, seaweed, other fish, and so on), which their bodies can metabolize. Farmed fish typically eat a non-native diet, which can include GMO corn, soy, and canola; and are exposed to antibiotics, hormones, neurotoxins, pesticides, and other toxins.[40]

One thing to keep in mind is that wild-caught fish can be contaminated by mercury, radiation, and other toxins in the water. In general, cold-water fish and smaller species, like sardines, may have fewer toxins.

Sustainability is an issue when it comes to choosing fish because many popular species are overfished and in danger of becoming extinct. While fishing practices and options can change over time, here are some guidelines as of the writing of this book[41]:

- *Some examples of overfished species are:* Atlantic salmon, grouper, Chilean sea bass, and bluefin tuna.

- *Examples of more sustainable fish are:* Atlantic bluefish, Pacific halibut, herring, sardines, Pacific albacore and yellowfin (ahi) tuna, and Alaskan salmon.

The fish industry is looking for ways to improve sustainability and farming methods, so it's useful to stay aware of fishing practices as they evolve. Many health-food stores with seafood departments can guide you to the best choices.

9. Processed Food and Food Additives

Foods that come in boxes, cans, and packages are processed, which means that something has been done to alter their natural form and get them ready for a longer shelf life. In addition, processed foods contain fewer nutrients, more sugar, and toxic food additives.

We are grateful that more companies are creating healthy, organic versions of processed foods today that do not contain toxic chemicals. However, there are still too many products on the market that have no nutritional value.

Keep in mind that food manufacturers aim to make a profit, and one of the ways they do so is to get you to eat more food. They hire food scientists to identify the precise balance of sugar, salt, and fat that will make you want to eat more.[42] In essence, these foods are designed to keep you in a state of craving. If you want to reduce cravings, stop eating processed foods and eat whole foods instead. Once you do, your body will come back into balance and you can start to trust your body's natural cravings.

While this is not an exhaustive list, we wanted you to have examples of some of the most prevalent food additives to avoid:

— **Food dyes.** Found in foods like fruit cocktail, pickles, chips, candy, maraschino cherries, American cheese, sports drinks, and pet food, these dyes are being found to contribute to cancer, as well as to ADHD and other behavioral issues. A 2007 British study found that six dyes, called the "Southampton Six," created hyperactivity in children: Red #40, Yellow #5, Yellow #6, Carmoisine (red color in jellies), Quinoline yellow, and Ponceau 4R (red coloring).[43]

Over the years, many food dyes have been introduced and then banned when adverse health effects occur, yet we still have food dyes on the market today. A recent study found that these dyes can enter the bloodstream through the skin or gastrointestinal tract, which was surprising to many scientists who thought the dyes would be blocked by the sun or destroyed in the digestive tract before being absorbed.[44] We recommend that you avoid all food dyes.

— **Sulfites.** Used to preserve food and prevent browning, sulfites can be found in wine, beer, dried fruit, and pharmaceutical medications. They have been linked to a variety of allergy symptoms that affect the lungs, skin, gut, and heart, such as asthma, rashes, and abdominal pain.[45]

Ingredients to watch for include[46]:

- Potassium bisulfite
- Potassium metabisulfite
- Sodium bisulfite
- Sodium metabisulfite
- Sodium sulfite
- Sulfur dioxide

— **Butylated hydroxyanisole (BHA) and butylated hydroxytoluene (BHT).** These compounds are used to preserve fats and have been linked to cancer and behavioral changes.[47]

— **Potassium bromate.** This is used in breads and flour products, and animal studies showing a link to cancer have led to bans in the European Union, Canada, and Brazil, but not in the United States.[48] Avoid this ingredient when looking for bread and flour products.

— **Azodicarbonamide (ADA).** Used as a chemical foaming agent in the plastics industry, this toxin is making its way into bread products at fast-food chains such as Subway, Wendy's, Starbucks, McDonald's, Burger King, and Arby's; and in bread products made by manufacturers such as Ball Park, Healthy Life, Jimmy Dean, Sara Lee, Little Debbie, and Wonder. You can go to the Environmental Working Group's website to learn more: EWG.org.

— **Brominated vegetable oil (BVO).** Used to stabilize citrus flavoring, BVO is often used in sodas and soft drinks like Fanta, Mountain Dew, and Gatorade. While safety issues got it banned in Europe and Japan, the United States FDA is allowing it to be used while more research is conducted.[49]

Read Those Labels! Here's What to Avoid at the Grocery Store

Sweeteners[50, 51]

- Acesulfame-K (Sunette, Sweet One, DiabetiSweet)
- Agave nectar—this is deceptive because it's sold in health-food stores, but it often has more fructose than high-fructose corn syrup[52]
- Aspartame (AminoSweet, NutraSweet, Equal)—also an excitotoxin
- Barley malt or malted barley— these may contain glutamic acid, an excitotoxin[53]
- Beet sugar
- Brown rice syrup or rice syrup— suspected of containing free glutamic acid, making it a possible excitotoxin for highly sensitive people
- Brown sugar
- Cane sugar
- Confectioners' sugar
- Corn syrup
- Dextrose
- Fructose
- Glucose
- High-fructose corn syrup (HCFS)
- Invert sugar
- Isomalt
- Lactitol
- Lactose
- Levulose
- Malt extract

- Maltitol
- Maltodextrin
- Maltose
- Mannitol
- Milk sugar
- Neotame (NutraSweet's new and "improved" artificial sweetener)
- Oligodextrin
- Powdered sugar
- Raw sugar
- Saccharin (Sugar Twin, Sweet'N Low)
- Saccharose
- Sorbitol
- Sucralose (Splenda, Nevella, SucraPlus)
- Sucrose
- Sugar
- Table sugar
- Turbinado sugar

Excitotoxins[54]

- Annatto—could produce a reaction in highly sensitive people
- Autolyzed yeast
- Bouillon or broth
- Brewer's yeast—may contain glutamate, or glutamate may be used in processing
- Carrageenan
- Citric acid
- Cornstarch—could trigger a reaction in highly sensitive people

- Fermented protein foods
- *Flavors* or *flavoring*—beware of words like this on labels, particularly if there is no indication of what the flavors or flavoring are, because they're often hidden chemicals
- Hydrolyzed protein—or anything hydrolyzed, for that matter
- Modified food starch
- Monosodium glutamate (MSG)—or anything with the word *glutamate,* like *potassium glutamate, natrium glutamate, glutamic acid,* and so forth
- Natural flavoring (including natural beef or chicken flavoring)
- Plant protein extract
- Protein concentrate
- *Seasonings*—when you see this word, it can mean that MSG or other chemicals are hidden
- Soy isolate
- Soy protein
- Soy sauce or soy sauce extract
- *Spices*—while natural herbs and spices are wonderful, beware if you only see the word *spices* with no identification about which spice it is because it could be MSG
- Stock
- Textured protein
- Vegetable gum
- Whey protein concentrate
- Whey protein isolate

- White vinegar—could produce a reaction in highly sensitive people

Gluten grains[55]

- Barley (and barley malt or barley extract)
- Beer
- Brown rice syrup
- Couscous
- Croutons (unless gluten-free)
- Durum
- Farina
- Faro
- Gluten
- Kamut
- Malt
- Matzo flour/meal
- Oats (unless labeled gluten-free)
- Orzo
- Panko
- Rye
- Seitan
- Semolina
- Spelt
- Thickeners
- Triticale
- Udon
- Wheat (including wheat bran, wheat germ, and wheat starch)

Other

- Azodicarbonamide (ADA)
- Brominated vegetable oil (BVO)

- Butylated hydroxyanisole (BHA)
- Butylated hydroxytoluene (BHT)
- Dairy (except for organic, raw, and grass-fed butter or ghee— if you can tolerate dairy, choose organic, raw, and grass-fed)
- Enriched foods
- Food dyes (look for a color and number, like Red #40, Yellow #6, Blue #1, and the like)
- Potassium bisulfite
- Potassium bromate
- Potassium metabisulfite
- Sodium bisulfite
- Sodium metabisulfite
- Sodium sulfite
- Sulfites
- Sulfur dioxide
- Ultrapasteurized (a process also known as ultra-heat treatment, or UHT)
- Wheat (gluten)

Fats and Oils—avoid fats and oils that are refined, hydrogenated, partially hydrogenated, or trans fats, such as:

- Canola oil
- Corn oil
- Cottonseed oil
- Fried foods or processed foods cooked in refined or hydrogenated oils heated to high temperatures
- Margarine
- Peanut oil
- Rice bran oil
- Safflower oil
- Salad dressings—most have low-quality fats, so see the "Unrefined Fats and Oils" section later in this chapter to learn more
- Shortening (Crisco)
- Soy oil
- Vegetable oil
- Vegetable shortening

Yes-Yes: Foods to Emphasize for Your Best Health

Now that you know what to avoid, here's the exciting part: what to eat to love your body to good health!

1. Whole Foods

Instead of processed foods, choose whole foods. Whole foods are fresh and mostly located in the outer aisles of the grocery store: the produce aisle, the fish and meat counters, and the refrigerated areas with eggs and butter. In the center aisles, you can look for products that have been minimally processed, like coconut flour;

raw, unfiltered apple cider vinegar (which we like better than white vinegar); and unrefined fats and oils.

There are more healthy packaged foods being manufactured today that are organic, non-GMO, and minimally processed. While we recommend home-prepared foods, healthier packaged foods can be better options than the highly processed conventional foods on the market today. Your local health-food store, food co-op, or farmers' market is likely to have more great options for healthier foods than many conventional grocery stores do.

The most important thing you can do when considering any packaged foods (even those from your health-food store) is to read labels and look for *organic* whenever possible. Do watch out for health claims on packages, too. Just because an item claims to be "gluten-free," have "0 trans fats," or be "fair trade" does not mean it is healthy. Always read labels and use the "What to Avoid" list from earlier in the chapter to make grocery shopping easier.

What about Grains, Meat, and Vegetarianism?

We are not proponents of the complete removal of any category of whole foods, unless you are working on a certain aspect of your health that requires it. In this respect, we agree with Hippocrates, "the father of medicine," who said: "Let food be thy medicine, and medicine be thy food."

Each decade, a new food is vilified as "bad for you." At some point, one can pick apart every food and find something that is "bad," until eventually nothing seems safe for eating. However, nature loves us and provides for us—food that grows has a wide range of nutrients delivered in a way our bodies can understand.

Now, certain health conditions may be best served by a grain-free diet, a vegetarian or vegan diet, a raw-food diet, or some other nutritional plan. And because health is dynamic, you may reintroduce those foods successfully and be on to the next phase in using your food as your medicine.

Your body will always guide you when it's time to adjust your diet. When in doubt, work with a health practitioner or nutritionist who understands the digestive tract and how food impacts health. If you follow other people's rules without listening to your body, you're telling yourself that you don't matter. Remember, what your body needs matters. We have clients who were vegetarians for ethical reasons who knew in the back of their minds that their bodies needed meat, or at the very least, supplementation of vitamin B_{12} and other nutrients missing from their bodies. When they finally listened, they began to heal rapidly.

Dr. Natasha Campbell-McBride, author of *Gut and Psychology Syndrome,* teaches that vegetables help cleanse the body and animal protein helps build it. If you use food as your medicine, you may find that addressing whether your body needs to cleanse (break down toxins) or build (strengthen) is an important consideration for your health.

For those who choose to eat animal protein, it is definitely possible to pick ethical sources. You can select meat, poultry, and eggs from farmers who raise their animals humanely and allow them to roam free, eating their native diets.

While all three of us have gone through vegetarian and raw-food stages in our lives, we do eat animal protein as a side dish for our mostly vegetables diet. After much experimentation and listening deeply, we have personally found that meat has helped build and strengthen our bodies.

We are not here to tell you to go vegetarian, vegan, Paleo, Primal, grain-free, or raw. Instead, we invite you to listen deeply to your own body and find what works for you. Rigid rules and dogma mean nothing to the body; they are only food for the mind. Be willing to explore what *your* body needs to heal.

2. More Vegetables

Just about every food expert would agree that we can all benefit from a diet rich in vegetables. Eating all the colors of the rainbow supports the body, and if you're focusing on healing, eating more dark, leafy greens is a great place to start. Here are some examples for eating a variety of colors of vegetables:

- **Red**—beets, red leaf lettuce, radishes, red Swiss chard, red onions, tomatoes, and red bell peppers. (Note that tomatoes and red bell peppers are in the family of nightshades, which are not well tolerated by everyone. If you experience digestive pain, reflux, tremors, or joint pain, you may want to avoid or eliminate these and reintroduce them after two weeks to see if you're sensitive to them.)

- **Orange**—carrots, pumpkin, sweet potatoes, and butternut squash.

- **Yellow**—summer squash, yellow onions, and corn. (Many people have corn allergies or sensitivities, so make sure you can tolerate corn and that you choose organic to avoid GMO corn.)

- **Green**—lettuce and leafy greens (romaine, green leaf lettuce, red leaf lettuce, cabbage, arugula, kale, collards, bok choy, Swiss chard, dandelion, watercress, and spinach), artichokes, broccoli, brussels sprouts, snow peas, snap peas, green beans, watercress, spinach, escarole, cucumbers, chayote squash, zucchini, sprouts, and microgreens; as well as fresh herbs such as parsley, cilantro, basil, and fennel.

- **Blue/purple**—radicchio, shallots, turnips, and eggplant. (Eggplant is a nightshade, so please see the previous note about tomatoes and red bell peppers.)

- **White**—cauliflower, garlic, white onions, white asparagus, mushrooms, and ginger.

Green-Powder Drinks: Veggies on the Go

Green powder is a supplement that can be added to water, shaken up, and consumed on the go. It's also a convenient way to add more of the health benefits of greens to your diet. While we do not recommend green powders as a substitute for vegetables, you may want to consider them as a supplement to your healthy diet or a way to get started adding more greens to your meals. Adding a scoop of green powder to your daily smoothie can really boost the nutritional value.

Green powders vary in terms of quality. Look for a variety of organic cereal grasses such as wheatgrass, barley grass, and oat grass; and other concentrated nutrients like algae and chlorella. Avoid green powders with gluten, soy, sugar, or artificial sweeteners (see the list of foods to avoid in this chapter). Ahlea's favorite is Premier Greens by Premier Research Labs because it is organic and free of sugar, gluten, and other fillers.

Not many people love the taste of green powders, unless their taste buds have acclimated to healthy eating. You may want to mix the powder in a smoothie or add some honey or stevia to your green-powder drink to improve the taste. But give your taste buds a chance—they do change—eventually, you may find that you love the taste of greens!

---

3. Develop a Love Affair with Herbs and Spices

One of our favorite books is *Healing Spices: How to Use 50 Everyday and Exotic Spices to Boost Health and Beat Disease,* in which author Bharat B. Aggarwal, Ph.D., outlines the nutritional, medicinal, and culinary use of herbs and spices. Herbs and spices are concentrated sources of phytonutrients, which means they are concentrated sources of life-giving antioxidants. For example, 1 teaspoon of oregano or ½ teaspoon of dried cloves on their own have more antioxidants than ½ cup of blueberries.[56]

Imagine what kind of health benefits you can get from sprinkling these tasty antioxidant powerhouses into meals and desserts. They can be used to make your meals delicious and help resolve health conditions—which is truly using your food as your medicine!

Herbs are the green, leafy parts of a plant used to season foods. They're not the main ingredient of a dish (like kale or lettuce, for example); instead, they're flavor enhancers. Herbs are used either fresh or dried, and examples include:

• Basil	• Lemongrass	• Rosemary
• Bay leaf	• Marjoram	• Sage
• Chervil	• Mint	• Savory
• Cilantro	• Oregano	• Tarragon
• Dill	• Parsley	• Thyme

Spices are dried and come from a plant's root, stem, flower, fruit, seed, leaf, or bud. They are concentrated, flavorful, and aromatic. Examples include:

• Ajowan	• Clove	• Ginger
• Allspice	• Coriander	• Horseradish
• Aniseed	• Cumin	• Mustard seed
• Black pepper	• Curry	• Nutmeg
• Cardamom	• Fennel	• Saffron
• Cinnamon*	• Fenugreek	• Turmeric

---

*If you are a cinnamon lover, we recommend seeking out Ceylon, the "true cinnamon," instead of cassia cinnamon because cassia could have health risks if consumed in large quantities. You can find organic Ceylon cinnamon at: MountainRoseHerbs.com.

We will share ideas with you about using herbs and spices in the next chapter, and you'll also see that they're used plentifully in the recipes we included in this book. Soon you will be making fantastic health-packed meals, snacks, and desserts that your body and taste buds will love!

4. Natural Sweeteners

Nature has provided us with the sweet taste for a very good reason! In both Chinese and Ayurvedic medicine, two systems of health and healing that are thousands of years old, practitioners know that a balance of tastes is important. Chinese medicine talks about the importance of five tastes (spicy, salty, sour, bitter, and sweet), while Ayurveda talks about six tastes (astringent, salty, sour, pungent, bitter, and sweet). In both honored systems, the idea is that balancing all of these tastes is important for feeling satisfied during and after eating. In other words, balancing the tastes can ward off cravings!

In the U.S. in particular, our manufactured-food industry weighs heavily toward the sweet and salty tastes because they tend to increase the appetite and, in turn, increase profits for those companies. Home cooks have an advantage in that they can make foods with a balance of tastes for better health and satisfaction.

For the moment, let's look at the sweet taste. It's not something to be shunned, because it has many benefits. According to Chinese medicine, nutritionally dense sweet-tasting foods—called "full sweets"—provide soothing, strengthening, and nourishing actions for the muscles, nerves, and brain; they also provide energy for all bodily functions.[57] Examples of these foods are naturally sweet vegetables such as carrots and onions and whole-food sweeteners, which we will outline on the following pages. (The recipes in Chapter 10 will give you many options for meals with balanced tastes. We also provide dessert recipes that use whole-food ingredients, including sweeteners, and a balance of tastes.)

On the other hand, when it comes to junk foods with little to no nutritional value (called "empty sweets"), the natural balance is upset—they can shock the stomach and pancreas and can deplete the body's minerals.[58] Examples of these types of foods are refined sugar; artificial sweeteners; and processed cookies, cakes, and the like.

The sweeteners we recommend below are all-natural, whole-food options found in nature or minimally processed. Each of the sweeteners we recommend has nutritional value and when combined with healthy fats and proteins, can keep your body and blood sugar balanced.

— **Fruit.*** Fruit from nature is a great choice for the sweet taste. Some of our favorites are berries and green Granny Smith apples because of their high antioxidant value and lower sugar content.

— **Dates.*** We love using organic Medjool dates in desserts because they're rich in fiber and potassium and provide vitamin B_6 and essential minerals like copper, manganese, and magnesium.[59]

— **Honey.*** Honey is made by honeybees, is a source of vitamins B_6 and C, and has antiallergy and antimicrobial properties. Some rarer forms of honey, like manuka honey and jujube honey, have been shown to combat bacteria and candida respectively.[60, 61] We recommend raw, unpasteurized honey, but ask you to keep in mind that babies under one year of age should not be fed honey at all.

— **Organic, Grade B maple syrup.** Researchers at the University of Rhode Island found that maple syrup has 54 health-providing compounds, including anti-cancer, anti-inflammatory and anti-diabetes properties.[62] A good source of antioxidants and minerals, maple syrup comes from the sap of trees and is lightly processed. Choose organic, Grade B pure maple syrup for the most minerals.

— **Organic, unsulphured blackstrap molasses.** Molasses is derived from sugar making, after the sucrose is extracted from sugar-cane juice. It is the most processed of all the sweeteners we're recommending here, but it does have some nutritional value.[63] Molasses is rich in iron, magnesium, potassium, manganese, zinc, and calcium. We don't use it often, but we consider it a reasonable choice for some uses.

---

*The Gut and Psychology Syndrome (GAPS) diet and the Specific Carbohydrate Diet (SCD) are healing diets for people with chronic gastrointestinal and energy- and mood-related symptoms. These diets allow fruit, dates, and honey because they are easily absorbed by the small intestine, which is responsible for 90 percent of digestion. However, if you have candida or bacterial overgrowth, you may want to use these foods sparingly or eliminate them until your symptoms begin to resolve.

— **Lo han guo.** Cultivated from the *Siraitia grosvenorii* vine, it's also called Buddha fruit, monk fruit, and longevity fruit. This fruit is a green-brown ball from China or Thailand, is 200 times sweeter than sugar, and has been used in China to combat diabetes and obesity.[64] The least processed version of lo han guo is the dried balls that you can simmer in tea for a sweetened beverage or grind up into a powder.

Be mindful that lo han guo is being manufactured into a highly processed form because it is calorie-free (examples are PureLo, Purefruit, and Nectresse). These highly processed versions have little to no nutritional value and may have an effect of tricking the body that could unbalance blood sugar in sensitive individuals.

— **Stevia.** This is a sweet leafy herb that is calorie-free, is 200 to 300 times sweeter than sugar, and has antioxidants and immune-system benefits.[65] Stevia undergoes various levels of quality and processing, so we recommend that you look for dry stevia leaves and use them to sweeten teas and sauces, or grind them and use the powder to sweeten foods. If you want to make a more concentrated liquid, you can take ¼ cup of ground stevia and add one cup of warm water in a glass jar. Put the lid on the jar and let it sit for 24 hours, then strain the liquid out. You can also simmer the liquid on low after straining to get a more concentrated liquid.[66]

You might also experiment with the purest form of stevia liquid you can find on the market. Keep in mind that some people report adverse blood-sugar or appetite-enhancing effects from stevia. We recommend that you listen to your body and do what feels best for you.

— **Xylitol and erythritol.** These two sugar alcohols are lower in calories than sugar and do not spike blood sugar—they're also used in natural dental products because they do not feed bacteria contributing to tooth decay. Some people like these sweeteners because they can be used in place of sugar with a taste that more closely resembles it; others find that like stevia, these sugars play a trick on their appetite and blood sugar. We recommend that if you do choose to experiment with these sweeteners, you listen to your body. If you find yourself craving more sweets, having adverse symptoms, or experiencing unbalanced blood sugar, these sweeteners are not for you.

In addition, a major downside to these sweeteners is their gastrointestinal effects. They can cause nausea, cramping, and diarrhea and are not recommended for people following a small intestine healing diet like the Gut and Psychology Syndrome (GAPS) diet and the Specific Carbohydrate Diet (SCD).

More Health and Less Cravings— Keeping the Sweet Taste Balanced

A great way to eat desserts and treats is to balance sweet foods such as honey, fruit, and dates with healthy nuts, seeds, fats, oils, and spices. Protein fats like coconut flour, nuts, and seeds—along with healthy fats and oils—boost mood while slowing the absorption of the sugars. Additionally, adding spices like cloves, cardamom, cinnamon, and ginger aids your digestion, adds antioxidants, and balances your gut bacteria. This is a great way to please your taste buds with dessert while balancing your body's response to these foods. It also helps to balance the five or six tastes to bring you more satisfaction overall.

The desserts we have provided in Chapter 10 are designed to delight your body and taste buds. You deserve delicious health!

---

5. Water

How much and what type of water to drink are topics of great debate among health experts and researchers. According to U.K.-based science journalist Caroline Williams, the guideline to drink eight, eight-ounce glasses of water per day came from a 1945 U.S. National Research Council recommendation that some experts say has no scientific foundation.[67] At the same time, many studies show the benefits of water. For example, it can increase metabolism and aids in digestion, circulation, and excretion.[68]

In work with their clients, Heather and Ahlea have found that a focus on water consumption has improved health across the board. This is not unusual—in fact, studies on water and food consumption in U.S. adults from 1999 to 2001 found that water consumers drink fewer soft drinks and fruit drinks and have healthier eating patterns, including more consumption of vegetables and fruits.[69]

Ahlea recommends her clients drink half their body weight in ounces. For example, a 150-pound person would drink 75 ounces of water, which is about 9½ cups. She also asks them to drink 20 ounces (2½ cups) of water first thing in the morning. While 2½ cups of water in the morning may seem like a lot, the body is better able to absorb a large amount of water first thing in the morning before any food is taken. If you choose to experiment with this, make sure to wait 30 minutes before eating breakfast.

It's very important to listen to your body when it comes to thirst because everyone's body is different. Depending on your size, level of activity, climate, and other factors, your body may need more water.

Freyedoon Batmanghelidj, M.D., author of *Your Body's Many Cries for Water,* says that symptoms of dehydration are wide-ranging, because water impacts all of the body's functions. Some examples are[70]:

- Allergies
- Arthritis
- Asthma
- Autoimmune diseases
- Cravings
- Fatigue

- Feeling unrested upon waking
- Hypertension
- Mood issues (phobias, irritability, anxiety, depression)
- Thirst perception
- Type 2 diabetes

So what type of water is best to drink? This is also cause for much controversy. Tap water contains aluminum, fluoride, and disinfectants that make it harmful to the body.[71] We recommend pure springwater as the best option because it comes from nature, but it's important to know the source of the springwater you choose. Some cities have delivery services that come in large reusable glass containers, which is healthier than plastic bottled water of any size (due to toxins in plastic bottles, even those that are BPA-free).

Other options to consider are a high-quality carbon filter or a reverse osmosis (RO) filter. If you are filtering your water, we recommend adding minerals back in. Consider adding real sea salt or pink Himalayan salt; aluminum-free baking soda; or our favorites—Polar Mins by Premier Research Labs, and Anderson's Concentrated Mineral Drops (also known as Anderson's CMD; you'll learn more about them in Chapter 6).

6. Unrefined Fats and Oils

In the No-No's section of this chapter, you learned why refined fats and trans fats are damaging to the body. While fats and oils were once vilified altogether, new studies have found that healthy, *unrefined* fats and oils have important properties for good moods, satiety (and therefore losing or maintaining healthy weight), and brain health.[72] Fats also help carry important vitamins like A, D, E, and K into the body.

Essential fatty acids—that is, omega-3 and omega-6 fatty acids—are important for the body and must be obtained from food. While omega-3 and omega-6 fatty acids are ideally consumed in the same ratio (1:1), Western diets often contain way too many omega-6 fatty acids (in a 16:1 ratio, or 16 omega-6 to 1 omega-3).[73] This can contribute to cardiovascular disease, cancer, inflammation, and autoimmune disease.

An abundance of omega-6 fatty acids are found in polyunsaturated oils, which are vegetable oils. To ensure you get a better ratio of omega-3 to omega-6 essential fatty acids, eat a range of organic fats from animals fed their native diets (grass fed, pasture fed), along with unrefined extra-virgin coconut oil and olive oil.

The healthiest fats are organic, grass-fed, or pasture-fed animal fats; and organic, unrefined plant fats and oils. Here are some examples[74]:

- Grass- or pasture-fed animal fats*—egg yolks; raw butter; ghee; lard from pork; tallow and suet from lamb and beef; and goose, chicken, and duck fat are all receiving new attention as experts realize their health value[75]

- Borage oil

- Coconut oil* (extra-virgin)

- Cod-liver oil*

- Flaxseed oil (choose high quality, store in the refrigerator, and use in small quantities)

- Hemp-seed oil

- Olive oil (extra-virgin)*

- Palm oil (please note that we do not recommend palm oil at this time because it is not sustainably harvested, which is adversely impacting the ecosystem and endangering animals, particularly the orangutan)

- Pumpkin-seed oil

---

*Emphasize these oils for a better balance of omega-6 to omega-3 essential fatty acid levels.

How to Use Fats and Oil for Your Best Health

Did you know that cooking with polyunsaturated vegetable oils causes them to turn rancid? Rancid oils create unhealthy conditions in your body, such as upsetting the cholesterol balance and promoting immune problems and heart disease.

Keep in mind that most oils are meant to be drizzled onto your food after cooking. For example, if you make grains or cook vegetables, drizzle some pumpkin-seed oil on them at the table for delicious flavor. The following fats and oils, however, are meant for cooking[76]:

- Animal fats—butter, ghee, tallow and suet (from beef and lamb), lard (from pigs), chicken fat, goose fat, and duck fat

- Coconut oil

- Palm oil (it is worth repeating here that although palm oil can be used for cooking, it is not sustainably harvested, and we recommend using other alternatives from this list)

- For deep frying—only use tallow or lard

- For temperatures under 400 degrees or for light sautéing— olive oil, avocado oil, macadamia nut oil, and sesame oil

7. Grains, Nuts, and Seeds

Currently, grains are on the firing line due to books like *Wheat Belly* and *Grain Brain*. Paleo and Primal diets, which essentially eliminate grains, are also receiving a great deal of attention. There is good reason for this: digestive diseases are on the rise, now affecting up to 70 million people in the United States alone.[77]

Grains are challenging for the small intestine to digest, so people working on gut health or insulin issues may want to remove them while they allow their digestive system to heal. Once healed, these folks can often reintroduce grains into their diet.

Whole grains (no part of the grain is removed in milling), as opposed to lower-quality processed grains, have many healing properties. Whole grains are a source of carbohydrates and protein; are rich in fiber, B vitamins, and minerals; can combat constipation; and boost serotonin, the body's happiness hormone.

If you are working on any healing protocol and want to include grains, it can be helpful to eliminate all packaged breads, crackers, and cereals, and focus on cooking whole grains instead. (We have some options for breads, crackers, and hot cereals in the recipes section that you can use to replace these processed foods.)

When it comes to eating grains, we recommend that you listen to your body and work with a health practitioner if you're uncertain about whether they are beneficial for where you are in your health journey. (Using the food-diary exercise at the end of this chapter will be helpful in identifying symptoms associated with eating grains and other foods, so you can learn the language of your body.)

If you do eat grains, we recommend organic whole grains that are gluten-free, such as: quinoa, buckwheat, millet, amaranth, and white basmati rice. Be aware that rice is known to contain arsenic, and brown rice contains significantly more of it than white rice does, according to Consumer Reports.[78] Soaking your grains before preparing them is a great way to boost their digestibility, and we will show you how to do this in Chapter 10.

Nuts and seeds are protein fats that can be a wonderful addition to your diet, making great desserts and on-the-go snacks. Full of antioxidants and fiber, nuts have been shown to reduce cholesterol, aid weight loss, and promote satiety, so you feel full longer.[79] While there are many delicious options for nuts and seeds, be aware that cashews, peanuts, and pistachios have been known to accumulate mold more easily and cause symptoms in sensitive people.[80]

It is important to listen to your body when eating nuts and seeds because eating too many can cause digestive symptoms. Learn to find the right level for you by using the food diary at the end of this chapter or working with a knowledgeable practitioner. We recommend choosing organic, raw nuts and seeds. Nuts and seeds that are already roasted upon purchase have a greater chance of being rancid; instead, you can roast them at home by placing them in the oven on the lowest temperature (make sure to see the instructions in Chapter 10 for how to properly prepare nuts and seeds before roasting them).

Remember to rotate your grains, nuts, and seeds, rather than eating just one type every day or even every week. If you eat a food too often, your body could develop a sensitivity to that food, and eating a wide range of foods gives you more nutrients.

8. Healing Elixirs: Homemade Bone Broths and Vegetable Broths

Making your own broth is much easier than you think, and the taste and health benefits are definitely worth it! These are some of the most affordable healing tools possible.

Homemade meat stocks and bone broths aid digestion and provide an easy-to-digest form of vitamins, minerals, and protein. Dr. Natasha Campbell-McBride teaches that bone broths help "heal and seal" the gut, and she recommends them as some of the best ways to heal the digestive tract and related immune and mood disorders.

If you have inflammation, arthritis, or joint pain, you will benefit from bone broth because it contains glucosamine and chondroitin sulfates, which you may see often in supplements for these conditions.[81] Here is yet another way our ancestors used food as medicine!

We highly recommend bone stock or broth as part of your regular health routine. Louise drinks bone broth two times per day to keep her nourished and energized. When she returns home from traveling, she always has bone broth and soups for several days to nurture her body back into balance after being away. It is one of her biggest health secrets!

If you're a vegan or vegetarian, you can benefit from making vegetable stock or broth. The great thing about any homemade stocks and broths is that they're made with kitchen scraps that people tend to discard. Instead, you will be simmering these discarded bones and vegetable scraps with water and a touch of apple cider vinegar to pull out the nutrients. This easy combo creates a budget-friendly healing elixir that your body will love.

We have included recipes for bone stocks and broth and veggie stocks and broths in Chapter 10—you will love how simple they are to make!

Watch Cravings Fall Away

After a week to a month of eating healthy whole foods, your taste buds will begin to change, and you'll become more in touch with foods that nourish your body and seek out those body-satisfying tastes. In other words, your cravings change as your taste buds change.

Remember, too much of the sweet and salty tastes and chemical additives in processed food will prompt your taste buds and your body to crave more of the same. As you prepare more foods at home and make better choices when you're out to eat, you will start to see cravings falling away as your body is nourished and strengthened.

The more you listen to your body, the more you will understand the language of these cravings. If you've recently eaten, tune in to see if you're stressed, overwhelmed, nervous, sad, tired, or bored. Perhaps the food you just ate did not satisfy you or was unbalanced in some way (like so many fast and processed foods today) and your body is seeking more—maybe what you ate opened up your appetite instead of satisfying it. As you discover what works to truly nourish your body, cravings dissolve.

As Heather was recovering her health and learning to listen to her body after decades of being ruled by cravings, she realized that when she ate something that was too sweet and unbalanced, a buzz of energy would move up to her head, creating a kind of nervousness or restlessness. Yet when she ate a body-satisfying meal, it not only tasted good, but it created a calm, grounded feeling in the center of her body as well. This is how she started to evaluate how balanced her meals were. It's also how she started to create recipes—she wanted to make food that would be so balanced that it gave others a centered, satisfied feeling that then reduced or eliminated cravings at the physical level.

When it comes to cravings, which are rooted in the body and the mind, Louise's teaching is spot-on: everything is thoughts and food. Remember, whole foods and positive thoughts fulfill us at a very deep level. When we choose high-quality, nourishing thoughts and food, we are choosing to love ourselves. Our bodies can't help but respond to that!

Eating Healthy on a Budget

Louise once heard someone ask, "Why feed a sick body expensive healthy food?" This is not an uncommon question. After reading this book so far, you hopefully have a new understanding that healthy foods, just like healthy thoughts, have powerful healing properties.

Why would anyone deny themselves healthy food because it costs more than cheap, processed food? The first and most important thing to embrace is that you matter and are worth the investment of wholesome, healthy foods. The second thing to recognize is that there are several ways to eat healthy on a budget.

One thing Heather did when she wanted to invest in herself was to look carefully at the other things she was spending money on. When she finally decided that she mattered enough to heal, she realized that expenses like buying magazines, eating out at restaurants, and her monthly cell-phone plan could be reduced or eliminated. These were expenses that she didn't really value as much as her health, so it was easy to minimize them.

It's helpful to look at how you're spending your money versus the priorities that are most important to you. Perhaps there are things you're spending money on that don't matter as much to you; that money can be moved into your food budget. This can be a very eye-opening exercise.

Here are some ideas to save money on healthy, organic food:

— **Shop at your local farmers' market.**

— **Go to an organic farm and buy directly from the farmer.** Many organic farms sell direct to customers or have Community Supported Agriculture (CSA) programs where you can buy family-sized portions of vegetables, animal protein (like meat, poultry, eggs, and raw butter), and sometimes even fresh-cut flowers.

— **Buy in bulk online or in the store.** You can often get discounts when buying in bulk. Many health-food stores have 10 to 15 percent off cases, for example.

— **Get together with friends or groups and buy in bulk.** For example, a mom on a tight budget in San Diego began a Facebook group to reach out to people in her local area who wanted to buy healthy food at a discount. She contacted local and online sellers of organic foods and supplements and got wholesale prices, then started a shopping club. In this way, she and many other people in the community got to share in discounted prices. This is a great idea made much easier by social media.

If you don't have a large group to join, small groups of friends can get together to buy grass-fed meat, herbs and spices, and vegetables.

— **Investigate subscription programs.** Online stores like Amazon.com have monthly subscription programs where you can buy at a lower price.

— **Learn to garden, even indoors!** Both Ahlea and Louise have thriving, beautiful gardens, which are wonderful for growing organic, affordable food. Louise's pictures of her giant kale even got nearly 100,000 likes on her Facebook page!

If you have the space, gardening is a great way to connect with nature and eat well. Yet even if you have limited space or no outdoor space at all, there are wonderful options for gardening! Heather and her husband got an AeroGarden and grew plants hydroponically (that is, with organic liquid nutrients rather than soil) during the winter in Vermont. They set up a tiny room in their basement and were able to grow several types of lettuce, arugula, and basil so that they could have fresh vegetables all winter. Hydroponics allows you to grow vegetables quickly in small indoor areas.

Another option is to have an herb garden in your kitchen, near a window with plenty of sun.

— **Buy once and regrow your produce.** Certain vegetables can actually be regrown from the base that you often throw away! For instance, take the bottom (base) of a bunch of celery and place it, cut side facing up, in a bowl of warm water near a sunny window (change the water every two days). In about five to seven days, you will see yellow, then green, leaves sprouting. At this point, you can put the celery into a container with soil covering all but the small new leaves. Water generously and watch the new celery grow! Lettuce and bok choy can be regrown in much the same way.

Green onions are even easier: put the white bases in a jar of water, place in a sunny area, and watch as they regrow very quickly. Make sure to change the water every couple of days.

— **Stretch your food, like your ancestors did.** Our ancestors knew how to stretch food in ways most of us aren't taught today. Bone and vegetable broth is an example of stretching food: After eating meat or poultry, you take the bones and make a healthy, nourishing broth. The same is true for the vegetable scraps you can use in broths. What was once considered trash can actually be used to nourish the body. This is a great money-saving technique!

— **Love eating in.** Eating at home saves a lot of money, even when you're eating organically! Many restaurants serving non-organic food cost more than eating organic food at home. Have fun with home-meal preparation (we'll give you some ideas to make it easier in Part II).

— **Bag your lunch.** If you count up the money spent on eating out during your workweek, even for seemingly affordable lunches, you can see how easily you could set aside that budget for healthy food. Bagging your lunch takes planning, but the more you make home-cooked meals, the more leftovers you have to pack for the next day!

— **Make your own snacks and treats.** Snack food, bars, and desserts tend to be very pricey. It's much easier than you think to make your own! Plus, you can make extra and put them in your freezer to save time.

Take the Time to Nourish Yourself

When it comes to eating healthy, whole foods, one of the issues that comes up (in addition to money) is time: Many people feel they don't have the time to prepare foods. In addition, it can take time to learn the skill of healthy cooking.

Just as in the budget exercise a few pages ago, we invite you to look at how you're spending your time. Identify where time spent on your health and nourishing your body falls on your list of priorities.

As mentioned earlier in the book, while Heather was recovering her health, she was working 12-hour days in a competitive company. Changing her diet meant that she had to figure out how to spend time in the kitchen—to take that time for herself. As she looked at how she was structuring her days, she realized that she could actually make the time to prepare food, but she didn't think she was important enough. She realized that she placed more importance on her job than on herself. So she sought out a coach and learned how to work smarter, reduce her hours at the office, and spend more time in the kitchen.

Heather had to peel away a lot of limiting beliefs about taking time for herself. She realized that investing time in herself and her health actually improved her work performance; but more important, she discovered that the world didn't have to rest on her shoulders. She attributes time spent in the kitchen as one of the most healing steps she took because she learned how to deeply nourish herself and how to modify recipes to create the balance and energy she needed to feel her best.

Like Heather learned, you deserve to feel your best every day. In our modern times, it seems like feeling well is such a mysterious thing because the secret has been forgotten. In a world that emphasizes profitable companies making cheap, manufactured convenience foods that trick your taste buds and deplete your body, you may feel that you've moved so far away from true health that it is a challenge to find your way back. But it's easier than you think!

The real secret to feeling your best is taking time for yourself, and not just for meditating and doing affirmations. It's also time spent planning and preparing foods that nourish, strengthen, and energize your body. It's time spent in the kitchen preparing these whole foods in ways that delight your taste buds. It's time spent savoring the food with all of your senses. And when possible, time spent bonding with friends and family to embrace the connection that comes from shared meals. Louise said it best: "Everything is thoughts and food. When you get both right, you have the real secret for perfect health."

Later in the book, we'll provide ideas for fast, easy meals that can help you balance your busy life with a healthy body. We invite you to develop a love for time spent on nourishment—to prime your inner body with all of the nutrients it needs for your best life. You are worth it!

Exercises to Emphasize Food and Thoughts That Heal Your Body and Mind

The following exercises will help give you the key to unlock your inner journey, and remind you that you matter enough to nourish yourself both inside and out.

1. Listen to Your Body

While there are many wonderful doctors and experts who can give you guidelines for your diet, each body is unique. Because of this, it's incredibly important to learn to listen to your body. The more you do, the more you hear its unique needs, which makes it easier to nourish yourself in the way that suits you best. Dogma and rules live in your head and mean nothing to your body's true needs. The less you worry about rules and the more you honor what your body truly needs, the healthier you will be.

Chapter 4 is a great place to revisit if you want to practice listening to your body. In addition, the next exercise is wonderful to help you start learning how your body speaks to you and how it responds to food.

2. Food Diary

Ahlea and Heather use this with all of their clients as a way to learn the language of the body. The food you eat is so powerful that it affects your energy levels, your physical wellness, your thoughts, and your moods.

Here's how to do this exercise:

— **Write down all the foods you eat each day.** Use a notepad you can keep with you, your phone, or whatever is most convenient to capture this information easily.

— **During the day, write down any symptoms you experience, for example:**

- Energy—balanced, too wired, fatigue, improving
- Moods—happy, sad, anxious, content, good self-esteem, worried
- Sleep—restful, deep, restless, interrupted, insomnia
- Physical symptoms—reflux, joint pain, headaches, digestive upset, no symptoms, more allergies, fewer allergies
- Bowel movements—diarrhea, urgency, constipation, easy, felt fully evacuated

— **Review your list of food and symptoms every couple of days. Note the following:**

- Are certain foods triggering symptoms in the list above?
- Look over two or three days for patterns—food can have an effect over several days, so noticing patterns helps.
- Circle or write down the foods that seem to be triggers.
- After two weeks of writing down food and symptoms and recording patterns you notice, go to the next step.

— **Elimination experiment.** Now that you have noticed patterns, consider doing an elimination diet with the foods that you found to be triggers. We recommend eliminating one thing at a time, so that you'll know what is working. Eliminate that food for one or two weeks and see how you feel. Did the symptoms go away? Or improve in some way? Record what you learned. If your list is really confusing and you aren't sure how to proceed, we recommend working with a practitioner who has a good understanding of nutrition and the physical body. This can help shorten the process and make things even easier. Sometimes foods that trigger symptoms seem random, but have common links, like foods that trigger histamine intolerance symptoms. An experienced practitioner can spot patterns like this and help guide you.

3. Affirmations

Here are some great affirmations that relate to food and mealtimes. Continue to use your mirror, and repeat as many of them as you'd like throughout the day:

<u>Preparing Meals</u>

Planning healthy meals is a joy.

Hello, kitchen, you are my nourishment center. I appreciate you!

I have everything I need to help me prepare delicious, nutritious meals.

I am so grateful to be choosing food that supports my best health.

I can easily make a nutritious, delicious meal.

I love spending time in the kitchen!

I am worth the time and money I invest in my health.

Hi, body, what would nourish you today?

I love selecting foods that work in harmony with you, body.

I am so fortunate that I can choose healthy foods for my family.

My family loves to eat healthy food.

The kids love to try new foods.

I am learning new things that heal my body one step at a time.

Every time I prepare food, I am nourished by my connection to nature and other beings.

I am willing to take this time to nurture myself.

<u>Eating Meals</u>

I am so grateful for this wonderful food.

My body loves the way I choose the perfect foods for every meal.

All of my meals are harmonious.

I love taking time to eat mindfully and fully enjoy my meals.

I am well nourished in preparation for the day ahead of me.

My body heals and strengthens with every bite I take.

Mealtimes are happy times.

My family gathers together with great joy and love.

I bless this food and my body with love.

I listen for when I am satisfied and full.

I listen to my body as I eat.

I pay attention to all of my senses when I eat.

This food is healing me.

My taste buds are changing every day—I no longer crave foods that don't nourish me.

I listen to my appetite and it guides me with loving, nourishing choices.

I am willing to slow down and take this time to nourish myself.

Nourishing Food Is Part of Your Love Story

The food you eat is as important as the thoughts you think. We encourage you to make nourishing foods part of your love story. While it may seem challenging at first to change your food habits, you will find that small changes over time will allow your habits and taste buds to evolve in ways that support your optimal health. The results of more energy, better sleep, happier moods, and better health are worth it! As you adjust your eating habits, you'll see how truly healing food is.

In the next chapter, we'll share tips for healing foods and other natural remedies for physical and emotional symptoms you may be experiencing.

♥ ♥

Chapter 6

Step #6:
Empower Your Health—
Home Remedies for What Ails You

Did you know that a lot of remedies supporting health and healing can be found right in your garden or kitchen cupboard? In fact, today's modern pharmaceuticals have their history in medicinal plants. Up to the mid-1800s, drugs made of herbs, plants, roots, vines, and fungi were used exclusively, until the first synthetic drug was introduced in 1869.[1] Today, 70 percent of pharmaceutical drugs begin from or were inspired by nature.[2]

If science recognizes the medicinal benefits of plants, why did it move toward synthetics? One of the biggest reasons is the drive for profits—plants can't be patented or controlled the way synthetics can. Compounding the issue is the fact that it can take more than a decade for a pharmaceutical company to test a drug and get it to market, with a total price tag of over $800 million, which often means these drugs are rushed into production before the side effects are fully understood.[3]

In Chapter 2, you learned that properly prescribed pharmaceutical drugs were one of the leading causes of death in the U.S. The *Journal of the American Medical Association (JAMA)* reported that serious adverse drug interactions are found only after the drugs have been approved by the FDA.[4]

> "I lovingly do everything I can to assist my body in maintaining perfect health."
>
> — Louise

Keep in mind that we are not suggesting you ever ignore doctors' orders or stop using your prescription medications. If you have a serious health condition or are on medications, we recommend that you speak to your doctor and other practitioners you're working with before using the remedies or supplements in this chapter. Sometimes even natural remedies can have interactions with medications, so checking with your doctor will support you in taking responsibility for your good health.

The opportunity here is to open a dialogue about other options that may be available to you, so that you can discuss alternatives with your doctors and see what resonates with your health needs.

According to James Duke, Ph.D., one of the world's foremost authorities on medicinal plants, there are some very important reasons to look to herbal remedies as a legitimate health option when considering treatment protocols[5]:

- Ninety percent of plant-derived chemicals are cheaper both environmentally and economically to extract from whole plants than to synthesize.

- It can help the consumer to look at all the options so that the best choices can be made. For example, many herbal options can be just as helpful as pharmaceuticals, but with fewer serious side effects.

- Medicinal plants have preventive properties that can boost health and ward off disease.

This chapter is going to be fun because we're going to share some of our favorite home remedies, supplements, and ancient healing techniques that have stood the test of time. These are practices we use in our own homes and with our clients. (Please note that we recommend choosing organic herbs, spices, essential oils, food remedies, and teas whenever possible.)

What to Know Before You Start Taking a New Supplement

Before we jump into the remedies, there's something important to recognize: You are your best health advocate and the only one who lives in your body, so you know what feels and works best for you. The more you learn to listen to and trust your body, the more you will be guided well by its signals.

Some people like to experiment with remedies and supplements, while others require guidance from a doctor, nutritionist, or other health practitioner. Make sure you research the supplements you're considering and always listen to your body. If something you take makes you feel unwell, stop taking it and investigate why. Know that several things can happen when you start taking a new supplement:

— **You may kick off a detox reaction in your body.** Commonly called "die-off" or a "Herxheimer reaction," this is a very common response to starting a healthier diet or a new supplement that helps your body heal. It happens because bad bacteria and yeast die off and cause a variety of uncomfortable symptoms like gas, bloating, headaches, constipation, diarrhea, body odor, acne, fatigue, and more. You can generally tell it's die-off if you feel better in some ways, even though you're having other uncomfortable symptoms; for example, if you're sleeping much better or finding your discomfort alleviated in other ways. The key is, if the die-off symptoms are painful or uncomfortable, back off and listen to your body or seek support from a practitioner.

— **Your body may start working in ways it was unable to before.** Often referred to as "start-up symptoms," this is different from die-off in that the symptoms arise as your body starts healing. For example, children with autism who start getting methyl B$_{12}$ shots have been known to bite things, because the nerves in their mouth are healing and they experience a tingling effect. The tingling can be uncomfortable, but it's a sign that the nerves are healing. It's helpful to be aware of any potential start-up symptoms you might experience with a new remedy or supplement—because everyone is different, you can seek guidance from a practitioner or an online source that a trusted expert recommends.

— **Taking enough of one supplement may unmask a deficiency in others.** Heather experienced this when she started taking magnesium in the proper doses. She felt so much better that she knew it was working, but she also started to get periodic migraines, which she had never had before. She learned that taking magnesium in the right amounts can unmask a deficiency in its cofactors (the nutrients it needs to work well in the body), in her case, vitamin B$_6$ and biotin. As soon as she started supplementing with vitamin B$_6$ and biotin, the migraines went away completely, and her health moved to a much higher level. The key is that since Heather was listening to her body, she was aware that it would be important to note new symptoms and look into them. That made it easier to find a solution that supported her body.

— **The remedy or supplement may not be right for you for a variety of reasons.** One important reason could be that you're on medication that does not go well with the remedy. Remember to talk to your doctor first before using something new. Listen to your body, and stop taking something if it doesn't feel right.

The same can be said for foods that don't work for you. We are all unique, and your uniqueness deserves to be honored.

Guidance from professionals is incredibly helpful, and we always recommend working with someone who can partner with you on your health journey. Most of all, love yourself by taking active responsibility for your health. And always listen to and honor your body: A symptom is not a "bad" thing; it's a signal your body is using to speak to you. It's how your body loves you. How you respond is completely up to you because this is *your* health journey. Part of loving yourself is doing what feels right to you.

Loving Your Digestive System: Remedies for Your Digestive Health

Digestive issues can have a wide range of root causes, so we'll be focusing on some basic remedies that may be useful for 80 percent of cases. If you have chronic digestive issues that are not resolving with a healthier diet and lifestyle, your doctor or health practitioner is your best bet to address the root cause.

Constipation

Remember, constipation is related to diarrhea, so you'll notice that some of the remedies will be similar. See Chapter 3 for more information about constipation as well.

— **Herbs and spices**[6]:

- Aniseed

- Black pepper

- Caraway

- Cardamom

- Parsley

— **Castor-oil pack.** These have been used since ancient times for constipation, cleansing, and lymphatic drainage. Supplies you'll need are: castor oil (buy organic cold-pressed, rather than solvent-extracted or deodorized), a piece of cotton flannel (you can get this at your health-food store, or Amazon.com sells Heritage Products organic cotton flannel), a hot-water bottle, a towel, and some plastic wrap.

To administer the castor-oil pack:

- Apply several tablespoons of oil to several layers of cotton flannel.
- Place the oil-soaked fabric on your abdomen. You could concentrate on your lower abdomen (intestines) or your upper-right abdomen, near your liver and gallbladder.
- Place a layer of plastic wrap with a towel on top.
- Apply gentle heat with a hot-water bottle for 30 minutes to one hour.

— **Adequate hydration.** Make sure you're drinking enough water (see Chapter 5 for more on this subject).

— **Magnesium.** See the section on magnesium at the end of this chapter for more on why this mineral is so important for bowel health. Constipation is a sign of magnesium deficiency.[7]

— **Fiber.** As you eat a healthier diet, you will likely increase your fiber intake. For some, this alleviates constipation, while for others, it can create more challenges. If adding more fiber is constipating for you, avoid this and focus on the other remedies listed in this section. It's possible that fiber is more irritating for people with compromised small intestine health. If the other remedies listed in this section don't help, make sure to talk with your health-care practitioner.

Some popular options for supplementing your diet with fiber include:

- *Psyllium husks.* This is a natural source of soluble fiber that acts as a bulking agent in the body. There are organic psyllium husks on the market by brands such as Organic India and NOW.
- *FOS or inulin.* These are fructooligosaccharides, soluble fibers that are also used as alternative sweeteners because they have a naturally sweet taste. Derived from fruit and vegetable sugars, FOS and inulin are known as "prebiotics," which means that they feed good bacteria in your intestines. Some people do very well with them and others don't. This has led experts to be more cautious about FOS and inulin because newer evidence is showing that in cases of problematic bacterial overgrowth and small intestine challenges, FOS and inulin can feed bad bacteria as well as the good guys. You may want to avoid FOS and inulin if you have small intestine bacterial overgrowth (SIBO) or other chronic forms of bacterial overgrowth.

If you do choose to experiment with fructooligosaccharides, one study showed that inulin was the better option because it prompted the good bacteria to produce butyrate, a short-chain fatty acid responsible for cellular energy and reduced inflammation.[8]

- *Styrian pumpkin seeds.* Not your typical pumpkin seed, these hull-less seeds from Styrian pumpkins are larger and greener than most and gaining popularity among health enthusiasts because of their combination of fiber, magnesium, and zinc, all of which can be helpful for constipation. Pumpkin seeds make a great protein and mineral-rich snack on the go or you can grind them up to make your own pumpkin-seed butter, but do be sure to soak the seeds before consuming them (we'll show you how in Chapter 10). If you can't find organic Styrian pumpkin seeds in your health-food store, you can find them at: Vivapura.com.

— **Probiotics.** Learn more in the "Overall Digestive Support" section later in the chapter. (Note that the remedies in this section are all helpful options as well.)

— **Enema (or coffee enema).** If constipation persists, you may want to look into doing an enema. This inexpensive home remedy was a go-to cure dating back thousands of years. While there is a great deal of controversy about enemas, many well-respected medical doctors and naturopathic doctors still recommend them today. For example, in her book *Gut and Psychology Syndrome,* Dr. Natasha Campbell-McBride recommends that people with persistent constipation do an enema rather than staying chronically constipated because it's better for the body to eliminate the stored toxins.[9]

You can buy an enema kit with a stainless-steel bucket, medical-grade silicone tubing (as opposed to the lower-quality PVC tubing), and catheters at online retailers such as Amazon.com. When you receive your kit, you will have instructions for how to do the coffee enema as well. Always use clean, filtered water, and organic coffee that you have ground fresh in preparation for the coffee enema.

Diarrhea

Again, diarrhea is related to constipation, so some of the remedies will be similar. (See Chapter 3 for more information.)

— Herbs and spices[10]:

- Ajowan
- Cardamom
- Coriander
- Nutmeg

— Adequate hydration. Make sure you are drinking enough water (see Chapter 5 for more).

— Probiotics. Learn more in the "Overall Digestive Support" section later in the chapter.

— Foods to eat if you have diarrhea or are just recovering:

- Bananas and red-skinned potatoes without the skin are high in potassium and can help relieve diarrhea.[11] You can bake, boil, or mash the potatoes, preparing them without fats or oils or with just a minimal amount. You could put some chicken bone broth on the potatoes to flavor them, or add some ground coriander and/or ajowan to get the benefits of these spices as well.

- Organic applesauce. You can make this yourself by removing the skins of the apples and boiling or steaming them, and then mashing them. Add a little cardamom and nutmeg to get the spice benefits, too!

- Steamed chicken with no oils or fats added (fats and oils can be harder to digest if you have diarrhea or are just recovering).

- Chicken bone broth (see Chapter 10 for the recipe). Add some coriander seeds as you heat the broth, and sprinkle in some ajowan for added spice benefits.

- Blueberries. The tannins in blueberries are believed to be helpful for diarrhea.[12]

Gas, Bloating, or Indigestion

Note that Chapter 3 has more information on gas, bloating, and indigestion.

— **Herbs and spices**[13]:

- Aniseed
- Chamomile
- Coriander
- Fennel
- Peppermint. Try using therapeutic peppermint essential oil: Add 1 drop per teaspoon of carrier oil (such as unrefined organic almond oil or organic jojoba oil), and rub it into your abdomen. Studies show this can help alleviate cramps and abdominal pain associated with gas and IBS.[14]
- Turmeric

— **Castor-oil pack.** See the "Constipation" section earlier in the chapter for how to administer one of these packs.

— **Probiotics.** Learn more in the "Overall Digestive Support" section.

Acid Reflux, Heartburn, or GERD

While acid reflux and GERD (gastroesophageal reflux disease) can have a variety of root causes, some of these remedies may help. Keep in mind that reflux can be a sign of too much stomach acid or, paradoxically, too little. Chapter 3 talks more about how the sphincters, like the lower esophageal sphincter, can lose their ability to function properly. This is one of the reasons for heartburn, reflux, and GERD.

— **Herbs and spices**[15]:

- Caraway
- Fennel
- Ginger
- Parsley
- Turmeric

— Aloe vera juice. This has a long history of use as a folk remedy and continues to show promise today for reflux and GERD. If you decide to take this juice, do not use aloe gel directly from the plant (because it could contain latex toxins) or any preparation with laxative properties, including: aloe latex, aloin, or aloe-emoin.[16] Look for an organic juice with no chemical preservatives, such as Aloe Pro by Premier Research Labs.

— Magnesium. See the information on magnesium at the end of the chapter.

— Melatonin or L-tryptophan. Melatonin, the sleep-promoting hormone, has been shown in studies to alleviate GERD if used over an eight-week period. Additional studies had success with L-tryptophan (the amino acid precursor to serotonin, the happiness hormone) or a combination of melatonin and L-tryptophan.[17] This may be especially helpful for people who tend to have symptoms that increase from 4:00 P.M. on, or who feel energetically sensitive and have trouble breaking down stress hormones (that is, they feel overly stressed or anxious at night). Because there are some contraindications to using these supplements (for instance, if you're taking antidepressants), we recommend that you work with a health practitioner if you're considering this option.

— Foods for prevention. While foods and drinks such as tomatoes, coffee, tea, alcohol, carbonated beverages, citrus fruits, and chocolate can trigger acid reflux, heartburn, or GERD, a whole-food diet can help, with the following being especially helpful[18]:

- Bananas
- Leafy greens
- Melons

Remember to stop eating a few hours before bedtime so that your body has a chance to digest before you lie down.

— Digestive support. Since acid reflux, heartburn, and GERD are all symptoms of an overburdened digestive system, the remedies listed in the "Overall Digestive Support" section that follows can be very helpful. If you have persistent symptoms, though, make sure your doctor rules out candida with a stool test, small intestine bacterial overgrowth (SIBO) with a breath or urine organic acid test, and *H. pylori* bacterial infection with an *H. pylori* blood-antibody test or breath test.

Overall Digestive Support

Warm Mineral Bath

This is excellent for constipation and other forms of digestive distress. In a warm bath, place ½ to 1 cup of one of the following[19]:

- Epsom salts

- Sea salt (like Celtic sea salt)

- Raw, unfiltered apple cider vinegar

- Seaweed powder

Or use one of these products, in the amount listed, in the warm bath:

- 2 cups of Premier Research Labs Medi-Soak sea minerals

- ½ cup Magnesium Oil (from Health-and-wisdom.com), with ½ cup baking soda

- 1 cup Ancient Minerals magnesium flakes (from Ancient-minerals.com)

Soak for 10 to 30 minutes in the bath, and then rub castor oil or extra-virgin olive oil on the skin of your abdomen in a clockwise motion (starting from the right side of the body and moving toward the left in a circular motion).

Castor-Oil Packs

Castor-oil packs have many benefits, including: alleviation of constipation, arthritis, and lower-back pain; and cleansing the liver, kidneys, and other organs. (Learn more in the "Constipation" section earlier in the chapter.)

Digestive Enzymes

Digestive enzymes help supply your body with enzymes needed to digest protein, carbohydrates, and fats. Plant-based digestive enzymes tend to be a wonderful option to support digestion because they work well in both the stomach and intestines.[20]

We have had great results with Premier Digest by Premier Research Labs because there is a wide range of digestive enzymes and no toxic fillers. For example, Ahlea's client Marci was diagnosed with Hodgkin's lymphoma and had tumors throughout her digestive system. She had decided to do a mix of chemotherapy and natural-health protocols, and when she came to Ahlea, she was feeling very sick every time she took a prescription synthetic digestive enzyme. Ahlea switched Marci to Premier Digest and gave her a nutritional protocol that allowed Marci to feel better and save money. Marci's natural-health approach allowed her to go through chemo with no nausea or hair loss.

Probiotics

Probiotics literally means "for life," and the right supplement can help you add good bacteria and good yeast to your intestinal tract. Because of the wide use and sometimes overuse of antibiotics, researchers are exploring whether today's health problems stem from an unanticipated change in gut bugs—meaning that people's guts may have fewer good guys to help with health and digestion.

You learned about good bacteria in Chapter 3, so you know that they work hard to keep you healthy and strong. If you're experiencing immune or digestive-related disorders, probiotics are worth exploring. We tend to like the use of probiotics and have seen many of our clients benefit from them. Yet while many people have benefitted from using a probiotic supplement that has a wide range of good bacteria strains, new research is suggesting caution in their use. In cases of chronic digestive problems, it's important to talk to your practitioner, or carefully research the use of probiotics to make sure that they're right for you.

When choosing a probiotic, it may help to find one that contains a wide range of strains, is not fermented on dairy, and does not have any fillers. Custom Probiotics (CustomProbiotics.com) makes a variety of great ones, including 5-strain and 11-strain options. Another option is GutPro, which is recommended by Dr. Natasha Campbell-McBride for people with sensitive guts. (It can be ordered at: Organic3. com/gutpro.)

Improving Stomach Acid and HCl Testing

In Chapter 3, you learned about the importance of hydrochloric acid (HCl) for digestion. Produced in the stomach, HCl helps your stomach break down food and kills food-borne pathogens. If you don't have enough HCl, you can experience a variety of digestive issues, and studies have shown that it decreases with age.[21]

One easy way to check whether you have enough stomach acid is to do a test first thing in the morning, before eating or drinking. Mix ¼ teaspoon baking soda in six ounces of water and drink the whole glass. If you belch within two or three minutes, you likely have enough stomach acid; however, if you have not belched within five minutes, your stomach acid is likely low.[22] If you start belching quickly and continue belching often, you may have too much acid.

If your stomach acid tests low, you can consider the following options:

— **Drink four ounces of water with half of a fresh-squeezed lemon** about 15 minutes before eating a meal. This can boost stomach acid gently and naturally.

— **Put one tablespoon of raw, unfiltered organic apple cider vinegar** (such as those made by Bragg or Spectrum—you'll see debris floating at the bottom of the bottle) **into eight ounces of water.** Drink this about 15 minutes before eating a meal. Some people gradually add another tablespoon or two if they need more support. This is another natural, gentle way to boost stomach acid production.

— **Take digestive bitters.** Digestive or Swedish bitters have been used as a remedy in Europe for quite some time and are a natural way for stimulating HCl to aid digestion.[23] You can put ¼ teaspoon in water, or some in a spray bottle.

Most digestive bitters are made of a combination of herbs, such as: aloe, angelica root, manna, myrrh, saffron, rhubarb root, zedoary root, senna leaves, camphor, and others. We love the organic citrus bitters made by Urban Moonshine—you can get them online or in health-food stores in a glass bottle or purse-sized spray bottle. The ingredients are slightly different from Swedish bitters, and they are a little easier on the taste buds. They include: dandelion root and leaf, burdock root, orange peel, fennel seed, yellow dock root, angelica root, gentian root, and ginger root.

— **Take an HCl supplement.** The gentlest we've found is Premier HCl, by Premier Research Labs. While there are other supplements on the market, if you are very sensitive to HCl, you may get a burning reaction when you take it. We have seen the Premier HCl work gently for even the most sensitive people.

If you're uncertain about how to start, we recommend working with a health-care practitioner who can guide you. If you're not working with a practitioner, make sure to start gently, with just one capsule of HCl after each meal and build gradually. If, as you add more HCl, you begin to feel a warm burning that is uncomfortable, make sure to take one less than the amount that caused the burning. A little baking soda in water can stop the burning feeling.

Gallbladder Challenges (Including Removed Gallbladder) and Issues with Fat Digestion

At least 10 percent of adults (mostly women) have gallstones, and this number rises to 15 percent of men and 40 percent of women by the time they reach their 60s. In the U.S., gallbladder removal is one of the most frequently performed surgeries, with up to 700,000 removals per year.

Interestingly, we have heard anecdotally from countless clients that digestive symptoms return even after they've had their gallbladders removed. Too many patients are not given tips to support their bodies after their gallbladders are removed.

If you have the following symptoms after eating, you may benefit from gallbladder support: bloating, indigestion, fatigue, diarrhea, light-colored stools, trouble digesting fat, pain in the upper right side of your abdomen, sharp pain under your breastbone, pain between your shoulder blades, or pain in your right shoulder. Here are a couple of options[24]:

— **Ox bile.** This is especially important to take with meals if you have had your gallbladder removed. NutriCology brand is free of fillers and has two different strengths; start at a low dose and see how you feel. Work with a practitioner if you would like some guidance with this.

— **Bitter and sour foods.** These can aid your digestion. Some examples are dandelion greens, lemons, limes, and raw cultured vegetables (like sauerkraut) made without white vinegar. (Note that vegetables in white vinegar are typically pickled, which is different from fermentation, and white vinegar can act as an excitotoxin for sensitive individuals.)

You might also benefit from putting digestive bitters, lemon, or raw apple cider vinegar in your water (see the HCl testing section on the previous page). Raw apple cider vinegar is a fermented liquid made from apple cider that has many health benefits—it is very different from white vinegar, which is a fermented ethyl alcohol.

Cultured Vegetables

Real, raw cultured vegetables are made by shredding vegetables, mixing them in a brine, and allowing them to ferment in an airtight environment. During the fermentation process, the vegetables are broken down, making them easier to digest; the vitamins and minerals become more readily available to the body; and good bacteria form. Almost every culture in the world has a long history of using fermented foods—they provide a sour taste that's often missing these days, and are great antidotes to sugar and carbohydrate cravings.

When you first start eating cultured vegetables, you may experience some gas, which is normal as your good gut bacteria begin to repopulate in your intestines. One way to get started is to eat 1 teaspoon with your meals and build up to about ¼ to ½ cup with meals. Some people like to drink the juice that comes in the jars as well. While the majority of people experience health benefits when eating cultured vegetables, a small percentage of people cannot easily tolerate them for a variety of reasons. Listen to your body—if you can't tolerate them right away, you may find you do well with them once you improve your gut health.

You can make cultured vegetables yourself (we'll show you how in Chapter 10) or purchase them in a health-food store or online. If you do purchase them, be sure to look for those that are organic and have been fermented naturally in brine, not white vinegar. White vinegar can act as an excitotoxin; additionally, vegetables in white vinegar are often pickled and don't have the benefits of fermented vegetables. We also prefer glass jars instead of plastic bags or containers because toxins from the plastic can be leached into the cultured vegetables.

Food Combining

Food combining can be very helpful if you're experiencing gas, bloating, abdominal pain or cramps, fatigue after meals, belching, heartburn/reflux (or GERD), headaches, or any other symptoms of poor digestion that you have learned about so far. The basis of food combining is to remove stress from your digestive process by only eating together foods that digest in similar ways. Foods that require different speeds or enzymes for digestion can tax a weak digestive system, causing a wide variety of symptoms.

Food combining is particularly helpful if you're eating grains because they can be harder for a troubled small intestine to digest. Many people with digestive challenges choose to remove grains while they heal, and these folks tend to have fewer issues requiring food combining.

Here are the four basic guidelines of food combining:

1. Eat proteins with nonstarchy vegetables only. Protein foods include animal protein (meat, poultry, eggs, dairy, and fish) and plant proteins like nuts and seeds.

- *Proteins combine well with nonstarchy vegetables.* Examples are: arugula, asparagus, bell peppers, bok choy, broccoli, brussels sprouts, carrots, cauliflower, collards, cucumbers, kale, lettuce, spinach, and Swiss chard.

- *Proteins do not combine well with starches.* Examples of starches are: grains, bread, and crackers; and starchy vegetables like potatoes (white and sweet), winter squash, yams, parsnips, corn, and peas. In other words, you would not eat meat and potatoes or a hamburger with a bun. Instead, you could have meat with steamed broccoli or a hamburger on a salad or wrapped in a lettuce leaf. (We include food-combining guidelines in Part II so that you can learn more.)

2. Know that grains combine well with all—that is, starchy and non-starchy—vegetables.

3. Eat fruit alone, on an empty stomach. Fruit digests very quickly, so if you combine it with protein or carbohydrates, it can slow down in your digestive system, leading to internal fermentation and causing uncomfortable symptoms. Some people can tolerate fruit with nuts and seeds (like an apple and almond butter, for example), and these do combine well in your digestive system. However, always eat melons alone because they digest the fastest of all fruits and tend to combine poorly with other foods.

4. You can eat fats and oils with anything, except fruit. Check Chapter 5 for the healthiest options to choose for fats and oils.

Noteworthy Supplements for Overall Health

CoQ_{10}

Also known as ubiquinol or coenzyme Q_{10}, CoQ_{10} is an antioxidant found in every cell of the body. It's useful for improved immunity and energy and has properties that benefit the heart, muscles, and organs. CoQ_{10} is found abundantly in beef; sardines; and organ meats such as heart, liver, and kidney. Many people supplement with CoQ_{10} in recovery from chronic illness, cancer, or chronic fatigue.[25] Premier Research Labs is a great brand for pure CoQ_{10} supplements.

Vitamin C

Many people turn to vitamin C to support their health for colds and flu. However, it is an antioxidant vitamin with even more health benefits, including: the formation of collagen (the basis of connective tissue found in skin, bones, teeth, joint linings, and cartilage); support for the immune system, thyroid, and adrenals; aiding in cholesterol metabolism; and helping to burn fat.[26]

Keep in mind that ascorbic acid is only a part of the more important whole-food vitamin C molecule, and we recommend avoiding ascorbic acid in your supplements because research is showing that it may have adverse health effects. Instead, choose a whole-food form of vitamin C, such as rose hips, camu camu, or Innate Response Formula's Vitamin C-400.

Vitamin B_{12} and B Complex

B-complex vitamins include: thiamine (B_1), riboflavin (B_2), niacin (B_3), pantothenic acid (B_5), pyridoxine (B_6), biotin (B_7), folate, and vitamin B_{12}. You already learned about vitamin B_{12} (the "master key" vitamin) and how it helps almost every organ and system in the body. B-complex vitamins are helpful as a whole because they support moods, brain health, energy, and digestion. They dissolve in water, so excess is excreted in urine.[27] Make sure to look for a B-complex supplement that has the active forms of vitamin B_{12} (methylcobalamin and adenosylcobalamin) and folate (L-5-methyltetrahydrofolate or 5-mthf). Avoid folic acid, the synthetic form of folate, in supplements because over 40 percent of the population can't break it down, and it can become toxic to the body.

Triphala

Triphala is one of the most popular remedies used in Ayurvedic medicine, an ancient system of health and healing originated in India. Made of three fruits, *harada, amla,* and *bihara,* triphala is gentle, non-habit forming and has a wide range of benefits, including: helps tone and cleanse the bowel, improves overall digestion, reduces serum cholesterol, improves liver function, has heart- and eye-protective properties, and is antiviral and anti-inflammatory.[28] You can find organic triphala in powder form for use in teas or in capsule form at: MountainRoseHerbs.com. Organic India and Ayush Herbs brands can also be purchased online, at: OrganicIndia.com and Ayush.com.

Magnesium

In Chapter 3, you learned that researchers refer to vitamin B_{12} as the master-key vitamin when it comes to health and healing. We like to think of magnesium as the master-key *mineral.* Depending on which studies you read, magnesium is responsible for between 300 and 800 enzyme-driven processes in the body, such as[29]:

- Activates muscles and nerves
- Aids digestion
- Boosts moods (including reducing depression and anxiety)
- Can prevent blood clots
- Creates energy
- Helps with detoxification, including heavy metals
- May prevent or eliminate GERD/heartburn/reflux
- Protects bones and teeth
- Relieves headaches and migraines
- Prevents premenstrual syndrome (PMS)
- Promotes better sleep and may alleviate sleep apnea
- Supports kidney, bladder, bowel, and liver health

Magnesium is so important for so many functions of the body that you're likely to see it listed as a remedy for a wide range of health issues.

Magnesium: The "Master Key" Mineral

According to Dr. Carolyn Dean, author of *The Magnesium Miracle,* an estimated 80 percent of Americans are deficient in magnesium. This is no surprise when you learn that the mineral is burned big-time when you're under stress. The more stressed you are, the more magnesium you're likely to need.

Here are some important facts from Dr. Dean[30]:

— Magnesium is farmed out of the soil much more than calcium. As Dr. Dean explains, "A hundred years ago, we enjoyed a diet high in magnesium with a daily intake of 500 milligrams of magnesium in an ordinary diet. Today we are lucky to get 200 milligrams."

— People do need to supplement with magnesium. After all, two out of three Americans do not consume the Recommended Dietary Intake (RDI) for magnesium, which is 500 milligrams per day.

— Calcium has been touted as an important mineral to take regularly; however, many experts are backing off of that recommendation because new information is showing that we get enough calcium from food. These days, without supplementation, the standard diet is too low in magnesium and too high in calcium, making the amount of calcium ten times that of magnesium. This can contribute to a lot of health problems. Too much calcium with too little magnesium can lead to: arthritis, kidney stones, osteoporosis, hardened arteries, and heart disease.

— Vitamin D requires magnesium to be metabolized, so if you're taking a high dose of vitamin D and you're magnesium deficient, you could be putting your body into an even greater deficiency.

The following chart reveals the stages of magnesium deficiency, with stage 1 showing mild magnesium-deficiency symptoms, to stage 4, which shows life-threatening magnesium-deficiency symptoms. Circling any symptoms you have that appear on this chart can show you how serious a magnesium deficiency you may have. The good news is that once you're aware of this, there are steps you can take to replenish your body with magnesium.

Symptoms of the Stages of Magnesium Deficiency*

Stage 1: Mild Daily Challenge	Stage 2: Greater Daily Challenge	Stage 3: Severe Daily Symptoms	Stage 4: Life-Threatening Challenge
Fatigue	Anxiety & panic attacks	Arteriosclerosis	Alcoholism
Constipation	Arthritis	Blood clots	ALS (Lou Gehrig's disease)
Dizziness (vertigo)	Asthma	Bowel disease	Alzheimer's
Dysmenorrhea (excessive menstrual pain)	Attention Deficit Disorder	Calcified mitral valve (mitral valve prolapse)	Cancer (breast, colon, prostate)
Facial twitches	Backache, upper back: excess cortisol	CFS/ME (Chronic Fatigue Syndrome / Myalgic Encephalomyelitis)	Cardiac afibrillation
Food cravings (especially sugar, caffeine, simple carbs)	Backache, lower back: emotional	Celiac disease	Congestive heart failure
Headaches	Cystitis	Cerebral palsy	Eclampsia
Heart palpitations	Ear infections	Chronic kidney disease	Emphysema (COPD)
Hiccups	Gluten sensitivity	Concussion	Myocardial infarction
Hyperglycemia	Hyperlipidemia (high cholesterol, triglycerides)	Depression	Obesity
Hypoglycemia	Hypertension	Diabetes	Parkinson's disease
Irritability	Insomnia	Epilepsy/seizures	Renal failure
Loss of appetite	Insulin resistance (pre-diabetes)	Endothelial dysfunction (dysfunction of lining of blood vessels)	SIDS
Mood swings	Migraines	Failure to thrive	Starvation

*Chart reprinted with permission from Morley Robbins: GotMag.Org/magnesium-deficiency-101

Stage 1: Mild Daily Challenge	Stage 2: Greater Daily Challenge	Stage 3: Severe Daily Symptoms	Stage 4: Life-Threatening Challenge
Muscle cramps, spasms	Multiple pregnancies (exacerbates magnesium deficiency)	Heart arrhythmias	Stroke
Nausea	Nerve problems	Hormonal imbalance	Sudden cardiac death
Nervousness	Obesity	Hyperparathyroid	Ventricular fibrillation
Poor memory / concentration	Osteopenia (precursor to osteoporosis)	Hypothyroid	
Pregnancy (exacerbates magnesium deficiency)	PMS	Kidney disease	
Raynaud's syndrome	Poor concentration	Liver disease	
Weakness	Pre-diabetes; insulin resistance	Metabolic syndrome	
	Sinusitis	Miscarriage	
	TMJ disorder	Mitral valve prolapse (calcified mitral valve)	
	Weight gain (especially on waist)	Multiple sclerosis	
		Obesity, severe	
		Osteoporosis	

How to Get Your Magnesium Levels Tested

There are a couple of options for this. Given that it's important to look at your entire mineral status, we suggest you start by getting a hair mineral test. We highly recommend getting hair tissue mineral analysis (HTMA) from Morley Robbins at: GotMag.org. We have all had consults with Morley, who is known as the "Magnesium Man," and find him to be incredibly knowledgeable about how mineral imbalances create health conditions and how to correct it. We love that when Morley met with Louise months after she turned 87, he said that her mineral status was better than people half her age, and it was a testament to how she took loving care of herself with thoughts and food.

Another helpful test is a MagRBC test, which is a blood test to check your magnesium levels. If you get your HTMA first, Morley will let you know if this test is necessary for additional diagnostics. If you do want to get a MagRBC test, you can ask your doctor, or order online at: Requestatest.com and have your blood drawn in your local area (you will be able to choose a local lab from a list when purchasing your blood test).

How to Choose the Right Form of Magnesium for You

Morley Robbins suggests that you work with a wide range of magnesium, but remember to listen to your body when it comes to choosing the right form for you. The following chart, which we created with information from Morley, shows different forms of magnesium that might work for you.

Type of Magnesium	Typically Best For
Magnesium citrate or lactate	Intestines. Some people do very well on this and others do not. Magnesium citrate often comes in powder form and can be mixed into hot water or tea. Two popular brands are Natural Calm and NOW Magnesium Citrate (Pure Powder). Magnesium citrate has a laxative effect, so you don't need much, and while it works for many, it does not work for everyone.
Magnesium glycinate	This is a chelated form of magnesium that many believe is the most bioavailable and does not cause loose bowels. Be aware that in some sensitive individuals, this form of magnesium can convert to glutamate or oxalates. If you have an adverse reaction to magnesium glycinate, switch to another form.

Type of Magnesium	Typically Best For
Magnesium malate Magnesium taurate	According to magnesium expert Morley Robbins, these forms of magnesium are best for the heart.
Sea minerals that include magnesium—this gives you a natural, balanced form of magnesium, along with a broad spectrum of minerals	Morley Robbins and his colleagues have found that a supplement with a wide base of minerals and magnesium has prompted some of the best healing responses in people. His favorites are: Anderson's Concentrated Mineral Drops (also called Anderson's CMD) from Andersonscmd.com, and South Sea Minerals (Ocean Pure) from SeaMinerals.com
Magnesium orotate	Low doses have been found to be helpful in cases of multiple sclerosis (MS), mood disorders, alcoholism, radiation effects, and cancer.[31]
Milk of magnesia	If you feel you must use Tums, Morley Robbins suggests using milk of magnesia instead. He says you can get the same results without creating a magnesium deficiency from the calcium in Tums. The calcium-to-magnesium ratio in Tums is much too high at 300:1. Make sure to choose a brand of milk of magnesia that has only magnesium hydroxide and filtered water as ingredients, such as Good Sense brand original flavor, from Vitacost.com.
Magnesium oil	Magnesium oil is magnesium chloride in water, so it's not really oily. You spray this on your skin and rub it in. Because it is absorbed through the skin and does not need to go through the digestive system, it can be very effective for people with challenged digestive systems. Most people rub this on their feet. Ancient Minerals brand is respected by many experts, and you can purchase it online at Amazon.com and other vendors.

Type of Magnesium	Typically Best For
Magnesium bath flakes or Epsom salts	Magnesium bath flakes (magnesium chloride) are another good way to get magnesium in through your skin. You can use them for foot baths and full-body baths. Ancient Minerals is a respected brand that you can purchase online at: Ancient-minerals.com. Some people do well with Epsom salts for baths or foot baths. These are more affordable and work well for many people. However, if you are sensitive to sulfur or sulfates, Epsom salts may not be for you. Listen to your body. You can get Epsom salts in the grocery store, a health-food store, or online.
Avoid: Magnesium glutamate, magnesium aspartate, or chelated magnesium (e.g., magnesium with amino-acid chelates or magnesium chelate)	Dr. Carolyn Dean warns her readers not to take these forms of magnesium because they can act as excitotoxins and have adverse health reactions.[32] See Chapter 5 for more about excitotoxins.

Magnesium Contraindications

If you have kidney failure, bowel obstruction, heart blockage, or myasthenia gravis, do not take magnesium. Additionally, if you are on heart medication, talk to your doctor first before taking this mineral because it may reduce the need for your medication, and you'll want your doctor to help you track this.[33] Additionally, you may need to create a plan with your doctor for how much time to wait between taking your heart or blood-pressure medication and your magnesium.

How to Work with Herbs and Spices

Herbs and spices, chock-full of anti-oxidants and healing properties, can be wonderful healing tools in the kitchen. Here are some ideas to work with them:

— **Add fresh herbs to salads, smoothies, or cooked meals.** Herbs can be purchased fresh or dried. If you want the benefits of fresh herbs, you will find that many are included in the meals in our recipes section. Dried herbs and spices are also wonderful for your health, and you will find recipes for using these, too.

— **Heat dried herbs and spices in a healthy fat or oil first.** Gently heating your dried herbs and spices in a skillet with a healthy animal fat or coconut oil is a great way to release their aromatic taste and medicinal benefits. If a recipe calls for herbs and/or spices, heat them gently in a skillet for a few minutes and then continue with the steps in your recipe. As you get more comfortable with cooking, you might choose herbs and spices you want to work with for their health benefits and substitute those for the spices in a recipe. In general, the green herbs (rosemary, thyme, basil, parsley, and sage) are great for savory dishes; and spices like cinnamon, cardamom, ginger, cloves, allspice, and nutmeg are great for sweet dishes (although they can be used in curries and other delicious savory Indian recipes, too).

— **Sprinkle on and in foods.** Add fresh herbs or dried herbs and spices to soups, stews, salads or salad dressings, eggs, meat, fish, poultry, and any other foods you have already cooked. While they are best used during the cooking process, you can benefit from sprinkling them on for added flavor and medicinal benefits after cooking as well. You can even make a healthy popcorn with organic air-popped popcorn topped with melted coconut oil or raw butter and your favorite spices. Try fennel, fenugreek, sea salt and pepper, or turmeric and sea salt.

— **Make teas.** You can make your own healing teas with your chosen herbs (fresh or dried) and spices. The easiest way to do this is to purchase empty tea bags or re-usable organic muslin tea bags. It may be more convenient to make a quart of tea at a time and store it in a glass jar in your refrigerator. You can get quart jars very inexpensively at most supermarkets. You will use 4–8 tablespoons of herb/spice per quart (or 1–2 tablespoons per cup of water). Boil water and pour it into your glass jar, allowing your tea bag to steep in the water for 30–60 minutes. Remove the tea bag and store excess in the refrigerator. Reheat the tea or drink it room temperature or cold, if you like iced tea.

— **Chew seeds.** In India, Germany, and other cultures, people have been chewing seed spices, like fennel or caraway to aid digestion and reduce bloating, anise seed to freshen breath, and cardamom pods to stop cravings and freshen breath.

More Home Remedies to Love Your Body to Good Health

Health Condition	Remedies
Cravings	• Whole-food diet as a way of life (see suggestions for cravings in Chapter 5) • Sour foods (like cultured vegetables) • Bitter foods (dandelion greens, arugula, digestive bitters) • Spices—cardamom (sweet cravings), cloves and cinnamon (blood-sugar balance), turmeric (salty food cravings) • Magnesium • L-tryptophan (amino acid) when cravings are related to depression, worry, anxiety, SAD (seasonal affective disorder), or low self-esteem. Capsules come in 500 mg, so start there. Some people benefit with up to 1,000 mg. Do not take this if you are on anti-depressants, or talk with your doctor first. Pure Encapsulations has a pure form of L-tryptophan. • GABA (gamma-aminobutyric acid) for stress-related cravings or overwork/overwhelm-related cravings. Consider 100–500 mg. You can get this online or in a health-food store in pure powder form with no fillers. Source Naturals brand is an example. • Talk to your doctor or health practitioner about the amino acids: L-tyrosine (if you really need caffeine or have cravings related to needing an energy boost or lack of drive) or DL-phenylalanine (if you have cravings related to emotional pain or feel you need comfort or reward food). Both of these have contra-indications and are energizing, so it's important to know whether they will work for you before taking them. (Learn more by reading *The Mood Cure* by Julia Ross.) • 5-HTP—50 mg can help with evening cravings. This may not be suitable for long-term use. • See recipes section for more ideas on meals that support various cravings.

Health Condition	Remedies
Cholesterol Problems	• Shiitake mushrooms (you can purchase them in the produce aisle at your health-food store or take the medicinal shiitake mushroom supplement in capsule form) • Herbs and spices—basil, cinnamon, coriander, curry leaf, fenugreek seed, garlic, ginger, horseradish, oregano, lemongrass, mustard seed, turmeric • Seeds—pumpkin seeds (especially Styrian) and sesame seeds (make sure to soak them first; see Chapter 5 to learn how). • Triphala • Magnesium • Oil of oregano. (Premier Research Labs Oregano Oil or Olive Leaf Immune capsules are great options. Another option is Oregulin, from North American Herb and Spice: NorthAmericanHerbandSpice.com. Oregulin is an extract with a combination of oregano oil, cinnamon, fenugreek, cumin, and myrtle, giving you a nice dose of oregano oil and spices that aid with cholesterol and digestion.)
Headaches or Migraines	• Ginger • Peppermint essential oil (use a carrier oil, like almond oil or jojoba oil and rub onto the area of tension or rub on your belly) • Magnesium • Ice pack on your neck or head and hot-water bottle at your feet • Feverfew—studies have shown that 50–100 mg daily was successful with migraine headaches.[34] (MountainRoseHerbs.com carries an organic herbal extract of feverfew.)

Health Condition	Remedies
Insomnia, Sleep Apnea, and Sleep Problems	• Magnesium • Herbs and spices—coriander, lemongrass, saffron • B-complex vitamins • L-tryptophan, 5-HTP, or GABA (see the sections on cravings and moods to learn more about these supplements that also help with sleep). If you decide to take GABA, you may want to look into a supplement called ZenMind by Nutricology brand that has a combination of the amino acids GABA and L-theanine (a calming amino acid that is found in green tea). • Calming practices like meditation, deep breathing, and yoga are stellar ways to de-stress and allow your body to move into parasympathetic nervous system mode, necessary for good sleep.
Joint Pain and Arthritis	• Magnesium (several forms work; see information on magnesium oil in the previous section on magnesium, as it can be useful for spot-pain relief) • Medicinal mushrooms in capsule form, as tea, or add a teaspoon of powder to a smoothie—reishi, cordyceps. Paul Stamets, mycologist and author of *Growing Gourmet & Medicinal Mushrooms*, sells organic medicinal mushrooms online at: Fungi.com. • Herbs and spices—bay leaf, celery seed, fennel seed, ginger, rosemary, turmeric
Moods	• B-complex vitamins • L-tryptophan (amino acid)—see cravings section for more on L-tryptophan • 5-HTP—50 mg can help with mood[35] • Saint-John's-Wort—300 mg (you can find this in tincture form)[36] • Magnesium (depression, anxiety, irritability) • Herbs and spices for depression—black pepper, nutmeg, rosemary, saffron (also for PMS) • Herbs and spices for anxiety—lemongrass, mint, nutmeg, rosemary, sage, saffron

Health Condition	Remedies
Lack of Energy	• Green tea (switch from coffee to green tea or take the extract form, like Premier Research Labs Green Tea-ND) • L-tyrosine • B-complex vitamins • Herbs and spices for mental fatigue—saffron extract, sage • Herbs and spices for physical fatigue—pomegranate • CoQ$_{10}$ (see previous "Noteworthy Supplements for Overall Health" section)
Immune Deficiency	• Green tea (switch from coffee to green tea or take the extract form, like Premier Research Labs Green Tea-ND) • Magnesium • B-complex vitamins • Herbs and spices—almost all herbs and spices will support your immune system because they are rich in antioxidants. Some key players are: cinnamon, cloves, fenugreek seed, garlic, ginger, horseradish, oregano, parsley, rosemary, saffron, thyme, and turmeric.[37] • CoQ$_{10}$ (see previous "Noteworthy Supplements for Overall Health" section) • Medicinal mushrooms in capsule form, as tea or add a teaspoon of powder to a smoothie—reishi, cordyceps, maitake, agarikon, and shiitake. Paul Stamets, mycologist and author of *Growing Gourmet & Medicinal Mushrooms*, sells organic medicinal mushrooms online at: Fungi.com.

Love Your Body, Love Yourself

Finding natural remedies that work for you can be an exciting adventure if you embrace the joy of learning what supports you in feeling your best. The feeling of being healthy and well, balanced and joyful, is your natural state. The remedies in this chapter can coax your body gently back into your natural state of health. It's a beautiful act of self-love to listen to your body and give it what it needs!

Before we move on to the next chapter, take a moment just for you. Put one hand on the center of your chest and the other hand on your abdomen and say the following affirmations:

> *Every morning, I remind myself that I can make the choice to feel good.*
> *I love my body, and health is my natural state. I am always able to*
> *make the correct decision. I recognize my own intuitive ability.*

Now let's wrap up the first part of the book by giving you a road map to help lead you to your best health.

♥ ♥

Chapter 7

Step #7:
The Road Map for
Your Best Health

Take three deep breaths. As you exhale, let everything go . . . let go of every thought and idea about where you are right now. Let every symptom fall away, just for this moment. Imagine that you're a clean slate, starting fresh and new. Imagine yourself healthy, happy, and light. Remember, your body believes your mind, and with this practice, you're creating your best health.

Your future well-being is created in each moment with every thought you think, and the good news is that you get to choose your thoughts. It may not always feel easy, though. Change can feel scary because it's unknown territory, and your brain often fears what you don't know.

Here's the real secret: underneath all of the "problems" you carry around is just one belief: *I am not good enough.* When you believe you're not good enough, there's a kind of giving up that happens—a *Why bother?* attitude. It's easy to assume that things won't work out anyway.

The truth is that you *are* good enough. Now, what if you truly believed that? Resting on this one belief, you could start to change every other thought that is limiting your health and happiness. Resting on this one belief, you could start to change the thoughts that are no lon-

> "To create your best health, start with every thought you think and every bite you eat."
>
> — Louise

ger serving you. And as your limiting thoughts, beliefs, and habits dissolve, your health and happiness can blossom. As Lao-tzu, the father of Taoism, once said: "When I let go of what I am, I become what I might be."

In Taoism, an ancient philosophy about the way to live in balance with the universe, order and harmony is realized when humans align with nature.[1] To align with nature, we cannot force things to happen; we must allow them. Think of a seed, for example: It starts in a dormant state, small and dry. Inside it is enough information to grow a whole plant, but it needs tender loving care to do so. A seed needs to sit in a foundation of nutrient-rich soil, with enough sunlight and water to realize its growth potential as a plant. While sciencists have studied and documented seed growth, there is still much of this process that is a mystery to them. Indeed, this mystery of growth is fascinating to us all. And it is something we can never rush or try to find a shortcut for.

One of the most fascinating things about plants is that once they grow, they become the basis for nourishment and healing for all beings on the planet. Here's what Gary L. Wenk, a leading authority on brain health, has to say about plants in his book, *Your Brain on Food: How Chemicals Control Your Thoughts and Feelings:*

> How is it possible that plants and humans use such similar chemicals for normal, everyday functions? Plants produce chemicals that are capable of affecting our brain because they share an evolutionary history with us on this planet. Even primitive one-celled organisms produce many of the same chemicals that are in our brains. Therefore, whether you choose to eat a bunch of broccoli or a large pile of amoeba, the chemicals they contain may alter how your neurons function and, therefore, how you feel or think.

Nature has given us everything we need to be healthy and happy. When we nourish ourselves with natural foods, we are aligning ourselves with nature and creating balance. We humans lost our way a bit when we embraced science with more zeal than we did nature. Illness and dis-ease do not happen because of some uncontrollable force. They happen because we are being invited, by our bodies, to come back to nature. To natural food that grows with the goal to nourish us all. To thoughts and beliefs that allow us, like the dormant seed, to blossom into our best selves. We are being invited to step out of practices that create stress and overwhelm, and settle into a lifestyle that gives us the nutrients we need to feel happy, energized, and strong.

In order to find a space where you have the nourishment you need to heal, you may be asked to slow down and honor your humanness—to find a pace that feels soothing and nurturing, and to eat, sleep, move, and think in ways that allow you to blossom.

If You Experience a Health Challenge, Life Is Inviting You to Love Yourself

In a society that has forgotten the healing qualities of nature, we can sometimes be swept up in stress and worry. It happens to all of us as we focus on putting food on the table, caring for our loved ones, and making ends meet. The thing is, the more we step away from nature, the more we step away from ourselves as human beings.

We begin to think and feel like we're machines, capable of running nonstop to fulfill a to-do list, and we forget to honor ourselves. We think that if we're human or not perfect, we're not good enough, not worthy of love or acceptance. This is where things start to go wrong. This is where we rush through life, living and eating on the run—where we forget to love ourselves. Illness and dis-ease occur to remind us to come back to loving ourselves. Beneath all of the fears, doubts, and worry, we are encoded with the answers to blossom like the seed, if only we stop and listen.

As you learn to trust Life, love yourself, and listen to your body, you can come back into balance with what is natural for you. And you can build a life that nourishes and supports your health and happiness.

Every chapter in this book provides solutions to support you in doing this. Remember, it starts with learning to accept and love yourself. This is the rich soil in which everything can grow. From this place, you can begin to create habits that support you in blossoming.

Here is a summary of the 7 Steps to Eat, Think, and Love Yourself to Great Health:

— Step #1 is about **creating a new perspective on health.** Start the process of accepting and loving yourself—the mirror work and affirmations in Chapter 1 can support you in doing so. If change feels scary or uncomfortable, go back to the exercises in that chapter that focus on how to more easily move through change.

— Step #2 is about **loving yourself and your body.** The vision exercise at the end of Chapter 2 is a great way to create the blueprint for how you want your life and health to be. This is a powerful way to get clear about your goals and set yourself up for creating loving habits.

— Step #3 reminds you **how your body works** and why it needs nourishment from natural, whole foods in order to feel your best. Go back and look at why it's important to fuel your body well, so that your blood-sugar levels are strong and you have the willpower you need to stick to your new, healthy habits. Remember that what goes in your gut affects your brain, including your moods, memory, quality of sleep, and decision making.

— Step #4 teaches you to **listen to your body.** Experts are fantastic, but the rubber meets the road deep inside your body. How you feel and what you're being guided to do is just as (or more!) important as the guidance you get from others. Practice listening to your body and notice how much easier it is to trust yourself and to trust Life.

— Step #5 is about **choosing thoughts and food that heal your body and mind.** This is where you learn how to truly nourish yourself. Choosing healthy, whole foods may take some planning and adjustment, so give yourself the time and go at the pace that works for you. This is not about doing it all at once or becoming overwhelmed; rather, it's about taking baby steps and trusting that each step brings beautiful rewards. The exercise at the end of Chapter 5 will support you in making these changes.

— Step #6 is about **taking time to love your body with natural home remedies** for any physical or emotional symptom you experience. Any change you make—be it with food or lifestyle—tends to shake things up, and symptoms may show up as you let go of what is no longer serving you. This is a natural part of any cleansing or transformation process, and it sometimes causes people to retreat back into old habits. Instead, we provide you with natural remedies to support your body through this transition and any other transition you have in the future. Remember to see symptoms as signs—a language your body uses to communicate with you. Use these signs to listen to your body and take loving actions to move in the direction that Life wants you to move. The remedies in Chapter 6 can help soothe your body as symptoms arise.

— Step #7 is about **taking action to lovingly nourish your body.** In the next section, you will be provided with some ideas to take one step at a time and go at your own pace. Keep in mind that small steps can bring big rewards!

Now What? Taking Action to Lovingly Nourish Your Body

We invite you to begin gently on this journey of eating healthy, whole foods. Here is an outline to help you take the next steps:

Choose a Place to Get Started

— If you're brand-new to eating whole foods, start simply by adding one of the options below to your daily routine. It's up to you whether you want to use that option to replace a meal, add to a meal, or eat as a snack. This simple step will allow your body and taste buds to slowly adjust to a new way of eating. (Note that all recipes for these three food options are in Chapter 10.)

- **Bone broth.** This is particularly good for an energizing coffee replacement or a nourishing midafternoon snack; or as an addition to your breakfast, lunch, or dinner meal. Bone broth can be kept in a stainless-steel Thermos for a nice warm treat during your commute or workday.

- **Green smoothie.** This makes an ideal breakfast, but you can have one any time of day! You can often get a full day's serving of vegetables in a smoothie or two.

- **Blended soup.** Blended soups are like thick broths and so easy to digest—they're very healing and cleansing and can even boost your mood! These soups can make a great meal or snack, and eating soup for breakfast is a nice way to get vegetables into that meal.

— If you're used to eating whole foods and want to dive a little deeper, but perhaps you're busy and end up eating convenience foods more than you'd like, we have a solution for you. Chapter 10 is chock-full of meals that are fast and easy to make. Choose one new recipe and replace one of your convenience- or fast-food meals with this healthier option. Or perhaps you're pretty good with meals, but need snack or dessert options. That's a great place to start, too!

— If you have already jumped with both feet into a whole-foods way of eating, you may want to dive even deeper. Hooray! Again, the recipes in Chapter 10 will be very beneficial for you. Since you're likely used to making a lot of healthy meals already, choose the ones that appeal to you and start there, or follow the sample menus we've provided in Chapter 9 for inspiration.

Continue Your New Habits

— Part II contains a sample menu; a shopping list; and recipes for meals, snacks, beverages, and desserts. Have fun with these new recipes! No matter what you're shopping for, the Master Shopping List of foods to emphasize and those to avoid can help you at the grocery store. Make a copy of the list and take it with you, and you'll be a label-reading wizard!

— Have *fun* in the kitchen! Some people love to cook—if you have friends or family members who do, invite them over to cook with you. Everyone can contribute ingredients, and you can make delicious foods that each person can take home. If you make a lot, you can store it in the freezer for easy thawing later on. Ahlea has her toddler prepare foods with her, and he loves to help! Louise, Heather, and Ahlea often organize kitchen days together or with other friends to make meals or learn new recipes. These experiences have brought great laughter, bonding, and new skills to everyone involved. Magic happens when friends gather in the kitchen.

Heather and her husband also started having culinary date nights, where they'd pick a type of food and learn to make it together. While this is a popular activity at cooking schools, you can also do this at home with free YouTube videos or other online resources. Whether you plan this with a loved one or several friends, it can be a great way to make healthy food preparation fun!

— Continue to listen to your body! Remember how wonderful it feels to have a friend or loved one just listen to you with no judgment? And how incredible it is to feel loved and accepted? You are the only one who knows what you need the most. Listen to your thoughts, and listen to your body. The more you do, the more you'll understand what you need.

Along the way, continue to encourage yourself with mirror work and affirmations. You are tilling the soil you live in—creating a rich, fertile place so that you can blossom. This is how you love yourself. This is how you give yourself what you need to grow into your best self.

This Is Your Greatest Love Story

In this, your greatest love story, we invite you to love yourself a little more each day. That is the first place to start. Small, simple acts of love can go a long way toward creating habits that sustain your health for a lifetime.

You are not in a race with the people around you. No, this is your opportunity to write your love story *your own way.* To go at the pace that feels good to you. To listen to your body when it's time to take action or when it's time to rest. Nature teaches us to plant a seed, nourish it, and allow it to grow at its own pace, and this is what we invite you to do.

♥

We'd like to close Part I of this book with an affirmation treatment for your greatest love story. To get started, place one hand on the center of your chest and the other on your abdomen. Breathe deeply, in and out, and say the following words:

This is my love story. I only choose thoughts that create a wonderful future, and I move into it now. My heart is opening wider and wider. Love flows from and to me in ever-increasing amounts. Unconditional love and acceptance are the greatest gifts I can give and receive—and I give them to myself now. I am learning the secrets of Life. It is actually all very simple: The more I love myself, the more I feel Life loving me. The more I love myself, the healthier I am. The more I love myself, the more enjoyable my life gets.

I give myself the green light to go ahead, and I joyously embrace my new, loving habits of food and thoughts. The more I nourish myself, the more I am grateful to be alive. It is my joy and pleasure to live another wonderful day. Every person on this planet is interconnected with love, and it starts with me loving myself. I send loving thoughts to all. Love and forgiveness heals me and it heals us all. My life is balanced, and my immunity is strong. I am healthy, whole, and healed. I love Life, and Life loves me.

And so it is!

♥ ♥

PART II

I Love My Kitchen— How to Create Delicious, Healthy Meals

Chapter 8

Getting Started in the Kitchen

Having the right tools in your kitchen can make a big difference when it comes to making food preparation fun and easy. The key is to start with the basics and add more as you see a need. In this chapter, we'll share with you what we use and the brands we feel are worth the money. Of course, we want you to feel comfortable in your kitchen, so please use what works best for you.

If you're on a budget, know that there are many ways to get kitchen equipment affordably: thrift shops, eBay, Costco, garage sales, and swaps are all wonderful opportunities to treasure hunt for the most coveted kitchen gadgets.

The Basics for Every Kitchen

- **Cutting board.** (There are many affordable bamboo cutting boards available online and in kitchen stores.)

- **Peeler**—removes vegetable and fruit peels with ease.

- **Chef's knife.** If you only have one knife, this is the one to choose. It tends to be one of the most-used knives in any kitchen, and it's great for chopping fruits and vegetables.

- **Paring/boning knife**—to remove meat from bones or do detailed cutting work.

- **Stainless-steel or glass bowls** with airtight plastic lids, so you can prepare food and store it in your refrigerator.

- **Ball jars.** These are a great low-cost option for storing food or making cultured vegetables. We especially like the quart-sized wide-mouth jars. You can usually find these by the dozen in grocery stores. Alternatively, you could save glass jars from nut butters, raw cultured vegetables, and other foods and reuse.

The Stars: Helpful Kitchen Equipment We Use Daily

— **Food processor.** Your food processor can save you a lot of time. In fact, ours are the most-used pieces of equipment in our kitchens because they slice, dice, puree, and julienne in seconds. We have had good luck with our KitchenAid and Cuisinart brands.

— **Excalibur dehydrator.** Cookies, crackers, and snacks can be made in a food dehydrator and it's extra nice for people who don't want to watch over an oven, as there's no worry about things burning in a dehydrator. The nine-tray Excalibur food dehydrator is helpful if you have a family, or if you want to make a lot of snacks at once that you can then store in your refrigerator or freezer. There are also four- and five-tray options for smaller kitchens.

— **Vitamix blender.** Louise makes the best smoothies in her Vitamix each day. This is a high-speed blender that does more than an average blender and is worth the extra price. It is a workhorse that grinds nuts, seeds, herbs, and spices and also makes nut butters, smoothies, and soups. Look for deals on eBay or at Costco. You may even find one at a garage sale, like some lucky people we know.

— **Slow cooker.** Each of us has bone broths, soups, and dinners cooking daily in our slow cookers. They make life really easy and do all the heavy lifting of cooking with no worries about burning a meal. Heather swears by her Crock-Pot with a timer, which has lasted for more than a decade. It allows four-, six-, eight-, and ten-hour timed cooking options and goes automatically to warm once it's done. (The most handy slow cookers will have a timer feature like this.)

Be aware that there are some concerns that ceramic slow cookers may leach lead into food. Many of the manufacturers, like Hamilton Beach, are aware of this and have models they deem lead-free. You can also look into other options, like Instant Pot brand's IP-DUO or IP-LUX options (which have 18/8 stainless-steel bowls and pots and can be used to slow cook like a Crock-Pot; to brown, steam, or sauté; or to pressure cook). Or go to MiriamsEarthenCookware.com and ask about a lead-free clay insert for your existing slow cooker.

Other Appliances to Consider

— **Coffee grinder**—for grinding herbs, spices, or small seeds like chia or flaxseeds.

— **Juicer.** The juicer made by Jack LaLanne is popular because it's easier to use and clean than the Champion Juicer. However, the Champion is incredibly versatile and can make smoothies, nut butters, pâtés, and other foods. Some say it's one of the best and most versatile out there (and also easy to use).

— **Braun immersion blender.** At least 400 watts is strong enough to easily make soups and pâtés. This handheld blender also comes with an attachment so you can make smoothies, which is very handy if you want to make them while you're traveling.

Kitchen Tools

Instead of running out and buying everything you think you'll need, start preparing food and see what would be most helpful to you. Many of these pieces can be purchased in thrift shops or at garage sales if you like to treasure hunt for good deals.

- **Glass or Pyrex baking dishes** (avoid aluminum and nonstick bakeware)

- **Stainless-steel colander**

- **Garlic press**

- **Box grater or fine grater** (we recommend the Microplane brand). If you have a food processor, you may not need this often, unless you want to grate whole spices, lemon peel, or other small jobs.

- **Stainless-steel measuring cups and spoons**

- **Glass or stainless-steel mixing bowls** (avoid plastic). Get a really deep one if you will be using a hand blender. It might also help to get bowls with tops to store foods after blending them up.

- **Pyrex glass bowls** with plastic airtight tops for food storage

- **Silicone baking dishes.** Silicone baking sheets have many uses: If you have a food dehydrator, they are nonstick and can replace the toxic teflex sheets that come with the dehydrator. You can use them in your oven to line a cookie sheet or bake a bread or cake as well. There are also silicone waffle sheets, cake pans, and bread-loaf pans —all of which are very easy to work with and affordable.

- **Salad spinner**—to dry lettuce and vegetables after washing.

- **Silicone rubber spatula**—to scrape those last bits of sauce, batter, oil, and other goodies off the sides of bowls, your food-processor container, pots, and pans.

- **Fine mesh strainer.** Oxo and other brands make a fine, double-mesh strainer that is very helpful for draining soaked grains that could fall through the holes of a colander.

- **Whisk**—great for mixing things to a light and fluffy consistency.

- **Stainless-steel spatula.** This is a much better alternative than using plastic with hot foods, since plastic can leach toxins into your food.

- **A good set of knives**—consisting of a 5" serrated utility knife, 8" chef's knife, paring knife, kitchen scissors, and a knife sharpener.

- **Pots and pans.** While all pots and pans have pros and cons, we end up going to 18/10 stainless steel the most. It's lighter than Le Creuset (a really great option, but heavy!), affordable, and one of the least toxic options. Good chefs know you don't have to buy fancy brands like All-Clad to get great stainless-steel pans; look for deals on Cuisinart and Winware three-ply pans and skillets. The types of pans we use most often are: a braising pan, a skillet, and a saucepan. If you don't have a Crock-Pot, you will likely want a large stockpot for making bone broths and soups.

- **Cook-and-serve stovetop ceramic pots/bowls.** These are Ahlea's favorite time saver. Heat up soup or leftovers on the stovetop, and then eat right from the same soup pot—less cleaning! Xtrema brand makes ceramic 16-ounce soup pots and sells them in sets of four.

Avoid nonstick pans, but still get easy cleanup: We recommend avoiding nonstick pans because they're coated with toxic Teflon. You can clean up stainless-steel pans and skillets very easily by cooking low and slow. Even eggs come off easily if you cook them this way (which also makes them healthier and easier to digest!), and remove the eggs and allow the pan to cool a bit so you can safely touch it. Then use some hot water, dish liquid (we use Dr. Bronner's Magic Soaps to wash dishes), and a scouring sponge to clean off the eggs. They should come off quickly and easily, especially if you didn't overcook them. If you *did* overcook the eggs or used too high a temperature when cooking, add some soapy water to the skillet, put the pan with soapy water back on your stovetop, and put the heat on medium, allowing the water to heat up. Now use your stainless-steel spatula to scrape the pan and it should come right off!

Food Storage for Trips Away from Home

There are so many wonderful options these days for taking food with you to work or on trips or for carrying healthy sea salt, spices, and condiments to restaurants. We recommend looking for stainless steel, silicone, and glass wherever possible —although there are sometimes good reasons to use plastic containers, as long as you don't use them with hot foods. Here are some of our favorites that you can find at Amazon.com or in camping stores:

— **Silicone Go-Gear travel containers.** These two- or three-ounce containers are great for carrying healthy oils or pureed snacks, like Louise's Healing Asparagus Puree.

— **Stainless-steel containers with lids.** These come in a variety of sizes, from four ounces on up. The options with plastic lids are more airtight.

— **Wide-mouth insulated "bowl" containers.** LunchBots brand makes small wide-mouth insulated 16-ounce dishes so you can store warm breakfast, lunch, or dinner meals for hours on the road without any plastic touching your food. Carry burgers, soups, stews, grains, or anything you want to enjoy warm while traveling or at work.

— **Wide-mouth soup and beverage containers.** These are great for keeping soups, bone broths, veggie broths, and teas hot. Look for a stainless-steel or glass-inner container so that no plastic is touching your food. Some brands to check out are Thermos or Nissan, and for tea or broth, Klean Kanteen.

— **Insulated lunch bag.** There are many of these on the market today, and thankfully, some stylish ones as well. Heather's favorite is the black Crew Cooler

Jr. by eBags.com because it's a professional-looking lunch bag with extra compartments for water, supplements, cutlery, and napkins.

— **Spice jars**. These are great for carrying sea salt and fresh ground pepper for meals at work or restaurants.

♥ ♥

Chapter 9

Sample Menus and Meal Options

The options in this chapter have been created to show how some simple, healthy meals would look over the course of several days. Keep in mind that you may want to make extra food and eat leftovers for some of your meals. We did not account for this in the sample menus, but please feel free to do so when planning your own weekly meals. You can also freeze leftovers and heat them up at a later date.

In the beginning, you'll likely be most successful if you create a plan for as many of your meals, snacks, and desserts as possible. Making things ahead of time and even packaging them up in single-serving containers for school or work lunches can make things much easier. Be sure to set aside some time for yourself to do this. You may have to take something else off your schedule so that you can free up time for meal prep—adding it to an already-busy schedule can be overwhelming.

To keep things simple, one way to approach each week would be to plan four main dishes that you love and cook them ahead of time on a day that you have the time to do this. Many people have extra time on the weekend, so that's a good place to start. Invite friends over or cook with your family to make it fun. You can freeze meals you'll want to eat later in the week, and take them out to thaw the night before.

You may also want to wash fruits and vegetables ahead of time and even slice them up if you want. This way, you can grab snacks on the go if you're in a hurry.

About the Menus

The meal ideas and sample daily menus were set up to introduce some potentially new food habits into your routine, like vegetables for breakfast in the form of soups or smoothies.

The lunch and dinner options are interchangeable. If you're already eating meat, fish, and poultry for dinner and don't want a huge change in your routine right away, you might have the lunch meals for dinner and the dinner meals for lunch. If you're having digestive challenges, trouble sleeping, or symptoms that start or worsen at night (like abdominal pain, reflux, headaches, night sweats, and the like), consider following the menus as stated. They were designed to make the harder-to-digest meals (animal protein) at lunch, when your energy for digestion is stronger. At dinner, the meals are vegetarian so that your body will have an easier time digesting at night. On its own, this habit of eating may resolve many symptoms that start or worsen at night. (Note that the recipes mentioned can be found in the next chapter.)

Breakfast Ideas

— **Steamed apple slices and cinnamon.** Cut a green Granny Smith or Gala apple into slices and boil or steam in one cup of water. Drain the water, and sprinkle in one teaspoon of cinnamon. Eat as slices or puree into applesauce. You may want to add some coconut butter, a mixture of coconut oil and coconut meat that you can get online or in the health-food store. (Look for organic brands like Artisana and Wilderness Family Naturals.)

— **A bowl of fresh berries.** If you need a protein fat to keep your blood sugar strong, have some almonds or coconut butter with it.

— **Eggs.** For the easiest-to-digest options, try those that have been scrambled on low heat, poached, or soft-boiled.

— **Soup.** This is a great way to start eating vegetables for breakfast! Some great breakfast-soup options from our recipes chapter are: Kale Carrot Soup, Louise's Favorite Bone Broth or Veggie Broth, or Delightfully Sweet Zucchini Squash Soup.

— **Smoothies**—we have several delicious recipes in the next chapter.

— **Leftovers from yesterday's meal.** This is the true "fast food" in that you just heat it up and enjoy! Please avoid your microwave, though, as it radiates the food and decreases the nutrient value. You can get better-quality food almost as fast by heating it up in a saucepan or skillet. Or try Ahlea's favorite: little ceramic soup pots that can be heated on the stovetop and used as serving bowls to cut down on the number of dishes to clean (see Chapter 8).

— **Grain-free waffles or pancakes** with raw butter (or ghee or coconut oil) and maple syrup, honey, or berries.

— **Grain-free bread** with organic raw butter, coconut oil, or ghee. (See Chapter 10 for grain-free breads. The Gingerbread recipe makes a wonderful slightly sweet breakfast if you're used to eating doughnuts and want to change that habit.)

— **A bowl of quinoa flakes, buckwheat kashi (groats), cream of buckwheat, or gluten-free whole oats** (not quick-cooking oats). You can buy these in packages at health-food stores or online and follow the package instructions to make a breakfast that is like oatmeal. We recommend you soak the grains first (see how in the next chapter) and then follow the package instructions, reducing the amount of cooking water by ½ cup. You can make this slightly sweet or savory; or just add a little organic coconut oil, raw organic butter, or organic ghee.

— **Sweet Quinoa Bread.** Using the recipe in this book, you can also skip making this into bread and just make the pilaf and enjoy as a nice replacement to oatmeal.

— **Sweet Buckwheat Bread.** Using the recipe in this book, you can make this as a breakfast cereal instead of bread—it's similar to Cream of Wheat, only gluten-free!

Lunch or Dinner Ideas

— Chicken, turkey, lamb, or beef burgers with **Carrots and Greens Veggie Mash** and a chopped romaine lettuce salad

— **Crock-Pot Lamb Shanks** with **Green Beans and Leeks** and **Pickled Pink Cultured Vegetables**

— **Hassle-Free Fabulous Whole Chicken for Busy People** with steamed broccoli and **Celery Root Veggie Mash**

— **Magnificent Mahi Mahi Salad** with steamed zucchini and yellow squash

— **Short Ribs One-Pot Crock-Pot Meal**

— **Heavenly Haddock** and side salad or steamed chopped collards

— **Kale Carrot Soup** with **Grain-Free, Gluten-Free Rosemary Bread**

— **Thyroid Friendly Veggie Mash** with salad

— **Lovely Millet Loaf** with spring-mix salad

— **Good Luck Soup** with **Grain-Free, Gluten-Free "Rye" Bread**

— **Creamy Cream of Buckwheat** with sautéed brussels sprouts

— **Quinoa, Broccoli, and Leek Pilaf** with **Millet Pilaf—Super Thyroid Booster**

— **Outstanding Collards and Butternut Squash** with **Grain-Free, Gluten-Free Rosemary Bread**

Snack Ideas

— **Celery Basil Crackers** with **Pickled Pink Cultured Vegetables** (or purchase cultured vegetables at your local health-food store; be sure to look for real, raw cultured vegetables made in brine and not in vinegar) or **Mild Salsa**

— **Savory Beet Chips**

— **Savory Sweet Walnuts and Dates**

— **Tahini Crackers** with coconut oil or dipped in leftover **Carrots and Greens Veggie Mash**

— **Sunflower Granola Bars**

— **Almonds rolled in a piece of soft dulse.** This one needs no recipe because you just use as much dulse as you like with each almond. Dulse is a slightly salty, slightly sweet seaweed that is full of vitamins and minerals; it is wonderful for your adrenals and thyroid. You can get beyond organic soft dulse at: TheSeaweedMan.com.

— **A scoop of your favorite nut butter sprinkled with a little sea salt**

— **Apple slices with almond butter and a little sea salt**

— **Carrot and celery slices dipped in tahini and sprinkled with sea salt**

— A piece of **Grain-Free, Gluten-Free "Rye" Bread** or **Grain-Free, Gluten-Free Rosemary Bread** with coconut butter, coconut oil, raw butter, or ghee

— **Toasted nori.** There is no recipe for this, so we'll explain how to toast this tasty seaweed here. Nori seaweed is full of healthy minerals. Make sure to get it in its natural state, which is more like small strips and not in sheets—there are some who feel that nori sheets have arsenic and are best avoided. Once you've bought the nori in its natural state, place it in the oven on a cookie sheet, and bake at 200° F. The nori will get crispy and turn a slight green color. This will make it more like chips and turn it into a delicious snack! We love TheSeaweedMan.com as a source for beyond organic seaweed, including nori.

— **Real, raw green olives.** Choose a brand of cultured olives that uses real brine and not white vinegar (as we've mentioned, white vinegar acts as an excitotoxin in sensitive people and indicates a pickled product instead of a probiotic-rich fermented product). Divina brand and Essential Living Foods brand are two good options. Or try real, raw, dehydrated olives, like those made by Essential Living Foods.

Dessert Ideas

— You'll find several healthy dessert recipes in Chapter 10. As your taste buds change, you may begin to feel like you don't need a sweet dessert. A scoop of almond butter or tahini sprinkled with a little sea salt might be perfect for you, or perhaps some almonds with soft dulse seaweed will feel like dessert.

— An easy type of "fast food" dessert is to store some dates in your freezer, so you have them if you want the sweet taste, but don't have any prepared desserts on hand. One date may be all you need. Some people find even one date too sweet and like to combine it with some almond butter or tahini and a little sea salt. Another idea is to eat the date with a handful of almonds, walnuts, or macadamia nuts with sea salt.

Sample Menus for Five Days

These sample menus are designed to show you what all of your meals could look like over the course of five days. Keep in mind that they feature a variety of daily scenarios; in reality, you may decide you want to eat leftovers because it's a fast way to enjoy healthy eating. The easiest thing to do when you make a meal is to prepare extra and either eat the leftovers for various meals throughout the week, or freeze them and then thaw and heat when you want a fast meal.

If you don't mind eating the same meal for two or three days in a row, it can be nice to just grab something from the refrigerator and heat it up! To give yourself variety, though, you could change up the side dish (see the next chapter for fast options) or have a meal you originally made for lunch as a dinner or breakfast meal instead.

When it comes to desserts and snacks, you'll likely make one or two recipes at a time and either freeze or refrigerate them so that you have a healthy option whenever you need it. Remember, snacks can also be a small portion of any of your meals. The key is to listen to your body, and if you're hungry, keep your blood sugar balanced throughout the day. Keep in mind that balanced blood sugar means better willpower and decision making, not to mention a happier, healthier body!

Day 1

— **30 minutes before breakfast:** 1 cup of Louise's Favorite Bone Broth or Veggie Broth

— **Breakfast:** Quinoa Flakes (follow package instructions or use Sweet Quinoa Bread recipe and make the pilaf, but not the bread)

— **Midmorning snack:** Sweet and Savory Walnuts and Dates

— **Lunch:** Hassle-Free Fabulous Whole Chicken for Busy People with steamed broccoli (see recipe for Easy Vegetable Side Dishes) and Celery Root Mash

— **Afternoon snack:** Celery Basil Crackers with store-bought raw cultured sauerkraut (or use the Pickled Pink Cultured Vegetable recipe)

— **Dinner:** Creamy Cream of Buckwheat with steamed asparagus (see Easy Vegetable Side Dishes recipe)

— **Dessert:** Sweet Squash Pie

Day 2

— **1 hour before breakfast:** Great Green Smoothie

— **Breakfast:** Good Luck Soup and two slow-cooked scrambled or poached eggs. (Or if you want to do something fast and easy, crack two eggs in your hot-soup bowl and let the soup cook the eggs. When the eggs turn white and the yolk looks more cooked, your soup with eggs is ready to eat!)

— **Lunch:** Turkey burger with romaine lettuce, steamed green beans, and cultured vegetables

— **Afternoon snack:** 1 or 2 pieces of Chocolate Fudge

— **Dinner:** Lovely Millet Loaf with Kale Carrot Soup

— **Sweet-taste satisfier:** Ginger tea with 1 teaspoon raw honey

Day 3

— **Breakfast:** Grain-Free Waffles (topped with coconut oil, raw butter, or ghee; and either a touch of honey, maple syrup, or berries)

— **Lunch:** Magnificent Mahi Mahi salad with steamed slices of zucchini and yellow squash

— **Afternoon snack:** 1 cup of Louise's Favorite Bone Broth or Vegetable Broth with Savory Tahini Crackers

— **Dinner:** Quinoa Broccoli and Leeks Pilaf with spring-mix salad

— **Dessert:** Sweet Buckwheat Bread with a touch of honey or Raw Chocolate-Chip Cookies (if you are focusing on food combining and you eat dessert just after dinner, the Sweet Buckwheat Bread is a better option).

Following are sample menus for those who want to eat meat or fish for dinner:

Day 4

— **Breakfast:** Cinnamon Buckwheat Cereal

— **Midmorning snack:** Celery Basil Crackers with Mild Homemade Salsa

— **Lunch:** Joel's Surprisingly Delicious Sea Vegetable Soup

— **Dinner:** Simple Crock-Pot Lamb Shanks with Carrots and Greens Veggie Mash

— **Dessert:** Just Like Shortbread Cookies and holy basil hot tea (see next page)

Day 5

— **Breakfast:** Sweet Blueberry Banana Green Protein Smoothie

— **Lunch:** Millet Pilaf—Super Thyroid Booster on top of a salad

— **Afternoon snack:** Savory Beet Chips

— **Dinner:** Heavenly Haddock and Louise's Healing Asparagus Puree

— **Dessert:** Key Lime Pudding

Ideas for Beverages and Soda Replacements

— **Water:** Develop a love of water first and foremost! If you have an aversion to it, try adding lemon slices, the juice of half a lemon, or some organic pomegranate concentrate to an eight-ounce glass of water to make it more exciting to drink at first.

— **Herbal teas:** Nettles, dandelion, ginger, holy basil, peppermint, and chamomile are wonderful options.

- Here's how to make one of our favorite hot or iced teas (we like organic Krishna Holy Basil tea from MountainRoseHerbs.com): Take ½ cup loose tea and add to eight cups water in a saucepan. Bring water to a boil, and then turn off the heat and allow to simmer. Pour the water through a fine mesh strainer or cheesecloth (to strain out the tea leaves) into a two-quart-sized, wide-mouth Ball jar or a large glass pitcher. Drink warm for hot tea or store in the refrigerator and drink as iced tea.

— **Sparkling cherry or pomegranate drink:** To make one glass of this delicious fizzy soda replacement, start with six ounces of sparkling mineral water. Add four drops Urban Moonshine Citrus Bitters or use the juice from half of a fresh-squeezed lemon. Now add one ounce of organic cherry or pomegranate concentrate. Mix, add a wedge of lemon or lime, and enjoy!

Cravings: "Eat This Instead" Ideas

— **Bread.** Eat any of our bread recipes instead. Nuts are also a great bread substitute and may satisfy your craving—try Brazil nuts, macadamia nuts, almonds, or walnuts.

— **French fries.** Cut slices of red-skinned potatoes, drizzle with coconut oil, and bake in the oven at 350° F for 20 to 30 minutes, until the potato slices are soft. Or try any of the mashes in the next chapter. For a twist, try the Savory Beet Chips—you can make them in the shape of French fries, if you like.

— **Pasta.** One of the challenges with pasta is that it's made from flour and, very often, wheat flour. Any flour product, even if it's gluten-free, is not soaked and is therefore harder for the body to digest. As an alternative to pasta, try quinoa or millet with plenty of raw organic butter or ghee. Another option is to use spaghetti squash with homemade tomato sauce or an organic tomato sauce with good ingredients (read the label using the chart in Chapter 5). One of the red-skinned potato recipes may be a helpful comfort-food alternative to pasta as well. If all else fails and you really want pasta, consider the 100 percent buckwheat organic soba noodles sold in health-food stores (make sure to read the label because some soba noodles are a mixture of buckwheat *and* wheat).

— **Sweets.** Any of our dessert recipes will help satisfy your sweet tooth. The Delightfully Sweet Zucchini Squash Soup recipe is a naturally sweet soup that can be eaten as a snack to satisfy your sweet tooth as well.

To counteract a sweet craving, consider having a cup of hot tea with honey or stevia or some raw cultured vegetables. The sour flavor can help ward off a sweet craving—you can even take a sip of the brine of real, raw cultured vegetables.

— **Doughnuts.** Try the recipes for Grain-Free, Gluten-Free Gingerbread or Grain-Free, Gluten-Free Pancakes and Waffles.

— **Ice cream.** We've provided one Vanilla Spice Ice Cream recipe in the next chapter for those who want to put a little more effort into a recipe with big rewards! We even show you how to make it without an ice-cream maker. Another option is to put a banana or date in the freezer and take it out and mash it up when you're ready to eat it. Mashed frozen banana makes a really nice "ice cream."

Keep in mind that frozen foods can be challenging on the digestive system, so you can also consider the Raw Chocolate-Chip Cookies or Key Lime Pudding recipes, since they have a slightly similar smooth consistency to ice cream, but without the cold temperature. You might also like a scoop of nut butter with ¼ teaspoon of honey as a nice, smooth snack that can be enjoyed at room temperature.

— **Chips and salsa.** Use one of the homemade cracker recipes with the Mild Homemade Salsa recipe for a healthy version of this snack. You can also try a cracker recipe with some raw, cultured vegetables to get a great chips-and-salsa taste. See the recipe for Pickled Pink Cultured Vegetables or purchase them from a health-food store. Again, we want to emphasize that you make sure to buy real, raw cultured vegetables in brine, not white vinegar.

Recipe Shopping List

We have included this list as a helpful tool for meal planning when you're using recipes in this book. You may want to make a copy of this list and use it alongside the recipes as you plan meals for the coming week—once you've decided which recipes you want to make, you can use it to check off the food and ingredients you'll need to purchase.

For your ongoing shopping needs, we have also provided a separate Master Shopping List at the end of this chapter, which includes all of the No-No foods to avoid and Yes-Yes foods to emphasize. (Note that although these foods were already laid out for you in Chapter 5, we felt that having them all here for you again would be very helpful as you prepare to go to the grocery store, health-food store, or farmers' market to gather foods for the recipes.)

— **How to use the list:** This shopping list is set up with all of the ingredients from the recipes section of the book. It's important to note that you do not have to buy all of the ingredients on this list; you only need to purchase the ingredients for the meals you want to prepare. One great way to approach this is to plan the recipes you want to make, then check off the ingredients and write in the amounts you need on this shopping list.

— **How much to buy?** Since everyone cooks for different numbers of people in a household, you can go to each recipe and look at the serving sizes to identify how much of an ingredient you'll require.

Vegetables
(choose organic whenever possible)

- Asparagus
- Avocados (technically a fruit)
- Beets
- Bok choy
- Broccoli or broccoli rabe
- Brussels sprouts
- Burdock root (choose firm burdock root or purchase dried burdock root at: MountainRoseHerbs.com)
- Carrots
- Cauliflower
- Celery
- Celery root (celeriac)
- Cilantro
- Collards
- Cucumbers
- Garlic
- Green beans
- Green onions
- Herbs (fresh):
  - Basil
  - Chives
  - Dill
- Kale
- Leeks
- Lettuce:
  - Endive
  - Frisée
  - Green leaf

- Mâche (lamb's ears)
- Red leaf
- Romaine
- Spring mix (also called mesclun or mesculin)

• Microgreens (tiny, flavorful greens that are typically sold near the sprouts in the refrigerated section of the produce aisle)

• Mushrooms (shiitake and maitake)

• Onions (red, yellow, white)

• Parsley (flat, curly)

• Radicchio

• Red-skinned potatoes

• Seaweed: If you are making vegetable broth and haven't saved any vegetables, you could start by making an easy seaweed broth. If you do this, you just need one to three 6" strips of kombu, wakame, nori, or kelp. (You can also purchase bladderwrack, digitata, and soup mix from: TheSeaweedMan.com.)

• Shallots

• Sprouts (greens like broccoli sprouts, pea shoot sprouts, sunflower sprouts)

• Squash:
  - Acorn
  - Butternut
  - Chayote (green pear-shaped squash) or pattypan
  - Delicata
  - Kabocha
  - Spaghetti
  - Winter
  - Yellow

• Swiss chard

• Tomatoes (avoid these if you have issues with nightshades)

• Turnips

- Watercress

- Zucchini

- Cultured vegetables: If you are buying these instead of making them, look for organic raw cultured vegetables in a glass jar with no vinegar, like Gold Mine or Rejuvenative Foods brands. If you make them yourself, you will need (this is based on the recipe for Pickled Pink Cultured Vegetables in this book):

  - 4 sweet potatoes
  - 1 head red cabbage
  - 1 package fresh dill
  - 1 package kelp seaweed
  - ½ cup fresh basil
  - 1 cup red onion
  - 1 fresh ginger root

Fruit/Sweeteners
(choose organic whenever possible)

- Bananas (for smoothies, if you are starting with the fruit smoothie; or to freeze in your freezer to mash up and make "ice cream")

- Berries

  - Blackberries
  - Blueberries
  - Frozen berries (for smoothies)
  - Raspberries
  - Strawberries

- Blackstrap molasses

- Erythritol or birch xylitol (Globalsweet.com has these sweeteners if your health-food store does not, but you want to avoid these options if following GAPS, SCD, or any small intestine healing diet)

- Granny Smith apples

- Lemons

- Limes
- Liquid stevia (two popular brands sold in stores are NOW and SweetLeaf)
- Medjool dates
- Oranges
- Raw honey

Grains
(choose organic wherever possible)

- Buckwheat groats—raw or roasted groats are typically found in the bulk section or hot-cereal aisle (roasted groats are sometimes called kasha or kashi)
- Cream of buckwheat—typically found in the hot-cereal aisle or bulk section
- Millet—typically found in the bulk section
- Quinoa flakes—Ancient Harvest brand organic quinoa flakes are typically found in the hot-cereal section

Animal Protein—Meat, Poultry, Fish, Eggs
(look for organic, grass-fed/pasture-fed meat, eggs, and poultry; and wild-caught fish)

- Bones: If you want to make bone broth and don't have any bones saved from previous meals, you can purchase the bones of grass-fed animals from your butcher or in the meat department of your grocery store or health-food store. Ask the butcher for help finding bones. Other affordable and nutrient-rich options are chicken necks, chicken wings, or chicken feet (the meat department may have cleaned chicken feet, a delicacy in some countries). You only need about 2 lbs. of bones or other parts to make a bone broth.

- Eggs
- Ground meat (beef, lamb, chicken, turkey)
- Haddock
- Lamb shanks
- Mahi mahi
- Red snapper
- Short ribs
- Turkey parts, like legs, thighs, and breast
- White cod
- Whole fryer chicken

Nuts and Seeds
(see if you can get raw, organic nuts and seeds in the bulk section of your grocery store)

- Almonds
- Brazil nuts
- Flaxseeds (you can easily grind these to make your own flax meal, or purchase flax meal)
- Hazelnuts
- Hemp seeds
- Macadamia nuts
- Pine nuts
- Sesame seeds
- Sunflower seeds
- Walnuts

Nut Butters
(choose organic, raw, and sprouted whenever possible—sprouted nut and seed butters are harder to find and have a higher price, however)

- Almond butter

- Brazil nut butter

- Coconut butter

- Hazelnut butter

- Macadamia nut butter

- Tahini (sesame butter)

Sea Salt, Spices, and Ground or Dried Herbs
(choose organic whenever possible)

- Allspice

- Astragalus powder (if this is not in your health-food store, try: MountainRoseHerbs.com)

- Basil

- Bay leaves

- Black peppercorns

- Caraway seeds

- Cardamom (ground)

- Cayenne pepper

- Cinnamon (if your local store only has cassia, you can find ground Ceylon cinnamon at: MountainRoseHerbs.com)

- Cloves

- Coriander (ground)

- Cumin (ground)

- Curry (ground; check ingredients to make sure there are no artificial additives, and use turmeric instead if you can't find an additive-free curry powder)

- Dill
- Fennel (ground)
- Fenugreek (ground)
- Ginger (ground)
- Herbamare (blend of sea salt and organic herbs)
- Herbes de Provence (herbal blend)
- Kosher salt or rock salt (if you want to make the ice-cream recipe)
- Lemongrass powder (if you can't find this in the store, try: MountainRoseHerbs.com)
- Nutmeg
- Oregano
- Rosemary (dried leaves)
- Sea salt (Celtic Grey Sea Salt is a nice, all-purpose brand sold in most stores; or choose Sarah's Sea Salt, Selina Naturally Portuguese Sea Salt, pink Himalayan salt, or other sea-salt varieties)
- Thyme
- Trocomare (zesty version of Herbamare with some red pepper and horseradish)
- Turmeric
- Vanilla bean or pure vanilla extract

Condiments and Extras

- Almond flour
- Apple cider vinegar
- Baking soda (Bob's Red Mill brand is a great option)
- Cacao butter
- Chicken broth—organic, like Imagine brand (check ingredients to avoid sugar and other unwanted additives)

- Coconut flakes, shredded (Let's Do Organic brand is often sold in stores or online at: iHerb.com)

- Coconut flour

- Kuzu (typically comes in a small package in the ethnic-foods section or baking section, or buy online)

- Mustard (made with apple cider vinegar instead of white vinegar, like Whole Foods 365 brand)

- Raw cacao (healthy dark chocolate powder)

- Raw, cultured dehydrated olives (Essential Living Foods brand)

- Real, raw green olives in brine (Divina or Essential Living Foods brands are options with no white vinegar)

- Urban Moonshine Citrus Bitters (may be sold in the supplements section of your health-food store or check online at: Amazon.com or iHerb.com)

- Wheat-free tamari (this may not work well if you are sensitive to glutamates; if so, you can use apple cider vinegar and sea salt or ¼ tsp ground dulse seaweed in recipes instead)

- White cooking wine (organic)

Healthy Fats and Oils
(choose organic, unrefined oils)

- Borage oil

- Coconut oil (extra-virgin)

- Cod-liver oil

- Flaxseed oil (in the refrigerated section)

- Grass- or pasture-fed animal fats—such as raw butter; ghee; lard from pork; tallow and suet from lamb or beef; goose, chicken, or duck fat

- Hemp-seed oil

- Macadamia-nut oil

- Olive oil (extra-virgin)
- Pumpkin-seed oil (you may have to purchase this online if it's not available in stores)

Teas and Beverages
(choose organic where possible)

- Chamomile tea
- Dandelion tea
- Ginger tea
- Holy basil tea (or purchase loose holy basil Krishna tea at: MountainRoseHerbs.com)
- Nettles tea
- Peppermint tea
- Pomegranate concentrate (liquid)
- Sparkling mineral water
- Tart cherry concentrate (liquid)—you can get organic tart cherry concentrate in a glass bottle at: Amazon.com or iHerb.com

Supplements for Smoothie Recipes
(note that most can be purchased at Amazon.com
if you can't find them in your health-food store)

- NOW Organic Wheatgrass Juice Powder
- Organic elderberry extract
- Premier Research Labs Premier Greens
- Sunwarrior Protein Powder, Plain

Master Shopping List

This is a master shopping list for your ongoing shopping needs beyond our recipes. This list includes the No-No foods to avoid and the Yes-Yes foods to emphasize, as discussed in Chapter 5.

No-No's: Avoid These at the Grocery Store

Sweeteners

- Acesulfame-K (Sunette, Sweet One, DiabetiSweet)
- Agave nectar—this is deceptive because it's sold in health-food stores, but it often has more fructose than high-fructose corn syrup
- Aspartame (AminoSweet, NutraSweet, Equal), an excitotoxin
- Barley malt or malted barley—these may contain glutamic acid, an excitotoxin
- Beet sugar
- Brown rice syrup or rice syrup—suspected of containing free glutamic acid, making it a possible excitotoxin for highly sensitive people
- Brown sugar
- Cane sugar
- Confectioners' sugar
- Corn syrup
- Dextrose
- Fructose
- Glucose
- High-fructose corn syrup (HCFS)
- Invert sugar
- Isomalt
- Lactitol
- Lactose

- Levulose
- Malt extract
- Maltitol
- Maltodextrin
- Maltose
- Mannitol
- Milk sugar
- Neotame (NutraSweet's new and "improved" artificial sweetener)
- Oligodextrin
- Powdered sugar
- Raw sugar
- Saccharin (Sugar Twin, Sweet'N Low)
- Saccharose
- Sorbitol
- Sucralose (Splenda, Nevella, SucraPlus)
- Sucrose
- Sugar
- Table sugar
- Turbinado sugar

Excitotoxins

- Annatto—could produce a reaction in highly sensitive people
- Autolyzed yeast
- Bouillon or broth
- Brewer's yeast—may contain glutamate, or glutamate may be used in processing
- Carrageenan
- Citric acid
- Cornstarch—may trigger a reaction in highly sensitive people

- Fermented protein foods
- *Flavors* or *flavoring*—beware of words like this on labels, particularly if there is no indication of what the flavors or flavoring are, because they're often hidden chemicals
- Hydrolyzed protein—or anything hydrolyzed, for that matter
- Modified food starch
- Monosodium glutamate (MSG)—or anything with the word *glutamate,* like *potassium glutamate, natrium glutamate, glutamic acid,* and so forth
- Natural flavoring (including natural beef or chicken flavoring)
- Plant protein extract
- Protein concentrate
- *Seasonings*—when you see this word, it can mean that MSG or other chemicals are hidden
- Soy isolate
- Soy protein
- Soy sauce or soy sauce extract
- *Spices*—while natural herbs and spices are wonderful, beware if you only see the word *spices* with no identification about which spice it is because it could be MSG
- Stock
- Textured protein
- Vegetable gum
- Whey protein concentrate
- Whey protein isolate
- White vinegar—could produce a reaction in highly sensitive people

Gluten grains

- Barley (and barley malt or barley extract)
- Beer
- Brown rice syrup

- Couscous
- Croutons (unless gluten-free)
- Durum
- Farina
- Faro
- Gluten
- Kamut
- Malt
- Matzo flour/meal
- Oats (unless labeled gluten-free)
- Orzo
- Panko
- Rye
- Seitan
- Semolina
- Spelt
- Thickeners
- Triticale
- Udon
- Wheat (including wheat bran, wheat germ, and wheat starch)

Other

- Azodicarbonamide (ADA)
- Brominated vegetable oil (BVO)
- Butylated hydroxyanisole (BHA)
- Butylated hydroxytoluene (BHT)
- Dairy (except for organic, raw, and grass-fed butter or ghee— if you can tolerate dairy, choose organic, raw, and grass-fed)
- Enriched foods

- Food dyes (look for a color and number, like Red #40, Yellow #6, Blue #1, and the like)
- Potassium bisulfite
- Potassium bromate
- Potassium metabisulfite
- Sodium bisulfite
- Sodium metabisulfite
- Sodium sulfite
- Sulfites
- Sulfur dioxide
- Ultrapasteurized (a process also known as ultra-heat treatment, or UHT)
- Wheat (gluten)

Fats and oils—avoid fats and oils that are refined, hydrogenated, partially hydrogenated, or trans fats, such as:

- Canola oil
- Corn oil
- Cottonseed oil
- Fried foods or processed foods cooked in refined or hydrogenated oils heated to high temperatures
- Margarine
- Peanut oil
- Rice bran oil
- Safflower oil
- Salad dressings—most have low-quality fats, so see the "Healthy Fats and Oils" section later in this chapter to learn more
- Shortening (Crisco)
- Soy oil
- Vegetable oil
- Vegetable shortening

Yes-Yes!: Include These in Your Healthy Diet

Whole foods—typically found in the outside perimeter of the grocery store (produce; the fish and meat counters; some refrigerated areas)

Fruits and vegetables

- A rainbow of colored vegetables
- High-antioxidant fruits and vegetables:
  - Artichokes
  - Arugula
  - Dandelion
  - Green leaf lettuce
  - Kale
  - Red leaf lettuce
  - Romaine lettuce
- Fresh herbs, like basil, mint, parsley, rosemary, sage, and thyme
- Blueberries and black and dark red grapes

Animal protein

- Grass-fed and finished meats (organic preferred)
- Pasture-fed poultry and eggs (organic preferred)
- Wild-caught fish

Healthy fats and oils (choose organic, unrefined oils)

- Borage oil
- Coconut oil (extra-virgin)
- Cod-liver oil
- Flaxseed oil (in the refrigerated section)
- Grass- or pasture-fed animal fats—such as raw butter; ghee; lard from pork; tallow and suet from lamb or beef; goose, chicken, or duck fat
- Hemp-seed oil
- Macadamia-nut oil

- Olive oil (extra-virgin)
- Pumpkin-seed oil (you may have to purchase this online if it's not available in-store)

Whole-food sweeteners (organic preferred)

- Blackstrap molasses
- Fruit (like fresh apples)
- Grade B maple syrup
- Lo han guo
- Medjool dates
- Raw honey
- Stevia
- Xylitol or erythritol (see caveats for these sweeteners that may contribute to digestive symptoms)

Nuts and seeds (organic and raw, not roasted or salted)—most are great, although you may want to avoid peanuts, cashews, and pistachios due to mold contamination

Nut and seed butters—look for raw nut and seed butters, and make sure to read the labels to avoid unwanted additives (some companies, like Better Than Roasted, have presoaked or sprouted the nuts and seeds to make them more easily digestible)

Gluten-free grains (organic preferred)—amaranth, buckwheat, millet, and quinoa (and if you do eat rice, consider Lundberg brand Organic California White Basmati because it was found to be lower in arsenic than other brands)

Sea salt, spices, and ground or dried herbs—look for organic herbs and spices and real sea salt or Himalayan salt, and choose Ceylon cinnamon instead of cassia cinnamon

Chapter 10

Recipes

Before we get started with the recipes, we wanted to remind you that proper preparation for grains, beans, nuts, and seeds is key. These all have an antinutrient called phytic acid, which binds up the minerals in your body and can cause mineral deficiencies. Soaking first removes the phytic acid so you can more easily digest your nuts, seeds, grains, and beans.

How to Soak Nuts and Seeds

- Put the nuts or seeds in a glass or stainless-steel bowl. (Note that 2–3 cups of nuts or seeds at a time is useful for recipes, while 1–2 cups at a time is useful for snacks. If you want to make more and freeze them, consider up to 6 cups at a time when soaking.)

- Add enough filtered water to cover them.

- Add about 1 teaspoon sea salt per cup of nuts.

- Put a lid on if you have one (or cover with a plate) and leave on the counter for 8–12 hours. You can do this before going to bed.

- After 8–12 hours, drain the water, rinse the nuts or seeds, and either put them in the refrigerator (for 3 days to 1 week) or the freezer (lasts about 2 months).

- You can also dry or roast them: To dry them, put your oven on the lowest temperature and heat until dry. If you have a food dehydrator, set it to 115° F and dehydrate for 2–5 hours or until dry. They will last a couple of weeks in your refrigerator or several months in your freezer.

How to Soak Grains and Beans

- Put grains or beans in a glass or stainless-steel bowl (follow the same quantity guidelines as previously mentioned for nuts and seeds).

- Add enough filtered water to cover them.

- Add 1 tablespoon of apple cider vinegar and mix into the water.

- Cover with a lid or plate and let sit on your countertop for 8–12 hours for grains or 12–24 hours for beans.

- After soaking, drain and rinse the grains or beans.

- You can store the soaked grains or beans in your refrigerator for a few days before cooking them, or store them in your freezer for about a month before cooking them.

Easy Vegetable Side Dishes

Steamed, boiled, or sautéed veggie side dishes are easy to make and can often be cooked in 10 minutes or less. Here's how:

— Choose the vegetables you want to cook. You can use just about any veggie you'd like, but here are some fun options:

- Asparagus (cut off the denser ½ inch at the bottom of the spears and save for your bone or vegetable broth)
- Bok choy
- Broccoli or broccoli rabe
- Brussels sprouts
- Carrots
- Cauliflower
- Celery root (celeriac)
- Collards
- Green beans
- Kale
- Swiss chard
- Turnips
- Yellow squash
- Zucchini

— Wash and prepare the vegetables. Remember to save the ends and scraps for your bone or vegetable broth!

— Decide how you want to serve them:

- *Sliced, diced, or chopped:* You can slice them by hand or use a food processor if you have one. If you want slices or julienned vegetables, your food processor can do this in seconds with the right attachments (the long slits will slice, and the small holes will julienne). The S-blade will do either a rough chop of vegetables if you use the pulse button a few times, or finely chop or puree, depending on how long you let it run.

- *Mashed or blended:* If you want to make a mash, or blended vegetables with the consistency of mashed potatoes, chop up the vegetables first (any which way in large chunks), boil or steam them, then drain out the water, leaving about ⅓ cup of water for easy blending. Add sea salt, pepper, and chosen herbs or spices; then pour into your food processor and puree with the S-blade. Alternatively, you can use an immersion blender right in the same pan you cooked the vegetables in, which is fast and easy. If you don't have equipment, you can use a potato masher—just make sure your vegetables are softly cooked enough to do this.

— Directions for cooking:

- *Steaming or boiling option:* Place about 2–4 cups of vegetables in 2 cups of water, add ½ teaspoon salt and ¼ teaspoon pepper (and any other spices you're using). Boil or steam for 5 minutes or until your vegetables are as soft or firm as you like them. Drain water; add another ½ teaspoon sea salt and drizzle with your favorite healthy fat or oil (see Chapter 5 for ideas).

- *Sautéing option:* On low heat, place 2 tablespoons healthy cooking fat or oil (such as coconut oil or a healthy animal fat like raw butter, ghee, or our favorite, duck fat). Add ¼ teaspoon pepper, ½ teaspoon salt, and the herbs or spices you'd like to use, and allow the herbs and spices to get warm for about 2 minutes. Make sure the fat does not get too hot. Add the vegetables of your choice (see the list on the previous page for ideas) and turn the heat up to medium low. Cook for about 5 minutes or until the vegetables are as firm or soft as you like them. Remove from heat and serve.

— Taste your vegetables after you've cooked them, and add sea salt and/ or fresh ground pepper to taste. You might also feel that they need a little more of a healthy fat or oil after cooking. Some people like to have flaxseed oil, olive oil, or some other oil at the table so that people can serve themselves according to their own tastes. Pumpkin-seed oil makes a wonderful addition to cooked vegetables and can be a fun new twist to have at the table.

— Be creative. Most vegetables go beautifully with thyme, basil, and rosemary; alternatively, you could use a mixture of turmeric, allspice, and fennel powder (¼–½ teaspoon each). If you want to add these herbs or spices, feel free to experiment—and check Chapter 6 for herbs and spices that work on health issues you want to resolve!

♥

Carrots and Greens Veggie Mash:
A No-Starch Mashed Potatoes Alternative

Preparation time: about 20 minutes

This is comfort food at its best—hearty, warm, and deliciously healthy! This is your go-to for a no-starch alternative to mashed potatoes.

INGREDIENTS:

1 bunch carrot greens (about 2 cups chopped)

2 medium carrots

1 bunch asparagus

½ cup chopped onion

2 Tbsp. coconut oil

2 Tbsp. dried rosemary leaves

1 Tbsp. dried oregano

2 tsp. Celtic sea salt

2 tsp. lemongrass powder

1 tsp. black pepper

½ tsp. ground coriander

INSTRUCTIONS:

Bring 2 cups water to a boil in a saucepan, then add the carrots and boil for 3 minutes. Add the carrot greens and boil for 1 minute, then add the asparagus and boil for 2 minutes or until somewhat soft.

While this is boiling, put the coconut oil, onions, and all spices except the salt into a wok or skillet on medium heat. Lightly sauté until onions are translucent. Remove from heat.

Remove saucepan from heat and drain most of the water (leave 1" at the bottom of the pan), then pour the carrots and greens into the wok and put on medium heat. Toss the vegetables in the spices for 2 minutes, then remove from heat.

Using an immersion blender (or a high-speed blender or food processor with the S-blade), puree the mixture lightly if you like a somewhat chunky mash, or more if you like it smoother.

Serve over raw greens, with your favorite grains, on its own, or mixed with chicken for a delicious chicken potpie–type flavor.

Add sea salt or Herbamare herb sea salt to taste.

Celery Root Veggie Mash:
A No-Starch "Just Like Mashed Potatoes" Alternative

If you're following food-combining guidelines (see Chapter 6 for more information) or reducing starchy foods, you'll love this "mashed potato" alternative.

INGREDIENTS:

3 celery roots, peeled and chopped into large pieces (about 6 cups chopped)

4 cups water or bone broth

1 Tbsp. dried rosemary

1 Tbsp. dried thyme

½ Tbsp. dried dill

2 tsp. sea salt

2 tsp. fresh ground pepper

Optional: ½ cup diced red onion and 1 clove minced garlic

Optional: If you're serving this dish with meat, take about ½ cup of the meat drippings and add to the mash after draining out excess water.

INSTRUCTIONS:

Peel and chop celery root (you're going to boil the celery root, so you can rough chop it into halves or quarters).

Optional step to add more flavor: In a skillet on the lowest heat, add 1 Tbsp. coconut oil, raw butter, ghee, or fat from the meat you're using for the meal, and allow it to gently melt. Add all herbs, spices, and optional onions and/or garlic. Sauté gently for 3 minutes or until the onions are translucent. Add 1 cup water to the skillet, mix everything up, and put into the saucepan you're using to boil the celery root.

Bring water or bone broth to a boil. Add all ingredients and cook until the celery root is soft when you prick it with a knife or fork.

Drain all but ½ cup of water into a glass or stainless-steel bowl so that you can save this nutrient-rich liquid it for other meals (especially if you're boiling in bone broth!).

Mash up the remaining celery root and water. You can do this with a potato masher or large fork; or to make it much easier and faster, use an immersion blender right in the pan you cooked in, or transfer the celery root and ½ cup liquid into a blender or food processor and blend until smooth, like mashed potatoes.

Season with more salt, pepper, or meat drippings to taste.

Serve with meat, vegetables, or eggs, or as a comfort-food snack.

Louise's Healing Asparagus Puree

Servings: makes approximately 7 (2-oz.) servings

This recipe is not only delicious, it's very healing, too! This is the recipe Louise used as part of her nutritional healing regimen when she was diagnosed with cancer, and with great results—her healthy thoughts and food resulted in dissolving the cancer naturally!

INGREDIENTS:

2 cups chopped asparagus

Optional flavorings:

1 tsp. sea salt

¼ tsp. pepper

1 tablespoon coconut oil, raw organic butter, or ghee

INSTRUCTIONS:

In a saucepan, bring 1 cup water to a boil (you can use bone broth as another option).

Chop the tough ends off the asparagus (about ½" at the bottom of the spears) and save them for a future bone or vegetable broth (see the recipe of Louise's Favorite Bone Broth or Vegetable Broth in the Soups section).

Either boil or add a steamer basket and steam the asparagus until mushy (about 5 minutes). Drain the water (save it if you like and use to cook something else, like grains or more vegetables; or maybe add it to a bone or vegetable broth).

Allow the cooked asparagus to cool, and then blend it up to the consistency of mashed potatoes. You can use a potato masher, large fork, immersion blender, regular blender, or food processor.

Serving suggestion: Louise's practitioner suggested that she eat 3 (2-oz.) servings of this pureed asparagus each day. Louise put them in 2-oz. containers so that she could take them with her during the day, which was a great way to easily incorporate this into her routine. This puree makes a lovely veggie mash to accompany any meal or have on its own as a snack.

Roots and Greens Comfort Food

Preparation time: about 25 minutes

This recipe is comfort food at its best—delicious, hearty, and warms the soul. If you are experiencing the winter blues, this dish will pick you up!

INGREDIENTS:

10 small red-skinned potatoes

1 bunch watercress (2–3 cups)

¼ cup red onion, diced

2 burdock roots

2 Tbsp. ghee

1 Tbsp. coconut oil

1 Tbsp. dried rosemary

1 Tbsp. dried oregano

2 tsp. dried basil

2 tsp. herbes de Provence or Herbamare herb sea salt (you can use sea salt instead if don't have this on hand)

1 tsp. ground coriander

INSTRUCTIONS:

In a saucepan, add ¼ cup water, 1 tsp. ghee, the herbes de Provence, and all herbs. Simmer on low until the onions become translucent. Add 4 cups water and bring to a boil.

While water is coming to a boil, scrape off the skin of the burdock root with a butter knife. It's beneficial to leave some scraps of skin on, while removing most of it. (Burdock root, also called gobo root, looks like a stick and is best when it's firm, like a carrot. If you can't find it in your health-food store, you can buy organic dried burdock root at: MountainRoseHerbs.com.)

Slice up the burdock root. Once water comes to a boil, add the sliced root and reduce heat to simmer. Allow the water with burdock root to simmer for 5 minutes, then add in the potatoes, continuing to simmer on low heat.

Put the watercress into a food processor with an S-blade and pulse a few times to chop it up into small chunks/leaves. Set aside.

Once the potatoes are soft (a knife, fork, or spoon should easily slice through them), add the watercress and simmer for 1 more minute.

Drain the water and transfer the ingredients into a glass or stainless-steel bowl. Add ghee and coconut oil and mix in thoroughly.

Serving suggestions: Serve on a bed of greens that have been slightly chopped in your food processor with an S-blade or cut into bite-sized pieces with a knife. One suggestion is a chopped salad of red leaf lettuce, cilantro, and chives. Drizzle some flaxseed oil over each serving of green salad and put the potatoes on top of the greens. This makes a delicious fall or winter meal that will delight your family.

These potatoes also taste delicious with Creamy Cream of Buckwheat (see recipe later in the chapter) over a bed of greens.

Green Beans and Leeks

INGREDIENTS:

2 cups green beans, chopped up

1 yellow squash, sliced (2 cups)

½ leek, sliced thin (about 2 cups)

2 tsp. coconut oil

1 tsp. dried thyme

¼ tsp. Selina Naturally Portuguese
    Sea Salt (or any type of sea salt)

½ tsp. ginger powder

½ tsp. ground turmeric

⅛ tsp. ground cayenne

INSTRUCTIONS:

Using a skillet on your stovetop, set the temperature to low. Add in coconut oil, allowing it to melt. Add leeks and all herbs and spices (except the sea salt), and heat on low to allow them to release their aromas and medicinal properties.

Add in the green beans and squash and sauté together until the vegetables are soft. You may need to add more oil or some water if the pan becomes dry while you're cooking. Simmer on low heat for 5–10 minutes or until the green beans and squash are as soft as you like.

Remove from heat and serve alone or with your favorite main dish—it goes well with any meat, poultry, or grain recipe. Try drizzling flaxseed oil, olive oil, or pumpkin-seed oil over these vegetables for a delicious treat!

Naturally Sweet and Savory Mood Booster

Preparation time: 15 minutes   *Servings: 2–4*

If you're low in serotonin, the happiness hormone, your body may signal you with cravings for sweets and starchy foods (bread, bagels, cookies, and the like). In order to make serotonin, your brain needs your body to deliver to it the essential amino acid tryptophan. However, because other amino acids compete to get into your brain, the only way to deliver tryptophan to it is if you have insulin in your blood. This means you need a starchy snack.

Unfortunately, most people reach for unhealthy starches, which can fuel addiction, candida, and an eventual blood-sugar crash. Instead, you can support your body with a healthy starchy snack to boost serotonin without the crash.

This dish is designed for a meal or snack that is delicious, helps boost serotonin faster than grains, and doesn't feed candida. If you're having a stressful day, you may want to have this with your grain meal or as a late-afternoon or evening snack.

Heather used this recipe when she was transitioning to healthy eating because it was a great bridge from the taste of packaged foods to the taste of healthier foods. Your taste buds do change as your diet changes, and this recipe can help move you in the right direction!

INGREDIENTS:

4 red-skinned potatoes, cubed

4 carrots, sliced

¼ cup onions, diced

1 tsp. thyme

1 Tbsp. curry powder

1 tsp. Herbamare herb sea salt

2 tsp. ghee

INSTRUCTIONS:

In a saucepan, melt 1 tsp. ghee. Add spices and onions and sauté for 1 minute. Add 1½ cups water and bring to a boil. Add potato and carrots and cook until all ingredients are tender. Add additional ghee at the end of cooking.

Serve with cooked greens, like the Green Beans and Leeks recipe earlier in the chapter, or place over a raw spring-mix salad.

Outstanding Collards and Butternut Squash

Preparation time: 55 minutes   *Serves: 4–6*

This recipe is so delicious that even your non-health-nut friends and family will rave about it. Naturally sweet and rich, this dish is a perfect holiday meal or side dish, and makes a great cool-weather treat.

INGREDIENTS:

> 1 bunch collards (about 3–4 cups chopped)
>
> 1 butternut squash
>
> 1 Tbsp. coconut oil
>
> Herbamare herb sea salt, or regular sea salt, and pepper to taste

INSTRUCTIONS:

Preheat the oven to 350° F.

With a sharp kitchen knife, prick the squash to create a way for heat to escape during cooking. Place squash in a Pyrex cooking dish with 1" water in it, and bake for approximately 40 minutes. You'll know the squash is done when it feels soft and you can easily slice a knife into it.

Wash the collard leaves and then put them in your food processor and pulse a few times to chop it up a bit. You can also chop it up with a knife, into strips or bite-sized pieces.

When the squash is done, remove from the oven and put aside to cool. Once it's cooled, put the strips of collards into a steamer basket in a pan with 2 cups water. Steam collards until they're tender (about 5–10 minutes).

While collards are steaming, work on the squash. Slice it in half lengthwise and scoop it out with a spoon, discarding the seeds.

Transfer the steamed collards and squash to a pan with ½" water at the bottom, and set your stove to low heat. Add the coconut oil, black pepper, and Herbamare or sea salt and heat the whole dish up for 2–5 minutes.

Serve warm with other vegetables, sea vegetables, or a grain dish. Add Herbamare or sea salt to taste.

Salads

Salads are wonderful to have on hand for fast food! In her corporate days, Heather had a routine of making a salad and keeping it in a large glass bowl with a plastic airtight top. She could then grab the prepared salad from the refrigerator when she wanted it for a meal. She would also prepack a few days of salads in individual containers to take in her lunch bag during the workweek.

While salads seem like an easy health-food meal, some people do better with cooked foods, especially if digestion is compromised or the weather is cold. Many of the recipes in this book suggest adding a warm food on top of a salad. This lightly heats up the salad, making it more comforting for your body. If you're in a hurry and have a meat, poultry, or grain dish but no vegetables, try putting the warm food on top of a bed of lettuce for a more comforting meal any time of year.

Here's a general formula for making great salads:

— Use your favorite lettuce and rotate the types! Here are some fun options: romaine lettuce, spring mix, red leaf lettuce, green leaf lettuce, and endive.

— Add one to three additions to your salad: radicchio, carrots, green beans, snow peas, snap peas, green sprouts (sunflower sprouts, pea-shoot sprouts, and buckwheat sprouts are great options), microgreens, leeks, chives, parsley, cilantro, jicama, radishes, onions or shallots, yellow squash, and zucchini.

- For color, some great options are: radicchio, carrots, or radishes; or garnish with a little red bell pepper or tomato (remember that bell pepper and tomatoes are nightshades and may not work for everyone). Colorful lettuce is always an easy option, too, like red leaf lettuce, spring-mix salad, and colorful microgreens.

— Chop it up: Heather likes to put everything in a food processer and pulse 4–6 times so that no chopping is necessary. If you don't have a food processor, chop things up according to the size you want for your salad. There is no right or wrong way to do this! Some people love to be artistic when slicing vegetables and putting a salad together, while others want to go fast.

— Now add dressing. You can keep it simple and drizzle your favorite healthy oil on top, like hemp-seed oil, pumpkin-seed oil, extra-virgin olive oil, flaxseed oil, or macadamia-nut oil. Then, to get a balanced sour taste for the oil, add *one* of the following: a splash of apple cider vinegar, 1 Tbsp. raw cultured vegetables, 1 tsp. organic mustard (made with apple cider vinegar instead of white vinegar), or a squeeze of lemon.

Or make this healthy dressing:

- 1 cup of your favorite organic oil (see previous page for ideas)

- ⅓ cup apple cider vinegar

- ½ tsp. sea salt

- ¼ tsp. fresh ground black pepper

- Whisk all ingredients together, or place in a blender and blend well, and you have an easy, delicious vinaigrette!

- To experiment with different flavors, be as creative as you like: add a squeeze of lemon, a few drops of Urban Moonshine Citrus Bitters, a little mustard, or some dried basil or thyme for a variety of taste options.

Smoothies

This section contains a few simple versions of green smoothies that are easy to make and gentle on your digestive system. We've also included a fruit option that is sure to get anyone hooked on smoothies, kids included.

If you love smoothies, be creative with the vegetables and ingredients you use—they're a great way to incorporate your favorite vegetables, healthy fats, and healing herbs or spices into your meals. Some people also like to add their favorite protein powder or greens powder, which is a nice way to include more nutrients in your smoothie.

Great Green Smoothie (Easy to Digest)

Preparation time: about 10 minutes   *Servings: 2–4 people (about 4 cups of smoothie)*

Green smoothies may not sound too appetizing to the average person, and particularly not to kids used to eating the Standard American Diet! Yet this one is a gentle "entrée" into smoothies that will be kind to most people's taste buds.

The Granny Smith is a green apple that provides just the right amount of sweetness, and it combines well with vegetables from a food-combining perspective, which means it's easier for your body to digest. All other fruits are usually not as well tolerated when combined with vegetables, if you are experiencing gut issues and want to reduce the stress on your digestive system. Granny Smith apples also have the highest phytonutrients of any other apple.

Cinnamon aids digestion and is a natural anti-inflammatory. Have this for breakfast or a snack, and you're sure to get lots of easily digestible greens into your body!

INGREDIENTS:

2 cups filtered water

2 cups green leaf or red leaf lettuce

1 Granny Smith apple

4 carrots, peeled

2 large stalks celery

2 Tbsp. cilantro (fresh)—if you don't like cilantro, try flat leaf parsley, microgreens, your favorite green sprouts, or omit from recipe altogether

1 Tbsp. ground cinnamon

Optional: ¼–½ avocado. A healthy fat is a nice way to add satisfaction and sustenance to a smoothie; however, if you are having issues digesting fats or have other digestive challenges, try this smoothie without the avocado and have a meal or snack later, when you're hungry again.

Optional: Add a scoop of your favorite greens powder, like Premier Greens by Premier Research Labs or organic wheatgrass juice powder by NOW.

INSTRUCTIONS:

Core and slice the apple and combine it with all ingredients into your high-speed blender. (Vitamix or Blendtec blenders work really well for smoothies, but you can also use any blender or a NutriBullet. Note that some blenders that are not high speed may require you to chop your carrots, celery, and apple up a bit more.)

Blend all ingredients, until everything is completely smooth.

Pour into glasses and serve.

Serving suggestions: Add 4–6 drops of Urban Moonshine Organic Citrus Bitters per cup of smoothie and blend. This will add a nice flavor and help your body digest the smoothie. Add 2 drops of stevia per cup of smoothie if you want a sweeter taste.

Remember, digestion begins in your mouth! To get your digestive juices flowing, sip slowly and chew your smoothie.

Elderberry Fennel Immune-Boosting Green Smoothie

Preparation time: 5 minutes   *Servings: 4*

This smoothie is a rich orange color with a deeply nourishing sweet taste! The black elderberry is excellent as an immune booster to ward off colds and flu. The citrus bitters are a delightful, organic treat to help you digest better. If you don't have any citrus bitters on hand, use a lemon instead (see below).

The cardamom and fennel spices in this smoothie are great for digestion, and fennel is wonderful for eye health. The fenugreek also has eye-health benefits and helps to boost oxytocin, the love and social-bonding hormone responsible for feeling good!

INGREDIENTS:

4 stalks celery

3 large carrots

2 cups red leaf lettuce

2 cups filtered water

1 Tbsp. black elderberry extract or sambucus. (Choose those with no sugar, such as by the Nature's Answer brand, which you can get online at: Amazon.com or iHerb.com. This is great to have on hand during cold and flu season in general.) Use ½ of a Granny Smith apple if you don't have elderberry extract on hand, or omit altogether.

1 tsp. fennel powder

1 tsp. ground fenugreek

½ tsp. ground cardamom

Stevia to taste (approximately 4–6 drops per glass if you want a taste sweeter than the smoothie is naturally)

6 drops Urban Moonshine Citrus Bitters per glass (or juice from ¼–½ fresh lemon)

Optional: 1 Tbsp. coconut oil or coconut butter. (A healthy source of fat is a great way to add satisfying sustenance to a smoothie. If you have trouble digesting fats, you may want to try making your smoothie without a source of fat and have a snack or meal 30 minutes to an hour or so later, when you feel hungry.)

INSTRUCTIONS:

Put all ingredients except the stevia and citrus bitters into a blender and blend thoroughly. Pour into glasses. Add 6 drops citrus bitters per glass and mix up. Add stevia to taste.

Basic Green Vegetable Smoothie

½ small cucumber

½ cup fresh basil

1 cup cilantro—if you don't like cilantro, you could use a cup of your favorite dark green lettuce instead, like romaine, red leaf lettuce, or green leaf lettuce

½ avocado

2 cups fresh green beans

5 chive stalks

½ cup water

½ cup young coconut kefir—or if you don't have this, simply add either young coconut water or an additional ½ cup water and stevia to taste

INSTRUCTIONS:

Wash the vegetables and cut them up to prepare for blending.

Place all ingredients in a blender and mix until the consistency is smooth. Add more water if you want to thin out the consistency.

Pour into glasses and drink to your health!

Sweet Blueberry Banana Green Protein Smoothie:
A Great Entry-Level Smoothie

Servings: makes 2 large smoothies

Fruit smoothies are a wonderful way to get used to drinking smoothies if you're not yet ready for a green smoothie. It's also great for a person who is just starting to adjust to healthy eating, or for a milkshake lover who wants something on the sweeter side. Once you get used to smoothies, we recommend that you experiment with green smoothies for even more nutrients!

This recipe is how Heather got her husband started with drinking smoothies. It's an easy-to-make drink that is high in phytonutrients and protein, while feeling like a sweet treat to the person consuming it.

INGREDIENTS:

1 banana

1–1½ cups fresh or frozen organic blueberries (cherries make a nice alternative as well)

1 scoop Sunwarrior Classic Protein powder, natural flavor (you can get this at: Sunwarrior.com or Amazon.com)

1 scoop green powder—use your favorite green powder, or try one of these organic options: Premier Greens by Premier Research Labs or organic wheatgrass juice powder by NOW (note that wheatgrass is a green and not the same as wheat grain)

2–4 Tbsp. of your favorite nut or seed butter—tahini, sunflower butter, or almond butter are all great options

2 cups organic almond milk, plain flavor with no sugar (or make your own using our simple recipe in the Snacks section), or use 1–2 more Tbsp. nut or seed butter and 1–1½ cups water

INSTRUCTIONS:

Put all ingredients in a blender and blend well.

Pour into a glass and enjoy!

As you make any of these soups, feel the emotions of love and gratitude or say some of your affirmations. Every time you cook with or work with water, the energy of love and gratitude can transform the food and your health.

When you eat soup, smell the delightful fragrance. Eat or sip it with love and gratitude, and feel your body transform with radiant health!

Quick and Simple Bok Choy Soup

Preparation time: 15 minutes   *Servings: 2–4*

This soup is easy to make and surprisingly delicious! If you overindulged the day before, this is nice and easy on your digestive system. We've had clients double the recipe and eat this soup for an entire day if they're feeling the need to gently cleanse their system.

INGREDIENTS:

2 baby bok choy (chopped)

1 large or 2 small yellow summer squash (sliced)

1 tsp. coriander (ground)

1 tsp. fennel seeds

1 tsp. curry powder

1 tsp. Celtic sea salt

2 tsp. ghee

1 tsp. coconut oil

INSTRUCTIONS:

In a skillet, melt 1 tsp. ghee. Add spices and sauté for one minute.

Add 2 cups water and bring to a boil. Add bok choy and sea salt and simmer for 3 minutes, then add yellow squash and simmer for 2 more minutes.

Drain most of the water except for about 1" (½ cup). With a hand blender or food processor, blend the ingredients until smooth. This makes a soup with a nice consistency (not too watery and not too thick).

At the end of cooking, add additional ghee and coconut oil to taste.

Delightfully Sweet Zucchini Squash Soup (Crock-Pot Easy!)

Preparation time: 25 minutes   *Serves: approximately 6 people*

This soup is naturally sweet in a subtle, delightful way, and it's a great mood booster if you're feeling stuck or down in the dumps. The cardamom, fennel, and cumin help with digestion—these spices also help balance and reset the body and mind. Serve this soup to family and friends and they're sure to ask for more!

INGREDIENTS:

1 Tbsp. ghee or raw butter

1 cup onions, diced

4 cups butternut squash, cubed

1 large zucchini, sliced (about 1½–2 cups)

1½ tsp. ground cardamom

1 tsp. ground fennel

¼ tsp. cayenne pepper

¼ tsp. ground coriander

2 tsp. cumin seeds

2 Tbsp. fresh ginger, diced

INSTRUCTIONS:

Sauté onions and all spices (except fresh ginger) in ghee until the onions are translucent.

Put cubed squash, diced ginger, and sliced zucchini into a Crock-Pot and cover with water. You'll use approximately 6 cups of water, less if you'd like a thicker soup. We tend to like thick, hearty soups, although this is actually really wonderful as a thinner soup—experiment and see which you like best! If you don't have a Crock-Pot, put into a large soup stockpot (you'll simmer on the lowest temperature on your stovetop).

Add onions and spices to the mixture and simmer until the squash is soft. With a hand blender or food processor, blend the soup until it is pureed.

Add more raw butter or ghee and sea salt to taste. We like to let each person add the amount of ghee or raw butter and sea salt to their bowl according to their individual taste.

Good Luck Soup

Preparation time: 20 minutes if you have cooked butternut squash already; about 1 hour if you're making the butternut squash as well

Servings: 6–8

Heather's mother had a trick to get her kids to eat spinach noodles when they were little: she called them "good luck noodles." She was pretty smart when it came to tricking Heather and her sister into eating their greens. The name of this soup might help get your kids to eat their greens, too! It's so delicious, thick, and comforting that they're sure to like it.

INGREDIENTS:

3 cups sliced bok choy

2 cups leeks, thinly sliced

2 cups sliced zucchini

2 cups cooked butternut squash

2½ Tbsp. coconut oil

2 Tbsp. curry powder

2 tsp. Celtic sea salt

1½ tsp. ground black pepper

1 tsp. turmeric

1 tsp. ground coriander

1 tsp. cumin powder

Pinch each of: fennel powder, cinnamon, and ginger

INSTRUCTIONS:

If you don't have cooked butternut squash, take the squash, prick about 10 holes in it with a knife point, then put it in a baking dish with 2" water and cook for 45 minutes in the oven at 350° F. (Alternatively, you can cook it in a Crock-Pot while you're out during the day. Add 2–3" water to the Crock-Pot and put the pricked butternut squash inside, cover, and set your timer on the lowest setting. Cook until the squash is soft and you can easily put a knife into the center.)

Put 1 Tbsp. coconut oil into a saucepan on low heat. Add all spices, except for sea salt, and the leeks; sauté the leeks for 2–3 minutes.

Add 2 cups water into the saucepan and bring to a rolling boil. Add bok choy and zucchini and simmer on low for 3 minutes, adding sea salt while simmering. Remove from heat and add butternut squash.

With an immersion blender (or in your blender or food processor with the S-blade), mix all ingredients until you have a smooth, blended soup. Add coconut oil and mix again to evenly distribute it.

Serving suggestion: Drizzle a small amount of flaxseed oil onto the soup in each bowl. Mixing in the oil at the end makes for a delicious final taste!

Louise's Favorite Bone Broth or Vegetable Broth

Bone broth is a wonderful way to nourish and heal your digestive tract and energize your body; it provides an easily digestible source of vitamins, minerals, and protein. If you're vegetarian, you can leave out the bones and meat scraps and create a healing vegetable elixir to sip during the day.

You can also include just bones and no vegetables, if you like. This broth can be used to sip, or used in recipes for more flavorful grains, soups, and more!

Note: gather your ingredients at your own pace.

Take a large paper shopping bag; open and place it in your freezer drawer.

Over the course of the week or several weeks, throw all bones and meat scraps in the bag in your freezer drawer. Also add vegetable scraps, vegetable peelings, and the odds and ends that you chop off of vegetables. Some examples are: onion peels, the peeled skins of carrots, garlic skins, salad scraps, artichoke tips, the tough ends of asparagus, kale stems, and pea pods.

Add 1 or 2 (3") pieces of seaweed, like wakame or digitata, for extra minerals.

If you don't have enough meat and bones to get started with your broth, you can go to the health-food store and purchase the necks, feet, backs, and wings of a chicken (these are inexpensive parts of the chicken that have a tremendous amount of nutritional value). Other options are lamb neck, marrow bones, or beef bones. Add these to your bag until you're ready to make the broth.

Keep adding vegetable scraps, meat scraps, and bones to your bag in the freezer until it's full and you're ready to make your broth.

Vegetarian option: If you're a vegetarian, eliminate the meat and bones and use only vegetable scraps. If you are just starting and don't have any vegetable scraps yet, here's a fast way to get nutrient-rich veggie broth: start by making a seaweed broth; once cooked, set aside the seaweed to eat in other meals, like soups, grains, or salads (just chop it up). If you do this, you just need 1–3 (6") strips of kombu, wakame, nori, or kelp to 4 cups of water.

Put all of the contents of the bag in your freezer into a stainless-steel stockpot. Alternatively, you can use your Crock-Pot to make this even easier!

Pour water so that it just covers the top of your bones, meat, and vegetables. Add ¼ cup apple cider vinegar, to bring out the minerals from the bones.

Add sea salt and pepper to taste. Start with a small amount in the beginning (about 1 tsp. each) and add more if needed when the broth is finished.

Turn your heat to high, put a lid on the pot, and bring the water to a boil. As soon as it's boiling, turn the heat down to very low and allow the pot to simmer all night long. The longer it cooks, the more nutrients you'll bring out of the bones and vegetable scraps.

The next morning, strain the liquid out of the rest of the ingredients. You don't keep any of the meat scraps, vegetable scraps, or bones—your goal is to strain them out and keep the liquid, which is now full of incredible nutrition.

Put the broth into the refrigerator. When it chills, remove the fat layer that will accumulate on the top.

Now you have something to nourish your body. Drink one or two cups a day: Louise has a cup in the morning and a cup before bed. You can also use the broth to make delicious, flavorful soups and stews, or flavor and cook vegetables and grains. To do this, you will use the broth just as you'd use water when cooking.

To store for longer than 5 days: For any broth you're not using within a 5-day period, store the liquid in quart-sized containers and put in your freezer to thaw when you're ready to use them. You can also store the broth in smaller containers or even pour it into ice-cube trays to customize the amount you want to use in meals or recipes.

Start a new bag of bones and vegetable scraps in your freezer for your next batch of bone broth and repeat the steps. Your body will love you for continuing to nourish it in this manner!

Joel's Surprisingly Delicious Sea Vegetable Soup

Preparation time: 25 minutes—or one hour and 25 minutes if you're using digitata kelp, to allow time for soaking the kelp

Servings: 4–6

This is so surprisingly delicious that it will delight even those who aren't fans of the taste of seaweed—it has a delicate yet rich flavor that is as yummy as it is healing and strengthening. Sea vegetables are excellent for your thyroid, which helps your body create energy. If you love egg drop soup, you'll love this soup even more!

INGREDIENTS:

1 quart bone broth, or you can use 1 quart of Imagine brand's organic free-range chicken broth (check ingredients to make sure there is no cane juice or sugar, as sometimes they change the ingredients!)

¼ lb. wild-caught Pacific cod

2 organic pasture-fed eggs

1 cup sea vegetable soup mix (from TheSeaweedMan.com), or you can use kelp, digitata kelp, arame, or wakame seaweed from the health-food store. (Digitata is very rich in iodine, which makes it a nice choice if you have type O blood, want protection from radiation, or want to boost thyroid health. See the notes on the next page for more on using digitata kelp.)

2 Tbsp. wheat-free tamari (or more to taste) or apple cider vinegar

2½ Tbsp. organic unrefined coconut oil

INSTRUCTIONS:

On the stovetop, put the chicken broth in the pan and heat to just boiling; reduce to simmer. Add sea vegetables and let simmer for 15–20 minutes.

Add cod, tamari, and coconut oil and simmer for 3–5 minutes (until fish flakes or breaks up easily).

Remove from heat and add eggs. They will cook as the soup cools (you will see them changing color as they cook). This keeps the eggs from overcooking and becoming hard to digest.

Pour into bowls and enjoy!

Notes:

If you use digitata kelp, cut it up into small pieces and soak it for one hour before adding to the soup. Soaking it ahead of time allows it to soften up. Alternatively, you can soak it first and put it into a food processor with the S-blade to chop it up into small, bite-sized pieces. You can add the soak water to your soup or use it for other recipes (soups, cooking grains, and so forth).

You can also use salmon or any other white fish. You might want less tamari if you use salmon because of salmon's richer taste.

Kale Carrot Soup

Preparation time: 25 minutes   *Servings: 4*

This soup has a delightful, light-yet-hearty taste that is slightly sweet and great for all seasons.

INGREDIENTS:

1 bunch kale

2 cups water (add more or less depending on how thick you like your soup—2 cups provides a medium-thick soup that is not too watery)

2 large carrots, chopped

¼ cup onion, chopped

1½ Tbsp. coconut oil

1 tsp. thyme

1 tsp. Celtic sea salt

INSTRUCTIONS:

In a saucepan, sauté onions and ½ Tbsp. coconut oil until onion is translucent. Then add all ingredients except the remaining coconut oil and the sea salt. Heat to boiling, then reduce heat to low. Simmer for 15 minutes, then add remainder of coconut oil and sea salt. Simmer for another 5 minutes, and then blend all ingredients together with a hand blender or in your blender or food processor. If you like curry, add 2 tsp. for a delicious taste!

Serve warm and enjoy! Each person may want to add some Herbamare herb sea salt, ghee, or coconut oil to their bowl of soup to taste.

Turkey Stew or Bone Broth

This stew is reminiscent of Thanksgiving dinner, with *much* less work! It is a delicious comfort food that is ideal for cool weather or anytime you want a hearty meal.

INGREDIENTS:

2 lbs. turkey—dark meat is a delicious, healthy, and economical option, or you can use breast meat or a mixture of white and dark meat (use turkey bones if you just want to make a bone and vegetable broth; see directions on the next page)

½ cup diced red onion

1 cup leeks, thinly sliced

4 cloves garlic, minced

1 cup bok choy, thinly sliced

3 cups fresh broccoli

1 Tbsp. thyme

2 tsp. basil

⅓ tsp. cardamom powder

1 tsp. dill

1 Tbsp. ghee

2 tsp. Sarah's Sea Salt, Tuscan Blend. (This is a blend of sea salt and Italian herbs, tomato flecks, lemon peel, and rosemary that you can find online or in gourmet-food stores. If you don't have this delicious mixture on hand, use a blend of sea salt with some or all of these spices for the same effect. You could also just use sea salt.)

3 cups water

INSTRUCTIONS:

In a skillet, sauté the onion, leeks, garlic, and spices in ghee until onions are translucent (about 5 minutes).

Add 1 cup of water to the skillet. Add turkey, cover, and simmer lightly for 15 minutes, until the outside of the turkey is browned. This creates a concentrated soup-stock effect.

While the turkey and spices are simmering, bring 2 cups of water to a boil in a stockpot. Add broccoli and bok choy to the water and reduce heat to a simmer. Add the turkey-and-spice mixture; continue to simmer for 15–20 minutes, until turkey is fully cooked.

Add Sarah's Sea Salt about 5 minutes after adding the turkey-and-spice mixture into the broccoli and bok choy.

Serve warm in big soup bowls.

Variations:

For brilliant color, add 1 cup sliced carrots and/or 1 cup sliced red cabbage to the broccoli and bok choy.

You can make this into a kind of bone broth by using just turkey bones with a little meat on them, instead of the turkey. This will make a nice, easy-to-digest, and flavorful turkey and vegetable soup.

For those who are not food combining, this meal would be delicious with red-skinned potatoes (about a cup of diced potatoes). However, from a food-combining perspective, you would want to avoid combining a starchy vegetable (or any starch, like grains) with an animal-protein meal.

Fast, Easy Burgers (No Bun Intended!)

Forget fast-food restaurants—you can make healthy burgers quickly in your own home. If you haven't planned ahead, grass-fed and/or organic beef, chicken, lamb, or turkey are great to have on hand. Louise loves to buy ground meat or poultry, make it into patties, and put it in her freezer, so she can take a patty or two out at a time to thaw and serve. This is a great way to make sure you always have the option of a burger, even if you couldn't get to the grocery store!

Can I cook a frozen meat patty? Yes, you can. Put about 1" water or bone broth into your skillet and set your stove burner to low. Add in the frozen patty and allow it to slow cook. Once it is mostly thawed, you can add some healthy fat, like raw butter, or continue to cook the burger in water or bone broth. Bone broth is a wonderful way to add flavor to your burger!

What about the bun? Since most buns are made of flour that is hard on the digestive system, we recommend eating your burger without a bun. Instead, consider pairing it with our Grain-Free, Gluten-Free Rosemary Bread (see recipe later in the chapter) or putting it on top of a salad. Both options make for better digestion and food combining.

How to make a great beef, turkey, chicken, or lamb burger:

1 lb. ground meat makes about 4–6 burgers. Shape your meat into patties.

Put your skillet on low heat and add either bone broth or a healthy cooking fat, like raw butter, ghee, duck fat (wonderful for lamb burgers), or beef tallow, and let it melt onto the skillet.

Add herbs or spices of your choice. Some great options are: ¼ tsp. ground black pepper with ½ tsp. thyme, or ½ tsp. turmeric and ¼ tsp. cardamom or fennel. Allow the herbs and spices to warm in the bone broth or oil to release their medicinal properties.

Add the patties and cook on low or medium low, turning them when they lift easily from the pan with a spatula. As the meat cooks, it will shrink and plump a bit. When you touch it in the center, it will be a little bouncy and firm when it's done.

We actually like to put a knife or the edge of the spatula into the meat to see how ready it is. When it's cooked on the outside and still a little pink inside (rare), we take it off the heat and serve. If you like it cooked a bit more, keep checking the inside of the patty until it's done to your liking. (Keep in mind that meat cooked more rare is easier to digest.) This will take 5–10 minutes on low heat, which is a healthier way to cook meat. Allow more time for the extra steps above if you're starting with a frozen patty.

Serve with cultured vegetables, a salad, and mustard. (Look for a mustard made with apple cider vinegar instead of white vinegar. Whole Foods 365 brand has an organic German mustard made with apple cider vinegar and horseradish that tastes great with burgers!) If you must have bread with your burger, our Grain-Free, Gluten-Free "Rye" Bread and Rosemary Bread recipes are great options. They combine well with meat from a food-combining perspective, and while they're not going to hold your burger the way a bun does, they can be eaten with it on the side or with knife and fork.

Baked Stuffed Red Snapper

|||||||||||||||||||||||||||||||||||||||||||||||||||||||||||||||||||||||||||||||||||||||||||||||||||||||||||||||||||||||||||||||||||||||||||||||||||||||||||||||||||||||||||||||||||||

Preparation time: about 25 minutes for the stuffing and about 15–20 minutes for cooking the fish

Servings: 8

This recipe was modified from a very popular snapper recipe on Allrecipes.com. It's great for a dinner party or special meal, when you have a little more time to cook.

INGREDIENTS:

8 (4-oz.) fillets red snapper

8 oz. cooked baby shrimp

2 cup fresh maitake mushrooms, or reishi or shiitake mushrooms—if you can't find any of these preferred medicinal mushrooms, you could use portobello mushrooms

1 cup chopped red onion

1 bunch celery

1 bunch watercress

2 large carrots

4 cloves fresh garlic, minced

2 Tbsp. coconut oil

1 Tbsp. ghee

¼ cup organic white wine or apple cider vinegar

2 Tbsp. fresh parsley

1 Tbsp. fresh cilantro

2 tsp. oregano

1½ tsp. thyme

1 tsp. dill

1 tsp. Herbamare herb sea salt (if you don't have this around, use regular sea salt)

½ tsp. sea salt

⅛ tsp. ground black pepper

INSTRUCTIONS:

Preheat oven to 350° F.

To make the stuffing: Put all vegetables except for the garlic into a food processor (S-blade), and blend until the vegetables are finely chopped. Set this aside. Now, in a skillet, add the ghee, coconut oil, spices (oregano, dill, thyme, and pepper), and garlic. Let the ghee and coconut oil melt with the spices, and add the fresh garlic. Warm for 3 minutes, then add the vegetables, Herbamare,

sea salt, and vinegar. Let this mixture simmer on the lowest heat for 15 minutes. Remove from heat and let it cool; once cooled completely, add the cooked baby shrimp and mix thoroughly.

If you're making the stuffing ahead of time, put the mixture into the refrigerator until you're ready to make the fish. You might want to make the stuffing earlier in the day or the night before if you're having guests.

This allows the flavors to really come out and makes for a quick prep time when guests arrive.

Optional: Marinate the snapper for two hours in 6 Tbsp. olive oil, the juice of 1 lemon, and 3 cloves minced garlic.

To make the fish: In a baking dish, place snapper so that it's lying flat. Add a layer of stuffing on top. (If you have extra stuffing, you can thin it out with some water and make a wonderful stew or soup.)

Bake for 15–20 minutes or just until the fish flakes easily.

Heavenly Haddock

Preparation time: 15 minutes

Servings: 2

INGREDIENTS:

½ lb. fresh wild-caught haddock

1 Tbsp. coconut oil

1 Tbsp. curry powder

½ tsp. thyme

5 coriander seeds

Hemp-seed oil

Herbamare

INSTRUCTIONS:

In a saucepan, add 2 cups water and the haddock. Add in curry, coconut oil, thyme, and coriander seeds. Simmer for 5–7 minutes, until fish is cooked.

Serve over a bed of spring-mix lettuce with ½ cup cultured veggies for each person (our favorite with this meal is a blend of cultured daikon radish with ginger). Drizzle with hemp-seed oil and add Herbamare to taste.

If you'd like, you can use the broth for sea-vegetable soup: Remove the fish and add some digitata, alaria, or soup mix from Maine Seaweed (TheSeaweedMan.com). This family-owned company has the purest and best sea vegetables we've found.

Allow the sea veggies to soak in the broth while it's cooling. When you're ready to make or eat the soup, let it simmer for 5 minutes and add in vegetables of your choice, or simply enjoy with the sea vegetables and broth. You might also want to add some of the cooked haddock back into the broth at the end.

Magnificent Mahi Mahi Salad

Preparation time: approximately 25 minutes

Servings: 4

This is a delicious salad that has a delightful interplay of sweet and savory flavors.

INGREDIENTS:

1 lb. wild-caught mahi mahi

1 cup broccoli sprouts (or microgreens)

1 bunch broccoli (or use celery root, chopped into chunks)

1 head romaine lettuce

1 cucumber

1 avocado

1 onion

1" fresh ginger

2 tsp. dried basil

2 tsp. dill spice

Macadamia-nut oil (or flaxseed oil)

⅓ cup kimchee or cultured vegetables

INSTRUCTIONS:

Place mahi mahi in a baking pan with 2" water. Add sliced onion, diced ginger, and fresh cut broccoli; sprinkle dill and basil over the top. Cover and bake at 350° F for approximately 15 minutes.

While the fish is baking, prepare the salad: On each plate, arrange romaine lettuce, broccoli sprouts, thinly sliced cucumber, and sliced avocado.

Once the fish is cooked, cut it in quarters. Place one quarter of the fish on each plate, along with the cooked broccoli, ginger, and onions. Use a spatula or slotted spoon to drain out the water.

Add ⅓ cup kimchee or cultured vegetables with purple cabbage or carrots to add color and balance the dish with a sour taste.

Drizzle macadamia-nut oil over the salad. Add Herbamare or sea salt to taste, and enjoy!

Hassle-Free Fabulous Whole Chicken for Busy People

Preparation time: 20 minutes to prepare, 2–4 hours to cook   *Servings: 6–8*

Chicken, especially organic and pasture fed, is a wonderful, nourishing meal. While marketing will try to tell you that the white breast meat is the best, our ancestors knew that the dark meat is full of important fatty acids and nutrients, so go for *all* the meat and know your body will love you!

You can cook chicken so that it's fast, easy, and guaranteed to be moist—no more overcooked chicken done in the oven with a fear of burning. If you are pressed for time or want a sure thing in terms of tender chicken, this is the recipe for you!

If you buy chicken directly from the farmer—one you know has good practices, allows their chickens to run free and eat their native pasture diet, and does not feed them soy or any genetically modified (GMO) feed—you can get more affordable chickens *and* support your local farmer.

INGREDIENTS:

1 whole fryer chicken (between 4–5 lbs.), preferably
    organic pasture fed

½ cup organic extra-virgin olive oil (virgin unrefined
    coconut oil works well, too!)

4 cloves garlic, peeled and left whole

2 Tbsp. dried rosemary

2 Tbsp. dried thyme

2 Tbsp. dried basil

1 Tbsp. apple cider vinegar

½ tsp. sea salt

½ tsp. fresh ground black pepper

Optional: ½ cup sliced onions or 1 cup finely sliced leeks

INSTRUCTIONS:

Take the chicken and remove the bag of giblets and the neck from the interior cavity. Set these aside in the refrigerator because they are super nutrient rich and have important uses in other recipes! The neck can be used to make bone broth (see Louise's Favorite Bone Broth recipe earlier in the chapter), and the organs can be used to make delicious organ meat pâté (there are many great recipes online, especially if you do a search for "GAPS diet organ meat pâté recipe").

Rinse the chicken with filtered water and put it in your Crock-Pot. Add 1 cup of water to the bottom—you don't need more than that. Some Crock-Pot recipes say to brown the chicken first and not to use water. We've found that we can skip browning and add a little water to the bottom of the Crock-Pot for the best results. If you have the time to brown the chicken first and you love that, go for it! We find that it's not necessary for a flavorful, moist chicken.

In a small bowl, mix the olive oil, rosemary, thyme, basil, sea salt, and pepper. Take your hand and lift the skin at the edge of the chicken breast. See if you can gently push your fingers under the skin to make an opening between the meat and the skin. (It's usually pretty easy to do this with no or minimal breakage of the skin.) Now take some of the herb-and-oil mixture in your hand and rub it on the meat under the skin. We like to put it under the skin because it spreads the flavors right into the meat, but if you don't want to do this, you can rub the mixture on top of the skin. You should have some of the oil-and-herb mixture left over, and it can go on top of the skin or into the water in the Crock-Pot.

Add the apple cider vinegar to the water at the bottom of the Crock-Pot; set the timer to anything from 4 to 8 hours. The Crock-Pot will adjust the heat accordingly so that it's done. Our favorite is 4 hours—we put the chicken in around 8 A.M. and it's ready for lunch. If you're working, you could do 8 hours and cook it overnight so that you wake up to chicken you can grab for lunch that day. Or get it all together in the pot the night before, store the interior crock in your refrigerator, then take it out and set your Crock-Pot for 8 hours so that your chicken is ready for dinner when you get home! Your Crock-Pot will just go to "warm" once the cooking is done, so if you're not home within 8 hours, it will stay on warm until you return.

If you don't have a Crock-Pot, you can make this in your oven: Add the chicken to a glass or Pyrex baking container/large casserole dish with a good-sized lip. Put the water in the bottom of the baking dish. Preheat the oven to 350° F and bake until your meat thermometer reads 165° F (this should take about 1–2 hours). You could do this the night before and have the chicken for lunch and dinner the next day. Just grab a leg or two in the morning and go—it can make a great lunch or snack. Grab some spring mix, some avocado, and a little olive oil and apple cider vinegar, put it in a small container for transport, and you're good to go.

Serving suggestions: Serve with steamed carrots and broccoli. If you want, you can throw the broccoli right into the Crock-Pot with the chicken so you don't even have to cook it separately—it's all ready at once. How's that for convenience? Throw in some carrots, too, if you want some good color.

Simple Crock-Pot Lamb Shanks (with Bonus Lamb Bone Broth!)

This meal is so easy and makes incredibly tender lamb. You can make it overnight or in the morning so that it's warm and ready by lunch or dinner. As a bonus, you'll have delicious lamb bone broth to sip later or use in other recipes.

INGREDIENTS:

4 lamb shanks

4 cups filtered water

1 Tbsp. dried rosemary

1 Tbsp. dried thyme

1 Tbsp. dried basil

2 tsp. sea salt

1 tsp. fresh ground black pepper

1 tsp. ground allspice

INSTRUCTIONS:

Add all ingredients in a Crock-Pot. (If you don't have a Crock-Pot, you can make this dish in a braising pan or Dutch oven, on the lowest heat setting on your stovetop.)

Decide when you want your lamb shanks ready to eat: If it's morning and you want them done by lunch, set your Crock-Pot to high, medium high, or the 4-hour setting. (Check the directions on your Crock-Pot for timing—if you have one with the 4-6-8-10-hour settings, the 4-hour setting provides fall-off-the-bone lamb shanks by lunch.) If it's nighttime and you want to have your lamb ready to take to work by the morning—or if it's morning and you want it ready for dinner—use the lowest setting, or the 8- or 10-hour setting, depending on when you need it to be ready.

That's it!

Serve with steamed or sautéed vegetables for a delicious, easy meal. And remember to save the broth to sip or use for recipes!

Short Ribs One-Pot Crock-Pot Meal

Preparation time: 20 minutes to prepare ingredients and 8–10 hours to cook in your Crock-Pot

Servings: 6

If you want to make a special dinner or are having a dinner party when you're short on time, this is the perfect one-pot meal that will delight your family or dinner guests! Most short ribs served in restaurants have a lot of sauce and can even be heavy tasting. These short ribs are different—clean tasting, simple, fall-off-the-bone tender, and delicious!

INGREDIENTS:

4 lbs. short ribs

5 cups brussels sprouts

4 large carrots, sliced in rounds

1 bunch celery (about 8 stalks)

2 leeks (about 2 cups chopped)

4 Tbsp. coconut oil

4 cloves garlic, minced

2 bay leaves

1 Tbsp. thyme

1 Tbsp. rosemary

1 tsp. basil

2 tsp. pepper

2 tsp. sea salt

2 tsp. fennel, ground

1 tsp. paprika

2 cups bone broth—or filtered water, if you don't have bone broth

2 cups red wine

INSTRUCTIONS:

Optional first step: Put the coconut oil in a skillet on the lowest heat setting and allow to melt. Add all herbs and spices and heat for 2 minutes to release their flavors and medicinal qualities. You don't need to brown the short ribs, but if you want to do this for extra flavor, you can add them in and brown them on the top and bottom, then add them into the Crock-Pot. Add about a cup of the bone broth or water to the skillet and heat for 2 minutes, then put the liquid and spices into the Crock-Pot. This will boost the flavor of the meal.

Slice the carrots, celery, and leeks (to make this fast and easy, use the slicing attachment on your food processor, if you have one). Either slice the brussels sprouts or leave them whole.

Place all ingredients in the Crock-Pot. (If you don't have a Crock-Pot, you can make this dish in a braising pan or Dutch oven, on the lowest heat setting on your stovetop.)

Set your Crock-Pot to the lowest temperature or the 8-hour setting. You can slow cook this up to 10 hours for delicious, tender short ribs.

Cinnamon Buckwheat Cereal

Servings: 4 (make adjustments for number of people)

This makes a deliciously sweet breakfast that can be paired with a morning vegetable soup or smoothie. (Be sure to soak the cream of buckwheat or raw buckwheat groats the night before—see instructions on soaking grains, nuts, seeds, and beans at the beginning of this chapter.)

INGREDIENTS:

> 2 cups soaked cream of buckwheat cereal or
> raw buckwheat groats
>
> 1 cup water
>
> 1 Tbsp. cinnamon
>
> ½ tsp. sea salt
>
> 1 Tbsp. ghee or raw butter
>
> If you want this sweetened, add stevia, honey,
> or maple syrup to taste

INSTRUCTIONS:

Bring water to a boil. Add soaked cream of buckwheat or raw buckwheat groats; as this comes to a boil, reduce the heat to simmer.

Add cinnamon and sea salt and mix in grains. Simmer on low for approximately 10 minutes (15 minutes for groats) or until the water is soaked in. If the grains need more water, simply add another ¼–½ cup as needed until they're done. Add ghee or raw butter.

Add stevia, honey, or maple syrup to taste (optional)—each person can add their own when served, depending on taste.

Creamy Cream of Buckwheat

Preparation time: 8–10 hours to soak buckwheat (or soak overnight; see instructions at the beginning of this chapter) and 15 minutes to prepare.

This is a savory version of cream of buckwheat that makes a satisfying, comfort-food meal any time of day.

INGREDIENTS:

> 2 cups soaked cream of buckwheat cereal
>
> ½ Tbsp. turmeric powder
>
> ¼ tsp. coriander seeds
>
> 1 tsp. cumin powder
>
> ½ Tbsp. coconut oil
>
> ½ Tbsp. ghee or raw butter
>
> 1 tsp. Celtic sea salt

INSTRUCTIONS:

After the cream of buckwheat has been soaked, drained, and rinsed, follow package directions to cook it. Add in all of the spices. Just prior to all of the water being absorbed, add the ghee and coconut oil.

Serve with cooked greens and vegetables or place over a salad. Add Celtic sea salt or Herbamare to taste.

Delicate Quinoa with Chayote Squash

Servings: 4–6

Chayote, technically a fruit, is a green pear-shaped member of the gourd family and tastes like a cross between a potato and a cucumber. It's a lovely, delicate taste. You can substitute any winter or summer squash if you cannot find it in your local store.

Note that you may want to start soaking the quinoa the night before you want to make this dish (soak for 8–12 hours and see instructions at the beginning of this chapter). The recipe itself takes about 10 minutes to prepare and 15–20 minutes to simmer on the stovetop.

INGREDIENTS:

2 cups presoaked quinoa

2 chayotes (if they're not available in your local store, use delicata squash, pattypan squash, or acorn squash instead)

2 cups water

1 Tbsp. thyme

1 Tbsp. basil

2 tsp. ground fennel

1 tsp. ground coriander

2 tsp. Herbamare or Celtic sea salt

¼ cup ghee

½ cup red onion

INSTRUCTIONS:

Put 1 Tbsp. ghee into a saucepan and add all spices (except sea salt or Herbamare) and onions. Sauté and stir until onion is translucent.

Add water and bring to a boil. Add presoaked quinoa and allow to boil, then turn down the heat to simmer. Add chayotes; simmer until quinoa is translucent, adding sea salt or Herbamare just before it's done.

Turn off heat when quinoa is translucent, and add remaining ghee.

Serving suggestions: This dish is delicious with a side dish of vegetables and sea vegetables (seaweed). For one of our favorite serving suggestions, place the quinoa over a bed of romaine lettuce, with additional avocado chunks and a little extra-virgin olive oil drizzled over the whole thing for added flavor. Season to taste with sea salt and fresh ground black pepper.

Quinoa, Broccoli, and Leek Pilaf

Servings: 4–6

This recipe tastes delicious warm or cold. We use it as a staple for long day trips or air travel because you don't have to warm it up to enjoy it. On flights, when we can't bring olive oil or some other oil easily, we add extra ghee for healthy fat and delicious flavor. While cold meals for a full day of travel are not always pleasant, this one is really quite delicious and something to look forward to!

Note that you may want to start soaking the quinoa the night before you want to make this dish (soak for 8–12 hours and see instructions at the beginning of this chapter). The recipe itself takes about 10 minutes to prepare and about 15 minutes to simmer on the stovetop.

INGREDIENTS:

2 cups presoaked quinoa

1 Tbsp. ghee

½ cup leeks, sliced thin

1 cup broccoli florets, chopped small

2 tsp. curry powder

Sea salt to taste

INSTRUCTIONS:

Sauté ghee with leeks and curry powder for 3 minutes.

Bring 1 cup of water to a boil. Add quinoa, broccoli, leeks, and curry, and reduce heat to simmer until quinoa is cooked. This will take about 15 minutes—you'll know the quinoa is done when it looks more translucent and no longer has bright white spots in the center of the grains.

Add ghee and sea salt to taste.

Serving suggestions: When traveling, you can put this quinoa over romaine lettuce (romaine is a very hearty lettuce and travels well in an insulated lunch bag, even if you don't have ice to keep it cold due to being on a plane).

Lovely Millet Loaf or Pilaf

This dish can be cooked as a millet pilaf or a loaf of "bread" that is nutty tasting and satisfying, especially during cool fall and winter months.

Note that you may want to start soaking the millet the night before you want to make this dish (soak for 8–12 hours and see instructions at the beginning of this chapter). The recipe itself takes about 10 minutes to prepare and 15–20 minutes to simmer on the stovetop.

INGREDIENTS:

> 2 cups presoaked millet
>
> 2 cups water
>
> 2 Tbsp. dried burdock root (you can get organic dried burdock root from MountainRoseHerbs.com) or fresh burdock root, diced
>
> 1 Tbsp. coconut oil
>
> 2 tsp. thyme
>
> 2 tsp. basil
>
> 2 tsp. astragalus powder
>
> 1 tsp. sea salt

INSTRUCTIONS:

In a saucepan, bring water to a boil. Once it's boiling, add soaked millet and reduce heat to simmer. Add spices, sea salt, astragalus powder, and burdock root; simmer until millet is completely cooked and the grains are translucent and fluffy. Add coconut oil and stir thoroughly.

If you're eating this as a millet pilaf, it is now ready to serve with your favorite vegetable side dish.

If you're making millet loaf, let the cooked millet pilaf sit for 15 minutes to cool. Once cooled, transfer into a greased bread-loaf pan and cook in a preheated oven at 350° F for 15 minutes.

Remove from oven and cool. Slice like bread; spread on some coconut oil, raw butter, or ghee, if you like; and serve with salad and cultured vegetables or with a vegetable soup.

Millet Pilaf—Super Thyroid Booster

Servings: 6–8

Bladderwrack is a vitamin- and mineral-rich medicinal sea vegetable that has been known to help boost the thyroid and metabolism. Dr. Peter D'Adamo, a nutrition and blood-type expert, says that bladderwrack is especially good for weight loss for individuals with type O blood. If your energy is low or you have hypothyroid symptoms, this dish may give you the "get up and go" that you need, especially in the cold days of fall or winter!

While bladderwrack is known among the sea vegetable varieties to be strictly medicinal, rather than tasty, this dish actually brings the right blend of ingredients together to make it taste delicious. (You can find bladderwrack at: TheSeaweedMan.com.)

Note that you may want to start soaking the millet the night before you want to make this dish (soak for 8–12 hours and see instructions at the beginning of this chapter). The recipe itself takes about 10 minutes to prepare and 15–20 minutes to simmer on the stovetop.

Follow the instructions for the "Lovely Millet Loaf" recipe on the previous page, but prepare it as a pilaf (that is, do not cook in a bread-loaf pan). Then add the rest of the ingredients below.

INGREDIENTS:

> 6 cups pea-shoot sprouts (green sprouts—if you can't find these in the store, you can use 6 cups snow peas or snap peas)
>
> 6 carrots, washed and sliced (in rounds)
>
> 1 onion, diced
>
> 1 Tbsp. curry powder
>
> ½ Tbsp. coconut oil
>
> ½ tsp. bladderwrack seaweed per serving, ground up in a coffee grinder (this will give the dish a salty taste, so taste your meal before adding salt!)

INSTRUCTIONS:

Put 1" water into a saucepan; add carrots, onions, and curry powder; and simmer until the carrots are soft.

If you're using snap peas or snow peas instead of pea-shoot sprouts, add them in after 5 minutes of simmering the carrots and onions.

Add a pinch of sea salt and coconut oil. Add nutty millet loaf and simmer until warmed and set aside.

Serving suggestion: Put 2 cups of pea-shoot sprouts on each plate with some spring-mix salad and drizzle with hemp-seed oil. Add the millet pilaf over the fresh vegetables. Sprinkle ½ tsp. bladderwrack over the millet for each plate served.

Enjoy!

Grain-Free Rosemary Bread

Preparation time: 2 hours total—
15 minutes to prepare, 20–30 minutes to bake

Servings: Makes 2 generous-sized loaves

This is a very flexible, fast, and easy bread recipe with wonderful results! If going grain-free has made you miss bread, you now have a great substitute.

You can do a lot with this basic bread recipe: You could remove all the herbs and spices (rosemary, thyme, fennel powder, and pepper) and have a plain bread for sandwiches. Or you could make it sweet with cinnamon, cardamom, and a little more honey. Once you have experience baking this bread, let your creativity flow and create the tastes you love!

INGREDIENTS:

3 cups coconut flour

¾ cup almond flour

½ cup flax meal

¼ cup coconut oil

2 Tbsp. honey

2 Tbsp. apple cider vinegar

6 eggs

1 Tbsp. rosemary

1½ tsp. thyme

1 tsp. fennel powder

1 tsp. baking soda

½ tsp. sea salt

½ tsp. fresh ground black pepper

Water: You will likely want to add some water to the bread to get it to a consistency thicker than cake batter but a bit thinner than mashed potatoes. Start by adding a small amount and mixing in thoroughly, then add a bit more until you get the right consistency. The batter should pour easily into your bread loaf pan.

INSTRUCTIONS:

Preheat the oven to 350° F.

Grind up the dried rosemary leaves. Add all dry ingredients—including herbs, fennel powder, salt, and pepper—into a food processor with the S-blade and process until fully mixed. If you don't have a food processor, you can put all dry ingredients into a bowl and mix well with a spoon.

Now add wet ingredients—coconut oil, honey, apple cider vinegar, and eggs—to the dry ingredients and mix well. If you want, you can taste the batter and see what you think, as the baked bread will have a very similar taste. If you're an experienced cook or baker, you may want to tweak the herbs, salt, or pepper to your taste.

Put into a bread-loaf pan and bake for 15–30 minutes, making sure to check it at 15 minutes. As soon as you start to smell that baked-bread smell, it's time to check—so open the oven and see if the bread is starting to look browned on the top and edges. This bread can get quite brown before burning, but if you want a more moist loaf, you'll want to take it out when it's just starting to get golden brown or you see a little brown on the edges. Insert a clean knife in the middle and see if it comes out clean. If so, it's ready. You can also gently touch the top of the bread to see if it's firm with a little bounce. That is another indicator that your bread is done. Don't be afraid to make a cut in the bread and take a peek if this is your first time baking and you want to see if it's done! You can always pop it back in the oven if it needs a few more minutes.

Serving suggestions: Serve with raw butter, coconut oil, or your favorite all-fruit spread!

Grain-Free "Rye" Bread (Vegan)

Preparation time: 8–12 hours to soak the almonds and flaxseeds, 3 extra hours if you want to make your own almond flour (omit if you use store-bought almond flour), 15 minutes to make the bread, and 20 minutes to bake it

Servings: 6–8

This fast and easy recipe is a take on traditional rye bread, but without the gluten or grains! This bread is hearty and can be a meal in and of itself. Or you can slice it small and use it to dip into your favorite dip or pâté. You can even make small sandwiches with it—just don't overfill the sandwich.

Invent your favorite ways to serve this bread! It is grain-free, and if you soak the almonds and flax seeds first, the bread will be easier to digest.

We made this recipe without eggs, which are in typical Paleo, GAPS, and SCD baked goods, because we wanted to provide an option for people who have trouble digesting these foods or those who are vegan. We think that if you have trouble digesting typical Paleo, GAPS, and SCD baked goods with eggs, it's either because the nuts and seeds were not soaked first or because you may have issues digesting some high FODMAPS foods. It's worth exploring to see if one of these shifts makes it easier for you to enjoy baked foods!

What are high FODMAPS Foods? FODMAP stands for "Fermentable Oligo-Di-Monosaccharides and Polyols" and includes fructose, lactose, fructans, galactans, and polyols. For people sensitive to FODMAPS, foods like these (the list is longer) can create digestive symptoms: wheat, onions, garlic, honey, dairy, xylitol, erythritol, avocado, and even coconut milk and coconut flour. People with IBS (irritable bowel syndrome) are thought to be FODMAPS sensitive.

INGREDIENTS:

1 cup flax meal—you can purchase organic flax meal or use a mix of dark and golden flaxseeds, soaked and dehydrated, then ground into meal

⅔ cup almond flour

⅔ cup coconut flour

¾ cup water

4 Tbsp. caraway seeds

2 Tbsp. olive oil

1 Tbsp. honey

1 Tbsp. blackstrap molasses

2 Tbsp. apple cider vinegar

1½ tsp. ground cumin

1 tsp. sea salt

½ tsp. baking soda

INSTRUCTIONS:

Preheat the oven to 350° F.

Add all ingredients into a food processor with the S-blade and process until fully mixed. If you don't have a food processor, you can put all dry ingredients into a bowl and mix well with a spoon.

Put into a bread-loaf pan and bake for 15–30 minutes. Keep in mind that this bread does not rise the way breads with gluten do (even if you use eggs, it won't really rise much). So fill your pan up higher if you want a taller loaf that looks like sandwich bread when you slice it.

Make sure to check the bread at 15 minutes. As soon as you start to smell that baked-bread smell, it's time to check—so open the oven and see if the bread is starting to look browned on the top and edges. This bread can get quite brown before burning, but if you want a more moist bread, you'll want to take it out when it's just starting to get golden brown or you see a little brown on the edges. Insert a clean knife in the middle and see if it comes out clean. If so, it's ready. You can also gently touch the top of the bread to see if it's firm with a little bounce. That is another indicator that your bread is done. Don't be afraid to make a cut in the bread and take a peek if this is your first time baking and you want to see if it's done! You can always pop it back in the oven if it needs a few more minutes.

Serving suggestions: Serve with raw butter, coconut oil, or your favorite all-fruit spread (with no added sugar)! You can also serve this as an appetizer in small slices for pâté or even make little sandwiches with it. In addition, you can bake this bread recipe in little heart-shaped silicone baking cups for a wonderful snack on the go!

Easy Grain-Free Waffles or Pancakes

Preparation time: 10 minutes   *Servings: 6–10 pancakes or waffles, depending on size*

Who doesn't love pancakes and waffles? If you've gone gluten-free or Paleo, or you're jumping into healing diets like GAPS and SCD, don't despair—you can still eat this favorite breakfast and brunch dish! (If you are following FODMAPS and are sensitive to coconut flour, substitute with almond flour.)

These pancakes/waffles are delicious and will delight your taste buds. They will likely be loved by kids and adults alike. While not as fluffy as traditional pancakes/waffles, they come pretty close. The spices added help balance the recipe so that your body will feel more satisfied after just 2 or 3.

INGREDIENTS:

> 3 eggs
>
> 3 Tbsp. coconut oil (can also use butter or ghee)
>
> 3 Tbsp. coconut milk (see recipe for easy instructions to make your own coconut milk)
>
> 2 Tbsp. coconut flour (you can use almond flour instead, if you like)
>
> 2 tsp. cinnamon powder
>
> 2 tsp. cardamom powder
>
> 1 tsp. honey, or 3 dates
>
> 1 tsp. allspice
>
> 1 tsp. sea salt

INSTRUCTIONS:

You can make these pancakes or waffles on the stovetop or in the oven. If you make them in the oven, preheat to 350° F.

If you're using dates instead of honey, you can blend all of these ingredients in your food processor with the S-blade. Add the dates, coconut milk, coconut oil, and eggs in first, and blend them up well. You can then transfer to a bowl and whisk in the rest of the ingredients, or just add the rest of the ingredients to your food processor and blend well.

If you don't have a food processor, honey will be easier to work with. Melt your honey and coconut oil in a saucepan on low so that they are liquid and easier to work with.

In a mixing bowl, combine eggs, coconut milk, honey and coconut oil, whisking together well. Add in the rest of the ingredients, and whisk everything up.

Now you have a choice: pancakes or waffles? Pancakes are easy and just need to be ladled onto a warm saucepan (with butter, ghee, or coconut oil melted in the pan first to keep them from sticking) or on a greased cookie sheet to go into your oven. For waffles, Heather likes to use silicone waffle pans you can get at Amazon.com. She takes a couple of stainless-steel cookie sheets, puts the waffle pans on top of them (because the silicone is flexible and bendy), and pops them in the oven for 5–10 minutes.

Your pancakes or waffles are done when they're golden brown.

Pancake tip: If you make them on the stovetop, the time to flip them is when you either see little bubbles in the batter or they come up easily when you slide a spatula under them. A thin stainless-steel spatula works best for flipping your pancakes.

Waffle-maker tip: Most waffle makers have toxic nonstick coatings to make them easy to use. While waffle makers are fun and make a slightly more perfect waffle, you may opt for the silicone waffle pans instead if you're focusing on reducing toxic exposure.

Serving suggestions: These pancakes and waffles are delicious with maple syrup, if you are eating it. If not, you could use honey, plain butter, coconut oil, or fruit as a topping. Puree strawberries in your food processor as a replacement for maple syrup (add a couple dates if you want it really sweet). These are also delicious drizzled with Cinnamon Orange Coconut Butter (see recipe in the Gingerbread recipe that follows).

Grain-Free Gingerbread with Cinnamon Orange Coconut Butter

Preparation time: 20 minutes   *Servings: 8–10 slices*

This is a slightly sweet quick bread that is easy to make and makes a wonderful alternative to those standard breakfast standbys, muffins and doughnuts. Full of protein and mood- and digestion-boosting spices, this is a healthy, tasty treat for any time of day!

The bread can be enjoyed alone—or for a really wonderful fall or winter treat, add the Cinnamon Orange Coconut Butter topping, and you'll have a delicious dessert that will remind you of gingerbread.

INGREDIENTS FOR THE GINGERBREAD:

6 dates (about ¼ cup)—or use ¼ cup honey or 2 mashed bananas

¾ cup organic coconut flour

6 eggs

6 Tbsp. coconut oil

⅓ cup water

2 Tbsp. vanilla extract

¼ tsp. ground fenugreek

2 tsp. ground cinnamon

1 tsp. baking soda

1 tsp. sea salt

½ tsp. cardamom

¼ tsp. cloves

¼ tsp. ginger powder

INSTRUCTIONS:

Preheat the oven to 350° F.

Grease a bread-loaf pan (preferably glass or silicone) with coconut oil or raw, grass-fed butter.

Combine all ingredients for the bread and blend until thoroughly mixed and the coconut flour has absorbed all of the liquids. If you don't have a food processor or immersion blender, avoid using dates and instead use honey or mashed bananas for your sweetener. If you do have a food processor, put all ingredients in it with the S-blade.

Pour batter into your greased bread-loaf pan and bake for 30–45 minutes. You may want to check periodically with a toothpick or fork inserted into the middle of the bread. When the toothpick or fork tines come out clean, your bread is done baking. The bread will dry out if you leave it in too long; if you like it to be more moist, you can take it out earlier, at the 25–30 minute mark. Press the top of the loaf with your finger; if it's pretty firm, it's done. You can also take out the bread and slice it with a sharp knife to see if it is done to your liking.

When your bread is done, take it out of the oven and let it cool before removing it from the pan. Once it's cooled, slice and eat plain or add your favorite topping, like coconut oil, raw pasture-fed butter, or apple butter.

INGREDIENTS FOR THE CINNAMON ORANGE COCONUT BUTTER:

½ cup coconut oil (organic, unrefined/virgin)

¼ cup dates

2 Tbsp. vanilla

2 Tbsp. juice from a fresh orange

1 Tbsp. cinnamon

½ tsp. sea salt

INSTRUCTIONS:

Put all ingredients into a food processor with an S-blade and process until completely blended.

Serving suggestions: Drizzle this over the top of the bread and enjoy! It's even better if you warm up the bread slightly before serving: Just put the slices you're serving into your oven on the lowest temperature for about 5 minutes, then remove and drizzle with the topping. Garnish with orange slices and mint leaves.

Sweet Buckwheat Bread

Servings: 8–10 slices

This is a delicious, breadlike dessert. It is lightly sweet and satisfying and has received the stamp of approval from kids transitioning to a healthy diet.

Note that you may want to start soaking the buckwheat the night before you want to make this dish (soak for 8–12 hours and see instructions at the beginning of this chapter). Once soaked, it only takes 15 minutes to prepare and about 15 minutes to cook.

INGREDIENTS:

3 cups presoaked cream of buckwheat cereal

About 1 cup water (add more if needed)

1 Tbsp. vanilla extract

1 tsp. sea salt

2 Tbsp. organic cinnamon (add more if you really like it—
it has antifungal properties and is great for people who
love cinnamon tastes in their desserts)

1 Tbsp. organic ghee, coconut oil, or raw butter

Sweetener options: The recipe tastes the same warm or cold,
so add the amount of sweetener that works for you. You
can taste the cooked mixture before baking, to make
sure it's to your liking and add more sweetener if you
want. Choose either 35 drops liquid stevia extract (or you
can customize to taste; if you like the taste, stop adding
stevia) or ¼ cup raw honey.

INSTRUCTIONS:

Preheat the oven to 350° F.

Grease a bread-loaf pan with ghee, coconut oil, or raw butter.

Prepare cream of buckwheat cereal just as if you were making the "oatmeal-type" version of them—in a saucepan on the oven, following package instructions. (When you soak the buckwheat, there will still be water left over after draining the excess out. This is okay; the recipe takes that into account with a reduction in water to make the cream of buckwheat cereal.)

Add all ingredients and simmer until grains are cooked. Add the cooked buckwheat into the bread-loaf pan—make sure it's about 1" thick because it doesn't rise. Cook for 15 minutes. Remove and serve warm or cold. Refrigerate leftovers.

The longer you cook this bread, the drier it becomes. It you want a drier recipe, lower the temperature of the oven and leave it in longer. You can also take out the pan, cut up the squares, and put them in a food dehydrator to dry them out.

This recipe can be prepared as a flatbread by removing the cinnamon and sweetener and adding your favorite herbs and spices and more sea salt or Herbamare. It also makes a great flatbread sandwich or "toast" with butter or ghee.

Sweet Quinoa Bread

Servings: 8–10 slices

This is a delicious, breadlike dessert. It is lightly sweet and satisfying.

Note that you may want to start soaking the quinoa the night before you want to make this dish (soak for 8–12 hours and see instructions at the beginning of this chapter). The recipe itself takes about 15 minutes to prepare and 15–20 minutes to simmer on the stovetop.

INGREDIENTS:

3 cups presoaked quinoa flakes cereal

About 1 cup water (add more if needed)

1 Tbsp. vanilla extract

1 tsp. sea salt

2 Tbsp. organic cinnamon (add more if you really like it— it has antifungal properties and is great for people who love cinnamon tastes in their desserts)

1 Tbsp. organic ghee

Sweetener options: The recipe tastes the same warm or cold, so add the amount of sweetener that works for you. You can taste the quinoa flakes before transferring them into the bread-loaf pan, so you can add more sweetener if you like. Choose either 35 drops liquid stevia extract (or you can customize to taste; if you like the taste, stop adding stevia) or ¼ cup raw honey.

INSTRUCTIONS:

Preheat the oven to 350° F.

Grease a bread loaf pan with ghee.

Prepare quinoa flakes just as if you were making the "oatmeal-type" version of them—in a saucepan on the oven, following package instructions. (When you soak the quinoa flakes, there will still be water left over after draining the excess out. This is okay; the recipe takes that into account with a reduction in water to make the quinoa flakes.)

Add all ingredients and simmer until grains are cooked.

To make quinoa flakes pilaf instead of bread: Once the grains are cooked (it only takes a couple of minutes), they are ready to serve!

To make the bread: Add the cooked quinoa flakes into the bread-loaf pan—make sure it's about 1" thick because it doesn't rise. Cook for 15 minutes; remove and serve warm or cold. Refrigerate leftovers.

The longer you cook this bread, the drier it becomes. It you want a drier recipe, lower the temperature of the oven and leave it in longer. You can also take out the pan, cut up the squares, and put them in a food dehydrator to dry them out.

This recipe can be prepared as a savory flatbread by removing the cinnamon and sweetener and adding your favorite herbs and spices and more sea salt or Herbamare. It makes a great flatbread sandwich or "toast" with butter or ghee.

Simple Nut and Seed Milks

Servings: 4 cups

Nut and seed milks make a great alternative to dairy milk and can be used as a beverage, over the hot-cereal recipes in this book, in smoothies, in desserts, or to thicken soups. We don't include nut milks in many recipes, but we do include almond milk as an ingredient in the Sweet Blueberry Banana Green Protein Smoothie, so we wanted to give you a budget-friendly, healthy alternative to store-bought nut and seed milks.

With all of the questionable fillers—like carrageenan, gums, and unidentified "natural flavors"—buying premade nut milks can be challenging. The good news is that they are *very* easy to make! It's almost as simple as soaking nuts. (If you want to make your own coconut milk, check the instructions in the Vanilla Spice Ice Cream recipe later in the chapter.)

Note that you may want to start soaking the nuts or seeds the night before you want to make this dish (soak for 8–12 hours and see instructions at the beginning of this chapter). The recipe itself takes about 5 minutes to prepare once the nuts or seeds are soaked.

INGREDIENTS:

> 3–4 cups filtered water (you could start with 3 cups and add more if you want to dilute the milk a bit)
>
> 1 cup soaked nuts or seeds—choose your favorite, such as hemp seeds, flaxseeds, sesame seeds, sunflower seeds, walnuts, Brazil nuts, almonds, or hazelnuts
>
> *Optional:* sweeten with 1 tsp. honey, 1–2 dates, or a little stevia, if you want it sweet
>
> *Optional:* add 1 tsp. vanilla extract if you want a vanilla nut or seed milk

INSTRUCTIONS:

Add the soaked and drained nuts or seeds to 3 cups water in a high-speed blender and blend completely. Taste and decide if you want to dilute it with more water or add any sweetener or vanilla.

Get a stainless-steel or glass bowl or container to capture the milk, and pour the blender contents through a fine mesh strainer into the container.

Press the nut or seed pulp down into the strainer to squeeze all remaining liquid into the container. You can save the pulp for cracker recipes (see recipes in this section) or cookie recipes. Or you can add some herbs, spices, and sea salt to the pulp and dehydrate or bake it into a crunchy snack.

Store the milk for up to 4 days in your refrigerator in an airtight container. Freeze it if you don't think you'll use it all in that time.

Savory Sweet Walnuts and Dates

Servings: 6–8

Heather came up with this snack on a whim while she was particularly busy and wanted to stay grounded, yet open to her creativity. Food is a form of how she takes good care of herself so that she can stay calm during stressful times. And, of course, when things get busy, what's better than a fast, easy recipe that is also deeply grounding and satisfying? This recipe did the trick!

This snack is full of healing spices with some hints of India and Morocco. The spices in this recipe complement each other well, and all are anti-inflammatory. If you're experiencing PMS, joint pain, or other inflammatory condition, this could be the perfect snack for you!

Turmeric is wonderful as an anti-inflammatory if you're experiencing arthritis, swelling, or inflammation around your menstrual period or any other autoimmune-type symptoms. Incidentally, it's wonderful for your skin and a natural anti-wrinkle remedy. It can also protect against radiation from the sun or x-rays.[1]

Fennel is another spice that can help with arthritis. It can also help calm cramps (yes, including menstrual cramps) and colic, and is a powerful digestive aid and anti-inflammatory.[2]

Ginger is yet another anti-inflammatory spice that can help with arthritis, nausea, morning sickness, and migraines. It is also amazing for your digestion.[3]

Black pepper was considered the "king of spices" in the Middle Ages for good reason. Indian black pepper in particular is rich in nutrients that aid your digestion. If you have slow motility, pepper can help speed it up. It is also an anti-inflammatory, like the rest of its spice sisters in this recipe. And it just so happens that the hormonal shift women experience days before their periods can set the stage for inflammation—this is often behind PMS, menstrual cramps, swelling, and other menstrual symptoms.[4]

The sweetness of the dates in this recipe is mild and well balanced by the savory spices. So it's just enough of a treat to quell your sweet tooth, while keeping a grounding feeling in your body from the balanced taste of the spices.

Note that you may want to start soaking the walnuts the night before you want to make this dish (soak for 8–12 hours and see instructions at the beginning of this chapter). The recipe itself takes about 5 minutes to prepare once the nuts are soaked, and can be made with or without a food processor.

INGREDIENTS:

2 cups soaked walnuts

4 Medjool dates. (Add this only if you like a sweet and savory taste. Some people will just love the nuts with spices and not enjoy the added sweetness of the dates. This recipe is flexible—you can leave the dates out for a terrific savory snack or add them for a touch of sweetness. You can decide by making this without dates, then tasting the spiced nuts with a small piece of date to see what you think.)

½ tsp. Celtic gray sea salt

¼ tsp. turmeric

¼ tsp. ground fennel

¼ tsp. ground ginger

¼ tsp. fresh ground pepper

INSTRUCTIONS:

Add the spices to the soaked and drained nuts. You can now decide whether you want to chop your nuts or eat them whole. If you don't chop them, go ahead and slice up the dates into small pieces with a knife, spice grinder, or food processor (by pulsing the grinder or food processor until the date pieces are chopped a bit—it doesn't have to be perfect, just smaller chunks).

If you use a food processor with the S-blade, you can put all ingredients in it and pulse until you get the consistency you want. We sometimes like to pulse it until it's just short of a paste, so it's easy to digest. Do what you feel your own mouth and taste buds want at the time.

Now it's ready to eat!

Serving suggestions: Enjoy on its own or put a scoop in a small bowl and have it as a delicious snack to balance your blood-sugar levels, your taste buds, and your soul.

Savory Tahini Crackers

Servings: 15–24 crackers, depending upon size

This is a delicious cracker that will satisfy even your non-health-food friends. For people who are into making raw foods and have a dehydrator, you can make this recipe raw. For those who don't have a food dehydrator, you can make this in your oven, too.

If you've never heard of tahini, it's a sesame-seed butter that many people love as an alternative to peanut butter. You can get it in many stores in the ethnic-foods aisle, or in your health-food store in the aisle with nut butters. You can also purchase raw, organic tahini online at places like Amazon.com or iHerb.com.

Note that you may want to start soaking the nuts the night before you want to make this dish (soak for 8–12 hours and see instructions at the beginning of this chapter). The recipe itself takes about 5–10 minutes to prepare once the nuts are soaked.

INGREDIENTS:

> 1 cup raw soaked nuts—some great options
> are almonds, walnuts, or macadamia nuts
>
> ¼ cup unrefined coconut oil
>
> ¼ cup raw tahini
>
> 1 tsp. dried thyme
>
> 1 tsp. dried oregano
>
> 1 tsp. dried basil
>
> 1 tsp. sea salt
>
> Herbamare or added sea salt to taste

INSTRUCTIONS:

Take the soaked and drained nuts and put into your food dehydrator on 115° F for about 2–4 hours or until the nuts are dry. Alternatively, place them on a cookie sheet and dry them on the lowest temperature setting in your oven. It will go much faster in the oven, so check at 10 minutes and again at 15–20 minutes, and take them out of the oven when they're dry.

In a food processor with an S-blade, blend all ingredients except Herbamare. Taste them and see if you want to add more sea salt based on your taste.

Drop 1-Tbsp. scoops of the mixture onto silicone baking sheets, (like cookies). Add a dash of Herbamare or sea salt over the crackers.

Put in your food dehydrator at 115° F for 24–48 hours, or until they're as crisp as you want them. If you don't have a food dehydrator or want them ready faster, put them in the oven at 200° F (or your lowest temperature setting) until they're crispy like crackers, or take them out earlier and enjoy them soft. If you do make them soft, chill them in the refrigerator to stay cool and keep their shape.

Store for 2 weeks in the refrigerator, and up to 2 months in the freezer.

Celery Basil Crackers

This cracker recipe has more vegetables than nuts, making it a lighter and more balanced snack than your average raw-food cracker.

Note that you may want to start soaking the nuts and flaxseeds the night before you want to make this dish (soak for 8–12 hours and see instructions at the beginning of this chapter). You can combine the nuts in the same soaking bowl, but separate out the flaxseeds. When you soak flaxseeds, it creates a thick, pasty gel, which helps the crackers stick together. Once everything is soaked, this recipe takes 30 minutes to prepare, and either 20 minutes in the oven or 24–48 hours in the food dehydrator if you want raw crackers.

INGREDIENTS:

- 1 large bunch of celery (about 4–6 cups, chopped)
- 2 cups fresh basil
- 1 cup fresh chives or green onion
- 1 yellow summer squash
- 1 cup of any of these options: walnuts, sunflower seeds, macadamia nuts, or Brazil nuts (soaked)
- 1 cup soaked almonds
- 1 cup soaked flaxseeds
- 3 Tbsp. fresh ginger
- 2 tsp. Herbamare
- ½ cup water

INSTRUCTIONS:

Blend all ingredients up in a food processor, using the S blade or a high-speed blender.

Grease silicone baking sheets with ghee or coconut oil; spread mixture generously on the baking sheets (about ½" thick)

Set your dehydrator to 112–115° F and dehydrate for 24–48 hours or until the crackers are completely dried. If you want the crackers faster or don't have a food dehydrator, set your oven to the lowest temperature and cook until the crackers are dry and as firm as you like. This may only take 10–20 minutes, so watch the oven or set your timer.

To speed up dehydrating, you may want to flip the crackers over and remove the silicone baking sheets. If you do this, wait until the crackers are mostly dry and peel away from the silicone really easily. If they're too moist, they will stick to the baking sheet.

Pickled Pink Cultured Vegetables

Preparation time: 30 minutes   *Servings: 3 quarts*

Making your own cultured vegetables is easy and economical! Here's a great way to make a raw food that helps improve your digestion and boost your immunity. This is a slightly sweet (and sour) cultured vegetable recipe.

INGREDIENTS:

4 sweet potatoes

1 head red cabbage

1 cup fresh dill

½ cup kelp

½ cup fresh basil

½ cup red onion

2 Tbsp. fresh ginger

1 tsp. sea salt

Optional: While adding probiotics is not necessary, it can boost the health benefits of your cultured vegetables. There are many options to add probiotics:

• Add 3 oz. young coconut kefir or a probiotic liquid from the health-food store

• Use a culture starter packet from Body Ecology (which you can get at: BodyEcology.com)

• Add 3 oz. liquid from a previous batch of cultured vegetables

• Open 2 probiotic capsules or use ½ tsp. probiotic powder

INSTRUCTIONS:

Shred all vegetables (except dill and basil) in a food processor (usually you'd use the blade with tiny holes that makes julienned vegetables). Transfer to a large stainless-steel mixing bowl.

Make your brine: Take about 1 cup of the shredded vegetables, the sea salt, and the dill and basil and place in your food processor with the S-blade. Add filtered water (just keep adding filtered water so they blend completely) and blend until it's the consistency of guacamole.

Optional: Add in the probiotic starter of your choice. You don't need to add probiotics to cultured veggies, but it's highly recommended so that you get more consistent results.

Add the brine into the shredded vegetables and mix well. With a wide-mouth funnel, add your vegetable-and-brine mixture into quart-sized wide-mouth Ball jars (you can usually get these in the grocery store very inexpensively). Pack the vegetables down tightly.

Add some water to cover the vegetables (make sure they're not exposed to air). You can also put a rolled-up cabbage leaf at the top, to keep the vegetables well packed or to take up additional space between the vegetables and the top (if needed).

Screw on the top tightly and set aside for 3 days to one week at room temperature (72–75° F, but you can make these in warmer climates, too). You can take the top off and sample after 3 days. If you want them to have a more sour taste, let them ferment longer.

Notes:

If this is your first time making cultured vegetables, here are some things to know:

— Most people are nervous about making cultured vegetables at first. We're so used to refrigeration that it can feel weird to eat what may seem like "spoiled" vegetables. They are not spoiled, though! Fermentation is a way of preserving foods with good bacteria. The key is to "just do it" and see what happens. It's a great way to reconnect with a food-preservation technique our ancestors used.

— They do smell . . . sometimes you can even smell them while they're fermenting on your countertop. That's normal! They'll smell when you open them as well, but they're not as smelly once they are exposed to air and on your plate.

— Sometimes liquid does seep out of the jars during fermentation, so we like to put them in a shallow baking dish just in case.

— If your veggies look moldy at the top, they were likely exposed to some air during fermentation. It's okay to scrape the moldy part off the top, and if the vegetables underneath look good, you can still eat them. You can avoid mold by making sure your veggies are entirely covered with water, or use a rolled-up cabbage leaf to pack them down. You may need to discard the cabbage leaf if it gets moldy, but rest assured that your veggies will likely be fine underneath.

— The end result should be crisp and colorful. If your veggies taste swampy or look dull and colorless, they did not ferment well. Using Pro-Belly-Otic liquid (available at: RealFoodRealLife.tv) as a starter will aid the fermentation process by making sure you have a hardy source of probiotics to ferment the vegetables. Once you're more experienced at making cultured vegetables, you might try it without a starter. We like to use a starter to ensure that we get the most medicinal cultured vegetables.

— *Money-saving tip:* You can reserve 6 Tbsp. of your batch of cultured vegetables or liquid to create a new brine for your next batch.

— Expert cultured-vegetable makers have noticed that if they make their veggies while in a bad mood, the end result tastes bad, too. Play some music, make your vegetables with friends, or put a smile on your face and in your heart while making them. You'd be surprised at how great food can taste with this one little tip!

— Keep in mind that no experience or talent is needed to make cultured vegetables. Follow the instructions, and nature will do the rest! Experience and talent will certainly add flair to your end result, so keep practicing, and your taste buds will reap the rewards.

Savory Beet Chips or Slices

Preparation time: 15 minutes to prep and 20–25 minutes to cook   *Servings: 6–8*

This is a versatile recipe that you can use either as a side dish for a meal or turn into chips for a great on-the-go snack. These beets are a little sweet and a little savory—and best of all, they're ready in a jiffy!

INGREDIENTS:

> 6 medium-sized beets (you can clean them with a vegetable brush, but leave the skins on)
>
> 2 Tbsp. coconut oil
>
> 2 tsp. thyme
>
> 2 tsp. basil
>
> 1 tsp. sea salt
>
> 1 tsp. fresh ground black pepper
>
> *Optional:* 1 tsp. garlic powder, or 2 minced fresh garlic cloves

INSTRUCTIONS FOR SLICED BEETS:

Preheat the oven to 400° F.

If you want a nice, warm side dish to a meal with a firm, yet soft texture, you can make these beets in your food processor with the slice attachment (the round attachment with one long blade to do slices). This will make a thick sliced beet.

Slice your beets, put them in a glass pan, and mix up all of the ingredients well.

Bake for 15–20 minutes, or until beets are soft.

Instructions for beet chips:

Preheat the oven to 400° F.

If you want to make beet chips for a crunchy snack, use a mandoline at $^1/_{16}$" or as thin as you want the chips.

Slice the beets, put them in a bowl, and mix all of the ingredients well.

Using a glass pan or pizza stone, put the beets onto the pan in a single layer and bake until crispy, about 20–25 minutes.

Serving suggestion: These beets would be delicious as a side dish or chips with a grass-fed lamb burger (or beef burger!), chicken, or quinoa dish. They will store in your refrigerator for 4–5 days (softer beet slices) or up to 1 week for the chips. Freeze the chips if you want to make these in bulk and take them out for school lunches or a snack attack.

Easy Mild Homemade Salsa

Preparation time: 15 minutes   *Servings: 4*

Forget those jars of salsa that always seem to have sugar or agave! This is a delicious, naturally sweet and savory raw salsa that will be sure to please even those who don't like "healthy" food!

INGREDIENTS:

> 1 pint cherry tomatoes (remember, tomatoes are a nightshade vegetable and, therefore, may not work for everyone)
>
> ¼ cup red onion
>
> ¼ cup fresh dill
>
> ¼ cup fresh cilantro
>
> ⅛ tsp. cayenne powder
>
> ½ tsp. sea salt (it's even better to use "Herby" by Frontier Spices)
>
> *Optional:* ½ avocado
>
> *To make a medium or hot salsa:* add more cayenne powder or use chili powder or fresh jalapeño peppers

INSTRUCTIONS:

Puree all ingredients in a food processor with S-blade, a blender, or in a deep mixing bowl with your immersion blender.

After all ingredients are fully blended, serve in bowls at room temperature with raw crackers or vegetables. Add sea salt or an herb sea salt (like "Herby," Herbamare, or Trocomare) to taste.

Chocolate Fudge

||||||||||||||||||||||||||||||||||||||||||||||||||||||||||||||||||||||||||||||||||||||||||||||||||||||||||||||||||||||||||||||||||||||||||||||||||||||||||||

Preparation time: 15–20 minutes

This is an easy raw-food recipe—just mix the ingredients and chill in the refrigerator to firm up. The fudge freezes well, so you can make a batch, freeze it, and always have a healthy dessert on hand when you need it! The cinnamon and cardamom add balance to the sweetness of this fudge (to help satisfy without creating cravings!), and these spices also support your digestion and intestinal health.

INGREDIENTS:

 1 jar almond butter (16 oz.)

 4 Tbsp. raw cacao

 3 Tbsp. coconut butter

 3 Tbsp. coconut oil

 5 Tbsp. honey—if you like it sweeter, you might like to use ½ cup honey until your taste buds get used to a less sweet taste

 2 Tbsp. vanilla extract

 2 Tbsp. cinnamon powder

 1 tsp. sea salt

 1 tsp. cardamom powder

 Other options: 1 Tbsp. maca or 1 tsp. ginger powder

 And lots of love!

INSTRUCTIONS:

In a saucepan on low heat, add honey, coconut oil, and coconut butter, and allow to melt. Mix thoroughly and allow the mixture to cool to room temperature. This is important because if the ingredients are too warm, the oils can separate.

Add almond butter and mix thoroughly; add the rest of the ingredients and mix well.

Once you have blended all of this up, taste it and see what you think. You can add more sweetener, vanilla, or salt to get the taste you want. The finished fudge will taste almost exactly like the raw mixture, so making adjustments now for taste will give you a finished product you'll really like.

Press the fudge into a square or rectangular storage container with a lid, and chill in your refrigerator for at least an hour before serving. If you like, sprinkle the top with shredded coconut and goji berries and cut into squares for a pretty, dressed-up dessert.

Store in your refrigerator or freezer. This fudge will usually last up to 2 weeks in the fridge and several months in the freezer.

Serving suggestions: Cut in small pieces and eat by itself. You can also make the fudge into balls and roll them in shredded coconut for easy serving.

Halva

||||||||||||||||||||||||||||||||||||||||||||||||||||||||||||||||||||||||||||||||||||||||||||||||||||||||||||||||||||||||||||||||||||||||||||||||||||||||||||||||||||||||||||

Servings: makes about 20 pieces of halva cut in small squares, like fudge

Traditional halva recipes are often full of sugar and gluten flours. The bars in health-food stores are unfortunately the same.

This recipe makes a rich, delicious, chewy, and slightly crunchy dessert or snack. It needs to be chilled and stored in the refrigerator to get a fudge-like consistency.

Note that you may want to start soaking the sesame seeds and flax meal the night before you want to make this dish (soak for 8–12 hours and see instructions at the beginning of this chapter). Soak the sesame seeds and flax meal in separate containers. After soaking and rinsing the seeds, put them in your oven at the lowest temperature and roast them (about 10–15 minutes). Alternatively, you can dry them in your food dehydrator at 115° for about 2–6 hours.

The recipe itself takes about 15 minutes to prepare once the seeds and meal are soaked and the seeds are roasted.

INGREDIENTS:

> 1 cup organic ghee or raw butter
>
> 3 cups organic tahini
>
> 1 cup presoaked, roasted organic unhulled sesame seeds
>
> 4 cups presoaked flax meal
>
> 2 tsp. vanilla extract
>
> 1½ tsp. sea salt
>
> *Sweetener options:* The recipe tastes the same warm or cold, so add the amount of sweetener that works for you. Choose ½–1 tsp. stevia (or you can customize to taste; if you like the taste, stop adding stevia), ¼ cup raw honey, or 20 Medjool dates.

INSTRUCTIONS:

In a saucepan on low heat, add 1 cup of ta-hini with the ghee or raw butter, stir in flax meal, and gently heat while stirring constantly, until light brown. Then add the rest of the tahini.

Add sweetener and sesame seeds and mix well. If using dates, either make a date paste by soaking them in hot water for at least 30 minutes, draining and mashing up with a fork, or mash them up in your food processor. Once you're done making this, taste it to see if it's to your liking. You can add additional sweetener, sea salt, vanilla, or ghee if you want to shift the flavor to satisfy your taste buds.

Pour into a greased glass container with tall edges or a silicone bread-loaf pan (grease very lightly with raw butter, ghee, or coconut oil). Put in the refrigerator to chill, and cut as soon as it's solid enough. It will have the consistency of fudge.

The halva is best when kept refrigerated. Store in the refrigerator for up to 1 week, and in the freezer for up to 2 months.

Sunflower Granola Bars (Nut-Free Dessert or Snack)

These raw, no-grain, no-nut granola bars were inspired by Heather's friend Christina, who needed a nut-free, healthy granola bar for her son to take to school.

These bars are versatile, delicious, and nutritious. They're not too far off from those made by Lärabar, except that these bars have a more balanced sweetness that make them less triggering of cravings. We find Lärabars to be too sweet, and they're not always made with organic ingredients. They're also rather pricey, so our bars can save you money, too!

The ginger in these bars can help with digestion, morning sickness, migraines, arthritis and rheumatoid arthritis, cancer, cholesterol problems, and heart attack. Keep in mind that these bars are so versatile that you can add other spices instead of ginger or in addition to it. Cinnamon, cardamom, nutmeg, and cloves—some of our favorite powerhouse healthy spices would all work beautifully in this recipe. Get creative and play to your heart's content.

Note that you may want to start soaking the sunflower seeds and flaxseeds in separate containers the night before you want to make this dish (soak for 8–12 hours and see instructions at the beginning of this chapter).

For this recipe, Heather uses soaked and then dehydrated flaxseeds. You can try just soaking the flaxseeds without dehydrating them, or you can purchase already sprouted (soaked and dehydrated) flaxseeds from your local health-food store. These are great to have on hand for last-minute recipes in case you don't have time to soak and dehydrate. However, it's very easy to soak the flaxseeds, then dehydrate them until they're dry. They will stick together in the soaking water, like a gel (so you can't drain all the water out—and that's fine, because the gel keeps everything together!). Put the gel onto a silicone baking sheet in your dehydrator on 115° F for about 5–10 hours, then break it up, and put it in a container for use whenever you need flaxseeds! If you don't have a food dehydrator, you can put them in your oven on the lowest setting for about 30 minutes or so.

Once the seeds are soaked and dehydrated, it takes 10 minutes to prepare these bars.

INGREDIENTS:

2 cups presoaked sunflower seeds

1 cup coconut shreds (Let's Do Organic brand has a great finely shredded coconut that you can get in health-food stores or online at: iHerb.com or Amazon.com)

1 cup pitted Medjool dates

½ cup presoaked whole flaxseeds

2 tsp. ginger powder

1 tsp. Celtic sea salt

INSTRUCTIONS:

In a food processor with an S-blade, put in the dates and blend until mushy. Now add the rest of the ingredients and blend it up again. Keep blending until the mixture is completely smooth. If your food processor or blender is small, you can mix things up in two batches and then combine in a bowl afterward.

Taste the mixture and see if you like it: You can add more dates if you like a sweeter bar. Or if you want to use additional spices, like cinnamon, start with ½ tsp. and taste, then add more if needed. If you're adding more dates, start with 2 at a time and taste again until you reach the desired level of sweetness. You may need to add a little water to get them fully blended. Scrape the sides with a rubber spatula to keep things moving.

You can add things like raisins or goji berries if you or your family like chewy fruit pieces in the bars. If you want to do this, you can take out a few dates from the mixture, then remove the batter from the food processor, add the raisins or goji berries, and pulse a few times to get them into smaller chunks; then add to the batter and mix with a wooden spoon.

Scoop out the mixture with a tablespoon and flatten into bar shapes on silicone baking sheets. Put the baking sheets into your food dehydrator at 115° F for about 18 hours, or longer if you like a drier cookie. We like these a little moist and chewy, so we'll take them out before they get too dry or hard.

If you don't have a food dehydrator, put the bars on a glass or stainless-steel baking sheet greased with coconut oil, or on a silicone baking sheet over your cookie sheet (the silicone baking sheet does not need to be greased), and put it in your oven at the lowest temperature. Watch the oven for when you want to take them out. It should be anywhere from 30 minutes to 2 hours, depending on the lowest temperature of your oven and how dry you want them to be. Keeping your oven on the lowest temperature will be gentler to the nut oils.

Store in your refrigerator for a week or in your freezer for a couple of months. They will thaw quickly if you want to make more and freeze them for convenient snacks. Just pull a few out of the freezer, put into a baggie, and take on the go for a healthy snack or dessert on the run!

Serving suggestions: Serve as granola bars, or roll into balls in coconut shreds and serve immediately or after chilling in your refrigerator for 2 hours or more.

Key Lime Pudding

Preparation time: about 10–15 minutes   *Servings: 6–8*

This recipe makes a delicious key lime pudding that will have you wondering how avocados could taste so good!

INGREDIENTS:

3 ripe avocados

Juice of 4 limes

2 Tbsp. coconut oil

2 Tbsp. real vanilla extract

½ tsp. sea salt

½ cup natural sweetener—choose one of the following options:

- Organic erythritol or xylitol (made from birch) are great options that do not feed candida yeast, but should not be used if you are following GAPS, SCD, or any SIBO diet. (You can get organic erythritol and birch xylitol at: Globalsweet.com.)

- Raw organic honey

- Organic Medjool dates (if you use dates, remove pits and put them in your food processor first with ¼ cup hot water to make into a paste, then add other ingredients)

INSTRUCTIONS:

Cut the avocados in half, remove the pits, and place in your blender or food processor with the S-blade.

Add the rest of the ingredients and blend on high until it is a pudding-like consistency.

Taste—this part is important. Most likely, the recipe will turn out perfectly, but do taste it first to see if you may want to add more sweetener or vanilla, depending on your preference. Everyone is different!

Chill in the refrigerator for at least an hour and serve.

Alternatives:

— Garnish with berries, like strawberries, blueberries, or raspberries.

— Serve as pudding; it tastes great on its own.

— This makes a nice alternative to ice cream and junk-food puddings.

Sweet Squash Pie

Servings: 6–8

This is a wonderful pie that tastes almost like pumpkin pie and can be made with or without the crust.

Note that if you're including the optional crust, you may want to start soaking the millet the night before you want to make this pie (soak for 8–12 hours and see instructions at the beginning of this chapter). It then takes 45 minutes to an hour to cook the squash (you can make the optional millet crust while the squash is cooking) and 30 minutes to prepare and bake.

INGREDIENTS FOR THE PIE FILLING:

> 3 cups cooked, mashed kabocha squash
> (butternut is also an option)
>
> ½ cup water
>
> 2 Tbsp. kuzu
>
> 1 Tbsp. cinnamon
>
> 1 tsp. cardamom
>
> ½ tsp. sea salt
>
> ½ tsp. allspice
>
> ½ tsp. ground ginger
>
> ¼ tsp. cloves
>
> ¼ tsp. nutmeg
>
> *Sweetener options:* 2–4 Tbsp. raw honey
> or 10 Medjool dates

INGREDIENTS FOR THE OPTIONAL PIE CRUST:

> 1 cup soaked millet
>
> 2 Tbsp. raw butter, ghee, or coconut oil
>
> 2 cups water
>
> 2 tsp. raw honey (optional)
>
> 2 tsp. cardamom
>
> 1 tsp. sea salt

INSTRUCTIONS FOR MAKING THE FILLING:

Preheat the oven to 350° F.

To keep it simple, wash the squash and prick it several times with the tip of a knife to create holes where heat can escape during baking. Place in a baking dish with 2" water in the bottom, and bake for 45 minutes to an hour or when you can insert a knife easily into the squash.

Remove from the oven, allow the squash to cool, and then cut it in half lengthwise and remove the seeds. Then scoop out all the cooked squash.

In a saucepan on the lowest heat on your stovetop, dissolve kuzu in water. (Kuzu is a starchy vegetable root that is revered in Japan and is used as a natural thickening agent in cooking, and it can be purchased in your health-food store or online.) To dissolve the lumps completely, keep stirring while the kuzu thickens. Add pureed squash, natural sweetener, and spices.

If you're not using a crust, put the squash mixture in a greased pie dish and bake for approximately 25 minutes at 350° F (or 300° F if using a glass pie dish).

This recipe tastes great without a crust and can still be made in a pie dish and served like pie. But if you do want a crust, follow the instructions below.

INSTRUCTIONS FOR MAKING THE PIE CRUST:

In a saucepan, bring 2 cups water to a boil. Add millet and turn heat down to medium, cooking until the water absorbs into the millet and the millet becomes more translucent (with no hard yellow spots in the grain).

Turn off the heat and add raw butter, ghee, or coconut oil, and honey. Add spices and sea salt, and mix thoroughly.

Allow to cool, then transfer into a greased pie dish (glass Pyrex pie dishes work really well and are a great nontoxic baking option). Firmly pack the millet into the pie dish so that it is ¼" thick and goes up the sides of the dish a bit.

Cook the millet crust for 10 minutes at 350° F (or 300° F if using a glass pie dish). Then take out and add the squash filling; bake for another 25 minutes. Cool before serving.

Raw Chocolate-Chip Cookies

Servings: 15–20 small cookies

This is the closest Heather has been able to come to Toll House cookies—and it's really close! You can eat this as cookie dough, or dehydrate or bake it so that it's easy to take on the road. We like both options, but we love the cookie-dough version best!

Most other raw chocolate-chip cookie recipes tend to use cashews and oats. Because cashews can have mold, we often avoid them. And for those of you who are avoiding starches for health reasons, we wanted to offer an alternative recipe without the oats. The walnut-and-date combo has a nice hint of the taste from the brown sugar/white sugar combo used in Toll House cookies—but with much better health benefits!

Note that you may want to start soaking walnuts the night before you want to make these cookies (soak for 8–12 hours and see instructions at the beginning of this chapter). The recipe itself takes about 5 minutes to prepare once the nuts are soaked.

INGREDIENTS FOR OR THE COOKIES:

3 cups presoaked walnuts

3 Tbsp. coconut oil

1 Tbsp. ghee (or substitute with coconut oil)

2 Tbsp. vanilla extract

⅓ cup dates—taste after blending, and add
more if you like it sweeter

1 tsp. sea salt

INSTRUCTIONS FOR THE COOKIES:

Add walnuts, coconut oil, vanilla, and ghee to blender and begin on low speed. You can also use your food processor with the S-blade. Depending upon your blender or food processor, you may want to add a little water to get things blending smoothly: Start with 2 Tbsp. and add more if needed; you likely won't need more than ¼ cup. If you have a high-speed blender, like a Vitamix, you may only need 1 Tbsp. or less of water.

Remove to a bowl and allow to chill thoroughly (about 30 minutes). This mixture can get a little stiff in the refrigerator, so you may want to remove for 15–30 minutes before serving, unless you want a stiffer consistency.

If you want to make these into cookies, take a 1 Tbsp. measuring spoon and scoop the dough out onto silicone baking sheets. Flatten into cookie shapes and dehydrate on 115° F for about 8 hours. You want them to still be soft so that you can press the chocolate into them (see below).

If you want to make cookie dough instead, reserve the dough until the chocolate chips are ready.

INGREDIENTS FOR THE CHOCOLATE CHIPS:

½ cup cacao butter

¼ cup raw cacao powder made from freshly ground raw cacao beans (we grind the beans in a Blendtec blender, and it gives the raw cacao a really beautiful flavor—if you don't have beans on hand, you can use raw cacao powder)

¼ cup Medjool dates (if you don't have dates on hand, you can use 1 Tbsp. raw honey)

Pinch sea salt (about ¼ tsp.)

INSTRUCTIONS FOR THE CHOCOLATE CHIPS:

In a saucepan, heat the cacao butter on the lowest temperature on your stovetop.

Put the dates into a food processor with the S-blade or high-speed blender and blend until completely mushy.

Once the cacao butter is melted, add the raw cacao and dates and mix until blended. Remove from heat and allow to cool.

Two options—chips or chunks:

— *For chunks:* Line a cookie sheet with parchment paper or a silicone baking sheet. Spread the cooled chocolate out flat onto the parchment paper or silicone baking sheet and refrigerate until solid. Break apart into chunks with a knife.

— *For chips:* Once the chocolate is warm and semisolid, put it into an icing bag and pipe the icing onto a cookie sheet lined with wax paper or a silicone baking sheet. Put them into the refrigerator to harden.

INSTRUCTIONS FOR ASSEMBLING THE COOKIES:

Add the chocolate chips or chunks by pressing into the cookies while they're still soft.

For cookie dough, roll into balls of dough and refrigerate until serving.

For cookies, dehydrate them for 8 hours at 115° F and check to make sure that they're still somewhat soft. You don't want them to get too dry, or else you won't be able to press the chocolate chips into them. They should be easy to pick up and stay intact, but still soft. Remove them from the dehydrator, allow them to cool for 10 minutes, and press the chocolate chips into the top. You'll likely use about 5–6 chips for each cookie.

If you bake in your oven on the lowest temperature, check after 8–10 minutes to see if the cookies are still soft, while able to stay intact if you remove them from the cookie sheet.

For dough balls or cookies, store in your refrigerator for 2 weeks or in the freezer for up to a few months.

Vanilla Spice Ice Cream

Preparation time: 15 minutes to prepare, 2–6 hours to chill, and about 22–35 minutes in the ice-cream maker. If you don't have an ice-cream maker, you can look up instructions online for making ice cream without a maker, or follow our instructions below. This will take about 2–3 more hours in the freezer.

Servings: 6

This is a delicious twist on vanilla with some of your favorite Thanksgiving spices, like cinnamon, allspice, and cardamom. Easy to digest, dairy-free, and sure to delight!

INGREDIENTS:

> 1 (12-oz.) can of organic coconut milk (get a brand that is BPA free, or make your own by following the directions below)
>
> 1½ cups extra-virgin olive oil
>
> 10 dates
>
> 2 egg yolks
>
> 2 Tbsp. vanilla extract
>
> 1 Tbsp. cinnamon
>
> 2 tsp. cardamom
>
> 1 tsp. allspice
>
> 1 tsp. sea salt

INSTRUCTIONS:

To make your own coconut milk, get a bag of organic, unsweetened coconut shreds with no sulfites added. Boil 3 cups of water and allow to cool for 1 minute, then pour over 2 cups of shredded coconut. Let this sit until the water is lukewarm. Put it into a blender and blend for a few minutes. Strain with a very fine mesh strainer or through a nut-milk bag. You now have coconut milk! (Save the shreds to use as coconut flour.)

Put your coconut milk into a food processor with the S-blade and add the egg yolks. Blend for a couple of minutes, then slowly drizzle the olive oil into the food processor. Do this very slowly—take 2 full minutes to drizzle the oil in, practicing patience!

Once the olive oil is blended in, add the vanilla, sea salt, dates, and spices and continue to blend. Once this is fully blended, put your mixture into a glass container and chill in the refrigerator for at least 6 hours.

After it's been thoroughly chilled, place the mixture into your ice-cream maker and make the ice cream, according to the manufacturer's instructions; or follow the instructions for making ice cream without an ice cream maker that you find online. Or try this:

Take a large stainless-steel bowl and fill it halfway with ice. Add in some thick kosher salt or any coarse salt and mix it up. The salt won't be touching the ice cream—it's there to transfer cold from the ice into your dish of ice-cream mixture.

Put a smaller stainless-steel or ceramic bowl into the big bowl of ice and salt. Make sure it's set well into the ice, so that ice is going up the sides of the smaller bowl, but not into the bowl itself. Then fill the smaller bowl halfway up with ice-cream mixture.

Now take a handheld mixer or immersion blender with whisk attachment and mix up the ice-cream mixture for 10 minutes.

Take both bowls and put them in the freezer for 1–2 hours. Take the bowls out and use your hand mixer again for another 10 minutes.

Cover with some natural parchment paper (sitting directly on the mixture), then put a top on the smaller bowl and allow the ice cream to set in your freezer.

Serving suggestions: Serve on its own or with baked apples sprinkled with cinnamon.

Just Like Shortbread Cookies

Servings: approximately 24 cookies

If you love shortbread, you are going to love these cookies!

Note that you may want to start soaking the nuts and seeds the night before you want to make these cookies (soak for 8–12 hours and see instructions at the beginning of this chapter). Soak the pine nuts, Brazil nuts, and sesame seeds in separate containers.

The recipe itself takes about 5 minutes to prepare once the nuts are soaked and then 24–48 hours in the dehydrator (or 10–20 minutes in the oven), depending upon how crisp you want them.

INGREDIENTS:

2 cups presoaked sesame seeds

1½ cups presoaked pine nuts

1 cup presoaked Brazil nuts

½ cup coconut oil

2 Tbsp. vanilla extract

1 Tbsp. cinnamon

1 tsp. Celtic sea salt

½ tsp. ground ginger

½ tsp. ground fennel

⅓ cup natural sweetener—choose one:

- Organic erythritol or birch xylitol (Globalsweet.com has these sweeteners, but you want to avoid these options if you're following the GAPS, SCD, SIBO diets)

- Organic honey

- Organic Medjool dates (if you use dates, remove pits and put them in your food processor first with ¼ cup hot water to make into a paste, then add other ingredients)

INSTRUCTIONS:

Put the sesame seeds in the oven at 200° F until they're dry (this could take about 30–60 minutes—you could turn the oven up to 350° F to make it go faster). If you want to make raw cookies, put the sesame seeds in your food dehydrator until they're dry (115° F for about 5–6 hours).

Once the seeds are dry, add all ingredients into your food processor with the S-blade. Blend thoroughly.

With a spoon or 1 Tbsp. measuring spoon, scoop the dough onto silicone baking sheets (they don't need to be greased). Put in your food dehydrator at 115° F for 24 hours or until your cookies have the consistency you like (less time if you like softer cookies; more time if you like dry, harder cookies that taste like shortbread).

If you don't have a food dehydrator, put them in your oven on the lowest temperature and check after 10 minutes and again at 20 minutes. Test the firmness with your spatula and remove when they are as firm as you like them. If you like soft cookies, you'll take them out sooner.

Just Like Toffee Cookies

||||||||||||||||||||||||||||||||||||||||||||||||||||||||||||||||||||||||||||||||||||||||||||||||||||||||||||||||||||||||||||||||||||||||||||||||||||||||||||||||||||||||||||

Servings: approximately 24 cookies

Cinnamon, nutmeg, and rosemary make for some very good cookies—plus, they're packed with health benefits! These cookies have a wonderful taste that is a little like toffee.

Your roundup of healthy herbs and spices include the following:

Cinnamon is anti-inflammatory, helps promote healthy bacteria in your gut (those good guys that help you digest and assimilate your food), and keeps your blood sugar stable (which helps give you willpower!). It can also help with heart health and can prevent diabetes.[5]

Nutmeg has more benefits that you can count. Some of them are: protecting your skin from wrinkles due to the breakdown of elastin in the skin and skin-damaging ultraviolet (UV) rays, providing anti-anxiety and anti-depression benefits, and inhibiting the viral cause of diarrhea. And some studies have found that nutmeg has aphrodisiac activity and increases libido.[6]

Rosemary, another wonderful addition to these cookies, has been shown to reduce anxiety, reduce pain in arthritis, and lower blood sugar. Rosemary also helps improve your memory and protect your skin from the sun's UV radiation.[7]

Note that you may want to start soaking nuts and seeds the night before you want to make these cookies (soak for 8–12 hours and see instructions at the beginning of this chapter). Soak the nuts and seeds in separate containers. The recipe itself takes about 5 minutes to prepare once the nuts and seeds are soaked and 18 hours in the food dehydrator (or 10–30 minutes in your oven).

INGREDIENTS:

2 cups presoaked Brazil nuts

4 cups presoaked unhulled sesame seeds

4 Tbsp. vanilla extract

2 Tbsp. ground cinnamon

2 Tbsp. dried rosemary

2 Tbsp. unrefined virgin coconut oil

7 Medjool dates

2 tsp. sea salt

1 tsp. ground nutmeg

INSTRUCTIONS:

You can dehydrate the sesame seeds by spreading them out flat on a silicone baking sheet and dehydrating for 4–6 hours at 115° F. If you don't have a dehydrator, put the sesame seeds into a glass baking dish, making sure that they're spread out in a thin layer (you may need 2 pans). Put your oven on the lowest temperature and heat until dry and slightly brown. Set them aside until you're ready to make the cookies.

If your food processor or blender is small, you can cut this recipe in half and mix things up separately, then combine in a bowl afterward.

In a food processor with an S-blade, put in the dates and blend until mushy. Now add the soaked nuts and seeds, and blend again. Add the rest of the ingredients and keep blending until the mixture is completely smooth. Add a little filtered water as needed to keep everything blending up properly. Taste the mixture and see if you like it. You can add more dates if you like a sweeter cookie: Start with 2 at a time and taste again if you decide to add more sweetness. You may need to add a little water to get them fully blended. Scrape the sides with a rubber spatula to keep things moving.

Scoop out the mixture with a tablespoon and flatten it out onto silicone baking sheets. Put the sheets into your food dehydrator at 115° F. We like these a little moist and chewy, so we take then out before they get too dry or hard (about 18 hours). Leave them in longer if you like a drier cookie.

If you don't have a food dehydrator, put the cookies on a glass or stainless-steel baking sheet greased with coconut oil, or on a silicone baking sheet over your cookie sheet (the silicone baking sheet does not need to be greased), and put it in your oven at the lowest temperature. Watch the oven for when you want to take them out. It should be anywhere from 10–30 minutes, depending on the lowest temperature of your oven and how dry you want them to be. Keeping your oven on the lowest temperature will be gentler to the nut oils.

Store in your refrigerator for 1 week, or in your freezer for a couple of months. They will thaw quickly, so you may want to make more and freeze them for convenient snacks. Just pull a few out of the freezer, put into a baggie, and take on the go for a healthy snack or dessert on the run!

METRIC EQUIVALENT CHARTS

The recipes in this book use the standard United States method for measuring liquid and dry or solid ingredients (teaspoons, tablespoons, and cups). The following charts are provided to help cooks outside the U.S. successfully use these recipes. All equivalents are approximate.

Standard Cup	Fine Powder (e.g., flour)	Grain (e.g., rice)	Granular (e.g., sugar)	Liquid Solids (e.g., butter)	Liquid (e.g., milk)
1	140 g	150 g	190 g	200 g	240 ml
¾	105 g	113 g	143 g	150 g	180 ml
⅔	93 g	100 g	125 g	133 g	160 ml
½	70 g	75 g	95 g	100 g	120 ml
⅓	47 g	50 g	63 g	67 g	80 ml
¼	35 g	38 g	48 g	50 g	60 ml
⅛	18 g	19 g	24 g	25 g	30 ml

Useful Equivalents for Liquid Ingredients by Volume				
¼ tsp				1 ml
½ tsp				2 ml
1 tsp				5 ml
3 tsp	1 tbsp		½ fl oz	15 ml
	2 tbsp	⅛ cup	1 fl oz	30 ml
	4 tbsp	¼ cup	2 fl oz	60 ml
	5⅓ tbsp	⅓ cup	3 fl oz	80 ml
	8 tbsp	½ cup	4 fl oz	120 ml
	10⅔ tbsp	⅔ cup	5 fl oz	160 ml
	12 tbsp	¾ cup	6 fl oz	180 ml
	16 tbsp	1 cup	8 fl oz	240 ml
	1 pt	2 cups	16 fl oz	480 ml
	1 qt	4 cups	32 fl oz	960 ml
			33 fl oz	1000 ml	1 l

Useful Equivalents for Dry Ingredients by Weight

(To convert ounces to grams, multiply the number of ounces by 30.)

1 oz	1/16 lb	30 g
4 oz	1/4 lb	120 g
8 oz	1/2 lb	240 g
12 oz	3/4 lb	360 g
16 oz	1 lb	480 g

Useful Equivalents for Cooking/Oven Temperatures

Process	Fahrenheit	Celsius	Gas Mark
Freeze Water	32° F	0° C	
Room Temperature	68° F	20° C	
Boil Water	212° F	100° C	
Bake	325° F	160° C	3
	350° F	180° C	4
	375° F	190° C	5
	400° F	200° C	6
	425° F	220° C	7
	450° F	230° C	8
Broil			Grill

Useful Equivalents for Length

(To convert inches to centimeters, multiply the number of inches by 2.5.)

1 in			2.5 cm	
6 in	1/2 ft		15 cm	
12 in	1 ft		30 cm	
36 in	3 ft	1 yd	90 cm	
40 in			100 cm	1 m

ENDNOTES

Chapter 1

1. Theaston, Frank. "World Health Statistics 2008." World Health Organization. WHO Press, 2008. PDF file.

2. Zerhouni, Elias A. "Progress in Autoimmune Diseases Research." National Institutes of Health. Report to Congress, March 2005. Foreword. PDF file.

3. Nakazawa, Donna Jackson. *The Autoimmune Epidemic: Bodies Gone Haywire in a World Out of Balance—And the Cutting-Edge Science That Promises Hope.* New York, NY: Touchstone. 2008. Print.

4. Dugdale, David C. III. "Autoimmune Disorders." MedlinePlus Medical Encyclopedia. 2011. Web. 30 Dec 2013.

5. Acres, M.J., J.J. Heath, and J.A Morris. "Anorexia nervosa, autoimmunity and the hygiene hypothesis." *Med Hypothesis,* 2012 Jun; 78(6): 722-5. PubMed.gov. 2012. Web. 30 Dec 2013.

6. Alvord, Mary K., Karina W. Davidson, Jennifer F. Kelly, Kevin M. McGuinness, and Steven Tovian. "Understanding chronic stress." American Psychological Association. n.d. Web. 30 Dec 2013.

7. American Psychological Association. "Stress in America™: Missing the Health Care Connection." American Psychological Association. Feb 2013: 3–7. PDF file.

8. Gray, Kurt, et al. "More Than a Body: Mind Perception and the Nature of Objectification." *Journal of Personality and Social Psychology.* American Psychological Association (2011): 2. PDF file.

9. American Psychological Association. "Stress Weakens the Immune System." American Psychological Association, Feb 2006. Web. 30 Dec 2013.

10. Simon, Harvey. "Stress and Anxiety." *The New York Times.* Jan 2013. Web. 6 Jan 2014.

11. Zelkowitz, Rachel. "Your Brain on Stress." *Science.* American Association for the Advancement of Science. Nov 2008. Web. 5 Jan 2014.

12. Khanna, Vikas. *Return to the Rivers: Recipes and Memories of the Himalayan River Valleys.* New York, NY: Lake Isle Press, Inc. 2013. Print.

13. Lipton, Bruce. *The Biology of Belief: Unleashing the Power of Consciousness, Matter & Miracles.* Carlsbad, CA: Hay House, Inc. 2008. Print.

14. Hyman, Mark. "How to Stop Attacking Yourself: 9 Steps to Heal Autoimmune Disease." DrHyman.com. May 2013. Web. 4 Jan 2014.

15. Zelman, David. "What is Fibromyalgia?" WebMD. 6 June 2013. Web. 22 Jan 2014.

16. Oz, Mehmet. "Chronic Lyme Disease: Myth or Reality?" Oprah.com. n.d. Web. 22 Jan 2014.

17. Goldberg, Stan. "The 10 Rules of Change." *Psychology Today.* Dec 2012. Web. 4 Jan 2014.

Additional Sources:

• URMC Health Encyclopedia. "When the Immune System Chooses the Wrong Target." University of Rochester Medical Center. n.d. Web. 3 Jan 2014.

• Johns Hopkins Medical Institutions Autoimmune Disease Research Center. "Frequently Asked Questions." Johns Hopkins Medical Institutions. n.d. Web. 3 Jan 2014.

Chapter 2

1. Brennan, L., and W. Binney. "Fear, guilt and shame appeals in social marketing." *Journal of Business Research.* 63(2), 140–146. 2010. Web. 19 Jan 2014.

2. O'Reilly, Terry. "Shame: The Secret Tool of Marketing." *Under the Influence.* CBC Radio. n.d. Web. 20 Jan 2014.

3. Taylor, Eldon. *Mind Programming: From Persuasion and Brainwashing to Self-Help and Practical Metaphysics.* Carlsbad, CA: Hay House, Inc. 2009. Print.

4. Heldman, Caroline. "The Sexy Lie." TEDxYouth. San Diego, CA. 20 Jan 2014. MP4.

5. LaRosa, John. "U.S. Weight Loss Market Forecast To Hit $66 Billion in 2013." PR Web. 13 Dec 2012. Web. 20 Jan 2014.

6. "Overweight people in the world—definitions, sources and methods." Worldometers. n.d. Web. 20 Jan 2014.

7. Loyola University Health System. "Top four reasons why diets fail." ScienceDaily. 3 Jan 2013. Web. 21 Jan 2014.

8. Fitzgerald, Randall. *The Hundred-Year Lie: How Food and Medicine Are Destroying Your Health.* London, England: Dutton. 2006. Print.

9. Boyle, Matthew. "In the butter vs. margarine wars, butter is winning." *St. Louis Post-Dispatch.* 17 Jan 2014. Web. 21 Jan 2014.

10. Fitzgerald, Randall.

11. Critser, Greg. *Fat Land: How Americans Became the Fattest People in the World.* New York, NY: Houghton Mifflin Company. 2003. Print.

12. Sustainable Food Trust. "True Cost Accounting." Sustainable Food Trust. n.d. Web. 21 Jan 2014.

13. Lang, Tim. "Food and Public Health." Paper to Sustainable Food Trust True Cost Accounting in Food and Farming Conference. London, England: Royal Geographical Society. 6 Dec 2013. Print.

14. Strickland, Reata. *Interview with God*. New York, NY: The Free Press. 2001. Print.

15. Buettner, Dan. *The Blue Zones: Lessons for Living Longer from the People Who've Lived the Longest*. Washington, D.C.: the National Geographic Society, 2008. Print.

16. Crosta, Peter. "What is lupus?" Medical News Today. Aug 2013. Web. 21 Jan 2014.

17. Deardorff, Julie. "Prescription for nutrition." *Chicago Tribune*. 26 Mar 2013. Web. 22 Jan 2014.

18. Parker-Pope, Tara. "What Doctors Don't Know About Nutrition." *The New York Times*. 16 Sep 2010. Web. 21 Jan 2014.

19. Fox, Susannah. "Health Fact Sheet." Pew Internet & American Life Project. 16 Dec 2013. Web. 22 Jan 2014.

20. Weiss, Rick. "Prescribed Drugs' Toll Is Among Deadliest." *The Washington Post*. 15 Apr 1998. Web. 7 Feb 2014.

Chapter 3

1.   Neithercott, Tracey. "Food Cravings: Fighting the lure of sugar, salt, and fat." *Diabetes Forecast*. Mar 2012. Web. 2 Feb. 2014.

2.   Tannahill, Reay. *Food in History*. (p. 281). New York, NY: Three Rivers Press. 1988. Print.

3.   Ibid., 294.

4.   Ibid., 281.

5.   Fischler, Claude. "Food Selection and Risk Perception." Paris, France, n.d. Web. 3 Feb 2014.

6.   Braun, Ashley. "Americans need to stop multitasking while eating alone, argues French sociologist Claude Fischler." Grist. 16 Nov 2010. Web. 16 Jun 2014.

7.   Hurley, Dan. "Your Backup Brain." *Psychology Today*. 1 November 2011. Web. 10 Feb 2014.

8.   Lipski, Elizabeth. *Digestive Wellness: How to Strengthen the Immune System and Prevent Disease Through Healthy Digestion*. (p. 49). New York, NY: McGraw-Hill. 2004. Print.

9.   Ibid., xv.

10. Ibid., xv–xviii.

11. "Genes can be 'changed' by foods." BBC News. 17 Nov 2005. Web. 11 Feb 2014.

12. Lipski, Elizabeth. xviii.

13. "Healthy Digestion." How Stuff Works. n.d. Web. 4 Feb 2014.

14. Lipski, Elizabeth. 22.

15. Allbritton, Jen. "Modernizing Your Diet With Traditional Foods." The Weston A. Price Foundation. n.d. Web. 30 Mar 2010.

16. Palkovicova, Lubica, et al. "Maternal amalgam dental fillings as the source of mercury exposure in developing fetus and newborn." *Journal of Exposure Science & Environmental Epidemiology* 18 (2008): 326–331. 12 Sept 2007. Web. 05 Feb 2014.

17. Levine, Jonathan B. "Toxic Teeth: Are Amalgam Fillings Safe?" *The Doctor Oz Show,* 27 Mar 2013. Web. 10 Feb 2014.

18. Mercola, Joseph. "The International Mercury Treaty Is Finally Official!" Organic Consumers Association. 22 Oct 2013. Web. 11 Feb 2014.

19. Lipski, Elizabeth. 23.

20. Ibid.

21. Volkov, Ilia, and Yan Press. "Vitamin B12 Could be A 'Master Key' in the Regulation of Multiple Pathological Processes." *Journal of Nippon Medical School* 73 (2006): 65-69. Web. 14 Feb 2014.

22. Pacholok, Sally M., and Jeffrey J. Stuart. *Could It Be B12? An Epidemic of Misdiagnosis.* (p. 3) Sanger, California: Quill Driver Books/Word Dancer Press, Inc. 2005. Print.

23. Ibid.

24. Ibid., 18.

25. Ibid., 14.

26. Lipski, Elizabeth. 25.

27. Galland, Leo. "Do You Have Leaky Gut Syndrome?" The Huffington Post. 10 Sept 2010. Web. 12 Feb 2014.

28. "What is Pancreatitis?" WebMD Digestive Disorders Health Center. n.d. Web. 8 Feb 2014.

29. "Pancreas." Better Health Channel. State Government of Victoria, Australia, 31 Oct 2011. Web. 14 Feb 2014.

30. Lipski, Elizabeth. 29.

31. Boehlke, Julie. "Early Signs of Liver Problems." LiveStrong.com. 16 Aug 2013. Web. 15 Feb 2014.

32. Williams, David. "Symptoms of a Bad Gallbladder." DrDavidWilliams.com. 6 Feb 2014. Web. 14 Feb 2014.

33. Lipski, Elizabeth. 32.

34. American Society of Colon & Rectal Surgeons. "Constipation." ASCRS.org. Oct 2012. Web. 15 Feb 2014.

35. University of California San Francisco Medical Center. "Constipation Signs and Symptoms." UCSFhealth.org., n.d. Web. 15 Feb 2014.

36. Lipski, Elizabeth. 33.

37. Wong, Cathy. "Healthy and Unhealthy Stool." About.com. n.d. Web. 20 Feb 2014.

38. Basson, Marc D. "Constipation Clinical Presentation" Medscape.com. 21 Jan 2014. Web. 10 Feb 2014.

39. Heaton, K. W., et al. "Defecation frequency and timing, and stool form in the general population: a prospective study." *Gut.* 1992. 33, 818–824. Web. 11 June 2014.

40. Lewis, S. J., and K. W. Heaton. "Stool form scale as a useful guide to intestinal transit time." PubMed.gov. Sep 1997. Web. 31 May 2014.

41. Hyman, Mark. "Maximizing Methylation: The Key to Healthy Aging." DrHyman.com. 8 Feb 2011. Web. 17 Feb 2014.

42. Mullan, Nancy, and Amy Yasko. "Methionine and Methylation: Chicken or the Egg." Doctorsdata.com. n.d. Web 22 Feb 2014.

43. "The Meaning of Methylation." Autismnti.com. n.d. Web. 18 Feb 2014.

44. Hyman, Mark.

45. Lynch, Benjamin. "Improving Patient Outcomes: Identifying Methylation Polymorphisms." Presentation. www.youtube.com/watch?v=QRHif2aVPvw. 25 Apr 2012. Web. 19 Feb 2014.

46. Erlich,. Katherine. "MTHFR Basics from Dr Erlich." MTHFR.net. 01 Mar 2012. Web. 20 Feb 2014.

47. Lynch, Benjamin. "Improving Patient Outcomes."

48. Hyman, Mark. "Nutrition Tips: Folic Acid: Killer or Cure-All?" Huffington Post. 5 June 2010. Web. 20 Feb 2014.

49. Coghlan, Andy. "Stress can affect future generations' genes." *New Scientist.* 25 Jan 2013. Web. 21 Feb 2014.

50. Centers for Disease Control and Prevention. "CDC Grand Rounds: Additional Opportunities to Prevent Neural Tube Defects with Folic Acid Fortification." USA.gov. 13 Aug 2010. Web. 22 Feb 2014.

51. Smith, A. David. "Folic acid fortification: the good, the bad, and the puzzle of vitamin B-12." *The American Journal of Clinical Nutrition* vol. 85 no. 1 (2007): 3–5. Web. 22 Feb 2014.

52. "Unmetabolized Folic Acid (UMFA) Test – Serum – MetaMetrix." Seeking Health. n.d. Web. 18 Feb 2014.

53. George Mateljan Foundation. "Folate." WHFoods.com. n.d. Web. 21 Feb 2014.

54. Lynch, Ben. "Improving Patient Outcomes."

55. McDaniel, Laura. "What is the Gut-Brain Connection?" ConnectWC. The CCP Foundation. n.d. Web. 21 Feb 2014.

56. Ibid.

57. Hurley, Dan.

58. Nordqvist, Christian. "Eating Fat When Sad Really Does Lift Mood." Medical News Today. 26 July 2011. Web. 15 Feb 2014.

59. Hurley, Dan.

60. Ibid.

61. Ibid.

62. "What You Need to Know about Willpower: The Psychological Science of Self-Control." American Psychological Association. n.d. Web. 19 Feb 2014.

63. Baumeister, Roy F, and John Tierney. *Willpower: Rediscovering the Greatest Human Strength.* London, England: Penguin Books. 2011. Print.

64. Ibid.

65. Ibid.

66. Schwarzbein, Diana. *The Schwarzbein Principle II, "The Transition": A Regeneration Process to Prevent and Reverse Accelerated Aging.* Deerfield Beach, FL: Health Communications, Inc. 2010. Print.

67. U.S. National Library of Medicine, National Institutes of Health. "Cushing's disease." MedlinePlus Medical Encyclopedia. 11 Dec 2011. Web. 22 Feb 2014.

Chapter 4

1. Ridolfo, Heather, Amy Baxter, and Jeffrey W. Lucas. "Social Influences on Paranormal Belief: Popular Versus Scientific Support." *Current Research in Social Psychology* 15, no. 3 (2010). Department of Sociology at the University of Maryland. Web. 24 Feb 2014.

2. De Becker, Gavin. *The Gift of Fear: And Other Survival Signals That Protect Us from Violence.* New York, NY: Dell. 1998. Print.

3. Sidman, Amanda P. "Windows on the World Chef Michael Lomonaco Escaped 9/11 but Dedicates Cooking to Friends He Lost." *New York Daily News.* 11 Sept 2011. Web. 22 Feb 2014.

4. Winfrey, Oprah. "What Oprah Knows for Sure About Trusting Her Intuition." *O, The Oprah Magazine.* Aug 2011. Web. 21 Feb 2014.

5. Harris, Tom. "How ESP Works." HowStuffWorks.com. 3 Sept 2002. Web. 14 Feb 2014.

6. Science Channel. "Are dreams a window into our unconscious?" Curiosity.com. n.d. Web. 23 Feb 2014.

7. Zordich, Patti M. "Improve Communication—Listen with Your Heart." Triangle Psychological Services. 31 Jan 2014. Web. 15 Feb 2014.

Chapter 5

1. Genetic Science Learning Center. "PTC: Genes and Bitter Taste." Learn.genetics.utah.edu. n.d. Web. 20 Feb 2014.

2. Khanna, Vikas. "Window into Return to the Rivers: A Chat with Vikas Khanna Part 2." Interview. www.youtube.com/watch?v=4Cb-TF8aafE. 30 Jan 2014. Web. 19 Feb 2014.

3. Schmidt, Elaine. "This is your brain on sugar: UCLA study shows high-fructose diet sabotages learning, memory." UCLA Newsroom. 15 May 2012. Web. 20 Feb 2014.

4. Ng, Shu Wen, Meghan Slining, and Barry Popkin. "Use of Caloric and Noncaloric Sweeteners in US Consumer Packaged Foods, 2005–2009." *Journal of the Academy of Nutrition and Dietetics.* 25 June 2012. Web. 28 May 2014.

5. Casey, John. "The Hidden Ingredient That Can Sabotage Your Diet." MedicineNet.com. 3 Jan 2005. Web. 20 Feb 2014.

6. Lipski, Elizabeth. xxix.

7. Appleton, Nancy. "146 Reasons Why Sugar Is Ruining Your Health." BecomeHealthyNow.com. 12 Mar 2005. Web. 11 Feb 2014.

8. Farr, Gary. "What is Refined Sugar?" BecomeHealthyNow.com. 30 Dec 2002. Web. 11 Feb 2014.

9. Hyman, Mark. "5 Reasons High-Fructose Corn Syrup Will Kill You." DrHyman.com. 4 May 2013. Web. 14 Feb 2014.

10. Ibid.

11. Strawbridge, Holly. "Artificial sweeteners: sugar-free, but at what cost?" Harvard Health Blog. 16 July 2012. Web. 22 Feb 2014.

12. Ibid.

13. Pick, Marcelle. "Sugar Substitutes and The Potential Danger of Splenda." Women to Women. n.d. Web. 23 Feb 2014.

14. Blaylock, Russell. *Excitotoxins: The Taste That Kills.* Santa Fe, NM: Health Press. 1997. Print.

15. "Review of: Excitotoxins: The Taste That Kills." *Nutrition Digest Published by the American Nutrition Association:* vol. 36 no. 4. Web. 21 Feb 2014.

16. "GMO Facts." The Non-GMO Project. n.d. Web. 24 Feb 2014.

17. American RadioWorks. "History of Genetic Engineering." American Public Media. n.d. Web. 24 Feb 2014.

18. Arax, Mark, and Jeanne Brokaw. "No Way Around Roundup." *Mother Jones.* January/February 1997 issue. Web. 24 Feb 2014.

19. Bello, Walden, and Foreign Policy In Focus. "Twenty-Six Countries Ban GMOs—Why Won't the US?" *The Nation.* 29 Oct 2013. Web. 25 Feb 2014.

20. "Compost Tea Organic Farming and Liquid Organic Farming Fertilizers for Organic Gardening." Small-Farm-Permaculture-and-Sustainable-Living.com. n.d. Web. 20 Feb 2014.

21. Kasper, Lynne Rossetto. "Green Onions: The unheralded, phytonutrient-rich super food." The Splendid Table, American Public Media. n.d. Web. 24 Feb 2014.

22. National Foundation for Celiac Awareness. "Celiac Disease Facts & Figures." Celiaccentral.com. n.d. Web. 19 Feb 2014.

23. Oz, Mehmet. "Gluten Sensitivity Self-Test." DoctorOz.com. 25 Sept 2012. Web. 13 Feb 2014.

24. Campbell-McBride, Natasha. *Gut and Psychology Syndrome: Natural Treatment for Autism, Dyspraxia, A.D.D., Dyslexia, A.D.H.D., Depression, Schizophrenia.* (p. 49) Medinform Publishing. 2010. Print

25. Whitley, Andrew. "Bread—the staff of life or what makes us ill?" Foods Matter. n.d. Web. 20 Feb 2014.

26. Gentilviso, Chris. "The 50 Worst Inventions: Olestra." *Time.* 27 May 2010. Web. 12 Feb 2014.

27. "About Trans Fat." BanTransFats.com. n.d. Web. 11 Feb 2014

28. Enig, Mary. "Mary Enig On Saturated & Trans Fats." Presentation. www.youtube.com/watch?v=5dpFFqN94JE. 10 Sept 2012. Web. 19 Feb 2014.

29. "Understanding Trans Fats." WebMD: Food & Recipes. n.d. Web. 25 Feb 2014.

30. Fallon, Sally, and Mary G. Enig. "The Skinny on Fats." The Weston A. Price Foundation. 1 Jan 2000. Web. 24 Feb 2014.

31. ———. "The Great Con-ola." The Weston A. Price Foundation. 28 July 2002. Web. 11 Feb 2014.

32. The American Nutrition Association. "The Whole Soy Story." *Nutrition Digest:* vol. 36 no. 4. Web. 21 Feb 2014.

33. Ibid.

34. WGBH Educational Foundation. "Frontline Interview: Michael Pollan." PBS.org. n.d. Web. 24 Feb 2014.

35. Buford, Bill. *Heat: An Amateur's Adventures as Kitchen Slave, Line Cook, Pasta-Maker, and Apprentice to a Dante-Quoting Butcher in Tuscany.* New York, NY: Alfred A. Knopf. 2006. Print

36. Campbell-McBride. 95.

37. Weise, Elizabeth. "Sixty percent of adults can't digest milk." *USA Today.* 15 Sept 2009. Web. 14 Feb 2014.

38. Feblowitz, Joshua. "Milk Allergy: We answer your top questions about dairy allergy and lactose intolerance." *Living Without's Gluten Free & More.* Apr/May 2012 issue. Web. 10 Feb 2014.

39. Campbell-McBride. 96.

40. Ryan, Sheryl. "Health comparison: wild-caught fish vs. farmed fish." Greenopedia. n.d. Web. 14 Feb 2014.

41. "No Fish, Go Fish: A Guide to Responsible Eating." eNature NatureWatch. n.d. Web. 10 Feb 2014.

42. Kessler, David A. *The End of Overeating: Taking Control of the Insatiable American Appetite.* Emmaus, PA: Rodale Books. 2010. Print.

43. Fusaro, Dave. "When It Comes to Synthetic Food Colors: Beware the 'Southampton Six.'" *Food Processing.* 2010. Web. 11 Feb 2014.

44. Oaklander, Mandy. "A New Fear About Food Dyes." *Prevention.* Jan 2013. Web. 10 Feb 2014.

45. Grotheer, Paul, Maurice Marshall, and Amy Simonne. "Sulfites: Separating Fact from Fiction." University of Florida IFAS Extension. Publication #FCS8787. Web. 10 Feb 2014.

46. "Diseases & Conditions: Sulfite Sensitivity." Cleveland Clinic. 11 June 2010. Web. 10 Feb 2014.

47. Helmenstine, Anne Marie. "Chemistry of BHA and BHT Food Preservatives." About.com. n.d. Web. 10 Feb 2014.

48. Yoquinto, Luke. "The Truth About Potassium Bromate." Live-Science. 16 Mar 2012. Web. 11 Feb 2014.

49. Zeratsky, Katherine. "Should I be worried that my favorite soda contains brominated vegetable oil? What is it?" Mayo Clinic. 5 April 2013. Web. 9 Feb 2014.

50. Truth in Labeling Campaign. "Names of ingredients that contain processed free glutamic acid (MSG)." TruthinLabeling.org. n.d. Web. 25 Feb 2014.

51. Strawbridge, Holly.

52. Zerbe, Leah. "The 5 Best, and 5 Worst, Sweeteners to Have in Your Kitchen." Rodale News. 21 Feb 2012. 19 Feb 2014.

53. Truth in Labeling Campaign.

54. Ibid.

55. Lapid, Nancy. "Gluten-Free Diet Guidelines for Celiac Disease." About.com. n.d. Web. 27 Feb 2014.

56. Marley, Karen. "The Fantastic 5: Antioxidant Spice Heroes or how to Keep That Pesky 'Eat Healthy' Resolution!" Spice Sherpa. 26 Jan 2011. Web. 23 Feb 2014.

57. Pitchford, Paul. *Healing with Whole Foods: Asian Traditions and Modern Nutrition.* (p. 188). Berkeley, CA: North Atlantic Books. 2003. Print.

58. Ibid., 189.

59. Campbell, Meg. "Nutrition in Medjool Dates." SFGate Healthy Eating. n.d. Web. 23 Feb 2014.

60. Mandal, Manisha Deb, and Shyamapada Mandal. "Honey: its medicinal property and antibacterial activity." *Asian Pacific Journal of Tropical Biomedicine.* April 2011. Web. 14 Feb 2014.

61. Ansari, MJ, et al. "Effect of jujube honey on Candida albicans growth and biofilm formation." PubMed.gov. July 2013. Web. 23 Feb 2014.

62. University of Rhode Island College of Pharmacy. "URI Scientist Discovers 54 Beneficial Compounds in Pure Maple Syrup." URI.edu. 30 Mar 2011. Web. 24 Feb 2014.

63. George Mateljan Foundation. "Please Tell Me the Benefits of Unsulphured Molasses." WHFoods.com. n.d. Web. 25 Feb 2014.

64. Keith, Mary A., "One More New Sweetener—Monk Fruit." Penny Saver News, University of Florida IFAS Extension. 4 Apr 2013. Web. 10 Feb 2014.

65. Courtiol, Marc. "Stevia: The Best Natural Sweetener, or Just Another Fad?" Botanical.com. 28 July 2011. Web. 25 Feb 2014.

66. Curinga, Karen. "How to Use Stevia Leaves." SFGate Healthy Eating. n.d. Web. 23 Feb 2014.

67. 3B Scientific. "Health Myth: How Many Glasses of Water Should We Be Drinking?" Insights on Therapy & Wellness. 5 Sept 2013. Web. 22 Feb 2014.

68. Boschman, M., et al. "Water-induced thermogenesis." PubMed.gov. Dec 2003. Web. 23 Feb 2014.

69. Popkin, Barry M., Denis V. Barclay, and Samara J. Nielsen. "Water and Food Consumption Patterns of U.S. Adults from 1999 to 2001." *Obesity Research Journal:* vol. 13, issue 12 (2146–2152). Dec 2005. Web. 27 Feb 2014.

70. Batmanghelidj, Fereydoon. "Your Body's Many Cries for Water." Transcript of his lecture at "The Governmental Health Forum" in Washington, D.C. March 28–30, 2003. The World Foundation for Natural Science. Web. 27 Feb 2014.

71. Slovak, Robert. "Find Out the Naked Truth About What's In Your Water." Purative.com. 23 Jan 2012. Web. 28 Feb 2014.

72. Gómez-Pinilla, Fernando. "Brain foods: the effects of nutrients on brain function." PubMed.gov. July 2008. Web. 15 Feb 2014.

73. Simopoulos, AP. "The Importance of the ratio of omega-6/omega-3 essential fatty acids." PubMed.gov. Oct 2002. Web. 21 Feb 2014.

74. "Know Your Fats." The Weston A. Price Foundation. n.d. Web. 11 Feb 2014.

75. Schachter, Raluca. "Healthy Animal Fats." HandPicked Nation. 6 Sept 2012. Web. 23 Feb 2014.

76. "FAQ—Fats and Oils." The Weston A. Price Foundation. n.d. Web. 11 Feb 2014.

77. National Digestive Diseases Information Clearinghouse (NDDIC) "Digestive Diseases Statistics for the United States." National Institutes of Health Publication No. 13-3873. Sept 2013. Web. 12 Feb 2014.

78. "Arsenic in your food." *Consumer Reports*. Nov 2012. Web. 22 Feb 2014.

79. Young, Lisa. "Benefits of Nuts and Seeds: 7 Winners." The Huffington Post. 29 Nov 2012. Web. 12 Feb 2014.

80. Byrnes, Stephen. "Going Nuts! A Guide to the Wonderfully Nutritious World of Nuts." BecomeHealthyNow.com. 11 Mar 2002. Web. 11 Feb 2014.

81. "The Whole9 Bone Broth FAQ." Whole9Life.com. Dec 2013. Web. 10 Feb 2014.

Chapter 6

1. Jones, A.W. "Early drug discovery and the rise of pharmaceutical chemistry." *Drug Test Analysis*, 3: 337–344. June 2011. Web. 21 Feb 2014.

2. Hitti, Miranda. "Most New Drugs Tapped From Nature." WebMD: Information & Resources. 16 Mar 2007. Web. 22 Feb 2014.

3. Compton, K.C. "Choosing Between Natural Herbal Medicine and Synthetic Pharmaceuticals." *Mother Earth News*. April/May 2003. Web. 12 Feb 2014.

4. Ibid.

5. Ibid.

6. Aggarwal, Bharat B. *Healing Spices: How to Use 50 Everyday and Exotic Spices to Boost Health and Beat Disease*. (p. 298) New York, NY: Sterling. 2011. Print.

7. Dean, Carolyn. "The Magnesium Miracle." DrCarolynDean.com. n.d. Web. 10 Feb 2014.

8. Rossi, Maddalena, et al. "Fermentation of Fructooligosaccharides and Inulin by Bifidobacteria: a Comparative Study of Pure and Fecal Cultures." U.S. National Library of Medicine, National Institutes of Health. Oct 2005. Web. 15 Feb 2014.

9. Campbell-McBride. 225–228.

10. Aggarwal. 299.

11. U.S. National Library of Medicine, National Institutes of Health. "When you or your child have diarrhea." MedlinePlus Medical Encyclopedia. n.d. Web. 20 Feb 2014.

12. Bolen, Barbara Bradley. "Diarrhea: Top Eight Things to Eat When You Are Feeling Awful." About.com. n.d. Web. 21 Feb 2014.

13. Aggarwal. 295, 299, 301.

14. U.S. National Library of Medicine, National Institutes of Health. "Peppermint." MedlinePlus Medical Encyclopedia. n.d. Web. 14 Feb 2014.

15. Aggarwal. 301.

16. Wong, Cathy. "Heartburn Remedies: 7 Natural Treatments to Consider." About.com. n.d. Web. 21 Feb 2014.

17. Kandil, Tharwat S., et al. "The Potential Therapeutic Effect of Melatonin in Gastro-esophageal Reflux." Medscape. 2010;10:7. Web. 12 Feb 2014.

18. Oz, Mehmet. "Say Goodbye to GERD." DoctorOz.com. n.d. Web. 10 Feb 2014.

19. Campbell-McBride. 228.

20. Lipski. 194.

21. Kresser, Chris. "What Everybody Ought To Know (But Doesn't) About Heartburn & GERD." ChrisKresser.com. n.d. Web. 11 Feb 2014.

22. Debé, Joseph. "Stomach Acid Assessment." DrDebe.com. n.d. Web. 14 Feb 2014.

23. Lipski. 194.

24. Cabot, Sandra. "Things You Must Know If You Don't Have a Gallbladder." LiverDoctor.com. n.d. Web. 15 Feb 2014.

25. "Coenzyme Q10—Topic Overview." WebMD Heart Failure Health Center. n.d. Web. 20 Feb 2014.

26. Haas, Elson M. "Vitamin C." Healthy.net. n.d. Web. 24 Feb 2014.

27. "Vitamins." Harvard School of Public Health. n.d. Web. 25 Feb 2014.

28. Tierra, Michael. "The Wonders of Triphala." PlanetHerbs.com. n.d. Web 27 Feb 2014.

29. Dean, Carolyn. "The Magnesium Miracle."

30. ———. "Magnesium Is Crucial for Bones." The Huffington Post. 15 June 2012. Web. 12 Feb 2014.

31. Rosner, Bryan. *The Top 10 Lyme Disease Treatments: Defeat Lyme Disease with the Best of Conventional and Alternative Medicine*. South Lake Tahoe, CA: BioMed Publishing Group. 2007. Print.

32. Dean, Carolyn. "Glutamates in Magnesium Chelates." DrCarolynDean.com. 31 Jan 2011. Web. 23 Feb 2014.

33. ———. "The Magnesium Miracle." DrCarolynDean.com. n.d. Web. 10 Feb 2014.

34. "Feverfew." University of Maryland Medical Center. n.d. Web. 12 Feb 2014.

35. Ross, Julia. *The Diet Cure*. (p. 127) New York, NY: Penguin Books. 2000. Print.

36. Ibid. 127.

37. Aggarwal. 296.

Chapter 7

1. Hardy, Julia. "Human Nature and the Purpose of Existence." Religion Library: Taoism. Patheos.com. n.d. Web. 2 May 2014.

Chapter 10

1. Aggarwal. 241–250.

2. Ibid. 114–116.

3. Ibid. 135–139.

4. Ibid. 53–54.

5. Ibid. 79–82.

6. Ibid. 172–173.

7. Ibid. 202–204.

♥ ♥

GENERAL INDEX

♥   ♥

INDEX OF RECIPES AND MENUS

♥ ♥

ABOUT THE AUTHORS

Louise Hay, the author of the international bestseller *You Can Heal Your Life,* is a metaphysical lecturer and teacher with more than 50 million books sold worldwide. For more than 30 years, Louise has helped people throughout the world discover and implement the full potential of their own creative powers for personal growth and self-healing. Louise is the founder and chairman of Hay House, Inc., which disseminates books, CDs, DVDs, and other products that contribute to the healing of the planet. Visit www.LouiseHay.com

Ahlea Khadro is the founder and owner of Soulstice, a Center for Optimal Living & Rehabilitation through yoga, reformer Pilates, meditative practices, and nutrition. She specializes in: visceral manipulation, craniosacral therapy, holistic and nutritive support, emotional release techniques, and electromagnetic field (EMF) remediation. At an early age Ahlea could see the stories that lie beneath the surface of people's lives and under the layers of the human body. Coupled with a deep desire to serve others, her quest to translate these stories into healing protocols took her on a colorful, dynamic, and unconventional path to mastering the healing process. From mainstream hospital settings to the feet of yogic masters, Ahlea's unique path has allowed her to see new ways to heal your body and life. Visit www.AhleaKhadro.com

Heather Dane is a writer, researcher, and certified professional coach specializing in resolving chronic health conditions, addictions, eating disorders, methylation challenges, and out-of-balance lifestyles. After recovering naturally from so-called incurable chronic digestive disorders, bulimia, and depression, Heather discovered how to identify and solve symptoms at the root-cause level. She believes that there is no such thing as an incurable illness—there is only an invitation to come back to loving yourself. Heather has researched and worked with many of the great minds in medicine, natural health, nutrition, and energy healing. Her expertise in designing healing nutrition protocols led her to create hundreds of easy, delicious recipes (including desserts!) to transform the experience of "health food" into healthy gourmet. Visit www.HeatherDane.com

Hay House Titles of Related Interest

We hope you enjoyed this Hay House book. If you'd like
to receive our online catalog featuring additional information
on Hay House books and products, or if you'd like to find
out more about the Hay Foundation, please contact:

Hay House, Inc., P.O. Box 5100, Carlsbad, CA 92018-5100
(760) 431-7695 or (800) 654-5126
(760) 431-6948 (fax) or (800) 650-5115 (fax)
www.hayhouse.com® • www.hayfoundation.org

Published and distributed in Australia by: Hay House Australia Pty. Ltd.,
18/36 Ralph St., Alexandria NSW 2015 • *Phone:* 612-9669-4299
Fax: 612-9669-4144 • www.hayhouse.com.au

Published and distributed in the United Kingdom by: Hay House UK, Ltd.,
Astley House, 33 Notting Hill Gate, London W11 3JQ • *Phone:* 44-20-3675-2450
Fax: 44-20-3675-2451 • www.hayhouse.co.uk

Published and distributed in the Republic of South Africa by:
Hay House SA (Pty), Ltd., P.O. Box 990, Witkoppen 2068
info@hayhouse.co.za • www.hayhouse.co.za

Published in India by: Hay House Publishers India, Muskaan Complex, Plot No. 3, B-2,
Vasant Kunj, New Delhi 110 070 • *Phone:* 91-11-4176-1620
Fax: 91-11-4176-1630 • www.hayhouse.co.in

Distributed in Canada by: Raincoast Books, 2440 Viking Way, Richmond, B.C. V6V 1N2
Phone: 1-800-663-5714 • *Fax:* 1-800-565-3770 • www.raincoast.com

Take Your Soul on a Vacation

Visit www.HealYourLife.com® to regroup, recharge,
and reconnect with your own magnificence.
Featuring blogs, mind-body-spirit news, and life-changing
wisdom from Louise Hay and friends.

Visit www.HealYourLife.com today!

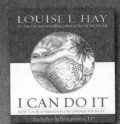
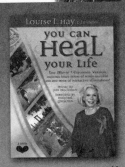
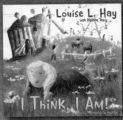

Free e-newsletters
from Hay House, the Ultimate
Resource for Inspiration

Be the first to know about Hay House's dollar deals, free downloads, special offers, affirmation cards, giveaways, contests, and more!

 Get exclusive excerpts from our latest releases and videos from *Hay House Present Moments*.

 Enjoy uplifting personal stories, how-to articles, and healing advice, along with videos and empowering quotes, within *Heal Your Life*.

 Have an inspirational story to tell and a passion for writing? Sharpen your writing skills with insider tips from *Your Writing Life*.

Sign Up Now!

Get inspired, educate yourself, get a complimentary gift, and share the wisdom!

http://www.hayhouse.com/newsletters.php

Visit www.hayhouse.com to sign up today!

 HAY HOUSE

HAYHOUSE RADIO)) *radio for your soul*

HealYourLife.com ♥

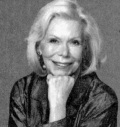
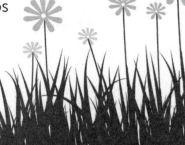